"Cooper's text is probably the most important statement on the connection between race, gender, and stress since the appearance of Alvin Poussaint and Amy Anderson's 2001 study on the biological, medical and mental health correlates of race-related stress."

William E. Cross Jr., Ph.D., *developer of the Black racial identity development model of Nigrescence, professor emeritus of Higher Education and Counseling Psychology, University of Denver*

BLACK MEN AND RACIAL TRAUMA

This volume comprehensively addresses racial trauma from a clinical lens, equipping mental health professionals across all disciplines to be culturally responsive when serving Black men. Written using a transdisciplinary approach, Yamonte Cooper presents a unified theory of racism (UTR), integrated model of racial trauma (IMRT), transgenerational trauma points (TTP), plantation politics, Black male negation (BMN), and race-based shame (RBS) to fill a critical and urgent void in the mental health field and emerging scholarship on racial trauma. Chapters begin with specific definitions of racism before exploring specific challenges that Black men face, such as racial discrimination in health care, trauma, criminalization, economic deprivation, anti-Black misandry, and culturally specific stressors, emotions, such as shame and anger, and coping mechanisms that these men utilize. After articulating the racial trauma of Black men in a comprehensive manner, the book provides insight into what responsive care looks like as well as clinical interventions that can inform treatment approaches. This book is invaluable reading for all established and training mental health clinicians that work with Black men, such as psychologists, marriage and family therapists, social workers, counselors, and psychiatrists.

Yamonte Cooper is a scholar, author, professor of counseling, adjunct professor of clinical psychology, clinical director of the West Coast Sex Therapy Center, licensed professional clinical counselor (LPCC), and certified sex therapist supervisor (CST-S). He is the co-editor of the book *Black Couples Therapy: Clinical Theory and Practice* (Cambridge University Press). As a Fulbright scholar, Dr. Cooper has exchanged best practices globally in career counseling and development.

BLACK MEN AND RACIAL TRAUMA

Impacts, Disparities, and Interventions

Yamonte Cooper

Routledge
Taylor & Francis Group

NEW YORK AND LONDON

Designed cover image: Jonathan Knowles © Getty Images

First published 2024
by Routledge
605 Third Avenue, New York, NY 10158

and by Routledge
4 Park Square, Milton Park, Abingdon, Oxon, OX14 4RN

Routledge is an imprint of the Taylor & Francis Group, an informa business

© 2024 Yamonte Cooper

Library of Congress Cataloging-in-Publication Data
Names: Cooper, Yamonte, 1974– author.
Title: Black men and racial trauma : impacts, disparities, and interventions / Yamonte Cooper.
Description: New York, NY : Routledge, 2024. | Includes bibliographical references and index.
Identifiers: LCCN 2023023367 (print) | LCCN 2023023368 (ebook) | ISBN 9781032554105 (hardback) | ISBN 9781032554112 (paperback) | ISBN 9781003430551 (ebook)
Subjects: LCSH: Race discrimination. | Men, Black.
Classification: LCC HT1521 .C6367 2024 (print) | LCC HT1521 (ebook) | DDC 305.8—dc23/eng/20230728
LC record available at https://lccn.loc.gov/2023023367
LC ebook record available at https://lccn.loc.gov/2023023368

ISBN: 978-1-032-55410-5 (hbk)
ISBN: 978-1-032-55411-2 (pbk)
ISBN: 978-1-003-43055-1 (ebk)

DOI: 10.4324/9781003430551

Typeset in Baskerville MT Std
by Apex CoVantage, LLC

This book is dedicated to my mother, Rosie, and father-in-law, Emory.

CONTENTS

ACKNOWLEDGMENTS

I must start by thanking E. Russell Walton for his unwavering support and encouragement, which were invaluable throughout the process of bringing this book to fruition.

I am forever grateful for the support of my dedicated review panel: Erica Holmes for your critical feedback; Jerel Lee and Jean Shirkoff for your time taken to review the early versions of this book and the feedback and encouragement. Thank you, James Wadley, for your support throughout this process and Sherrie Ross for your support over the years and the many expansive conversations about Black men.

A special thank you to Tommy J. Curry, William A. Smith, Les Greenberg, Sandy Darity, Thomas Parham, and William E. Cross for all your endorsements. Your expertise and continued support were valuable contributions to this book.

I also would like to thank the entire publishing team at Routledge, Heather Evans and staff, for your support with the publication of this book.

To my family, I appreciate your continuous love and encouragement.

FOREWORD

Black Male Vulnerability as a Conceptual Epidemiology: Black Male Studies' Interests in Trauma and Health

By: Tommy J. Curry[1]

For the last several decades, Black males have been bound by theories promulgated by academics and policymakers claiming they are culturally violent and that their peculiar Black masculinity makes them prone to rape, murder, and the abuse of women and children. This milieu of negation has insisted upon the need to label, incarcerate, and murder Black men and boys for the preservation of white civil society. This murderous attack on Black males that attempts to remove them from society (Stewart & Scott, 1978) has not only required the power and militarized might of white supremacist institutions such as the police and the complicity of various state apparati (e.g., courts, opinion-makers, etc.) but the at-large acceptance of neo-conservative logics which hold Black men to be deviants, criminals, and bad fathers (Stewart, 1994) within the guise of liberal politics proclaiming the inclusion of various classes of racial, ethnic, and sexual minorities as progressivism. The demonization of Black men within liberal politics has successfully integrated the image of the Black male deviant into contemporary theories of (toxic) masculinity and gender inequality and patriarchy (Curry, 2022a) ignoring the various forms of sexual and physical abuse at the hands of men and women over his life-course (Curry, 2019; Curry & Utley, 2018).

Black males are theorized as problems that must be disregarded in reality and through abstraction. Consequently, social problems that are often associated with external environmental factors or correlated to poverty and trauma such as intimate partner violence and various forms of interpersonal conflicts end up being explained almost solely by the internal constitution or pathological constitution of Black masculinity (hooks, 2004, 1990). The inability to theorize Black males as affected by ecological conditions and their exposure to trauma creates situations where clinicians and mental health practitioners are driven by their stereotypical views of Black males as violent and pathological. Said differently, the differential diagnoses proposed by mental health practitioners are not based on the clinical manifestations of behaviors but instead are the projections of clinicians upon Black male patients that allow their worldviews to cohere. Clinicians offer a diagnosis that fulfills the negativity required by their mind rather than seeking out explanations located in the communities, households, or patient history that could explain why *this particular* Black male exhibits certain behaviors.

Academic theory often seeks to replace the actual world and removes real people from the purview of the scholar and clinician alike. Motivated by the ideological foundations of feminism and class biases against the Black poor, the educated mental health practitioner endeavors to re-establish a norm of behavior and self-awareness (Wynter, 1992, 2006). The Black male patient is represented as a problem within the cognitive schema of the clinician or academic. He is studied as a problem and understood to possess deficits, so he is treated as the cause of the violence and instability he proclaims to be a victim of in his life. Quite often the presumptions of Black males are situated upon racist theories popularized under more commonly accepted tropes such as toxic masculinity or hypermasculinity (Pass et al., 2014). The tropes condition how the theorist and practitioner interpret the suffering of

---

1   Professor of Philosophy, Chair of Africana Philosophy and Black Male Studies, at the University of Edinburgh. He is the author of *The Man-Not: Race, Class, Genre and the Dilemma of Black Manhood* (2017) and *Another white Man's Burden: Josiah Royce's Quest for a Philosophy of white Racial Empire* (2018).

Black males and ultimately dictate how one rationalizes the imposition of death on the Black male patient. The death of Black males may be unfortunate, but the presumption of their guilt, aggression, and danger seems to make their elimination appear almost necessary to the preservation of civility and order. It is this dissonance expressed as

> our indifference to Black male death, our seeking recognition of "life" through our descriptions of him as barbarous, [that] fuels the necromantic rage of white supremacism – the sexual racism, the desire for the Black body, and the intellectual obsession with speaking of him as corpse.
>
> (Curry, 2017, p. 192)

ANALYZING TRAUMA: A WELCOME ADDITION TO BLACK MALE STUDIES

Yamonte Cooper's *Black Men and Racial Trauma* is a welcome contribution to Black Male Studies scholarship and theorization. His analysis argues for a reexamination of how trauma is an endemic feature of racist patriarchal structures in the United States that propagate various forms of self-negation and inferiority in the oppressed. Rather than simply approaching inferiority, or the inferiority complex, as a generalizable system of racial disputation concerning the humanity of Black people, Cooper's analysis extends the previous research on arbitrary-set discrimination (Sidanius & Pratto, 1999), racial battle fatigue (Smith et al., 2016), and misandric aggression (Curry, 2017, 2018) by showing how shame in-being-negated-by-man is a systemic existential invalidation of the Black male and the psychological representation he has of himself in the world. Cooper explains the following:

> The dominance and subordination of Black males is part and parcel of the patriarchal caste system. Black males are reminded daily of their undercaste status by the disgust and contempt that is directed towards them which demarcates their status. Black men are routinely exposed to degradation where their attempts to navigate the degradation can result in internalized feelings of inferiority (i.e., shame) and powerlessness. This author posits that shame contributes to the development and maintenance of racial trauma where the routine societal devaluation (i.e., BMN) of Black males can leave them feeling defective and without agency.

This negation of the Black male self aims to decimate the psychological resources of the individual, and this is extremely important – the society has to explain the disposition the world has towards Black men and boys. In *The Man-Not: Race, Class, Genre, and the Dilemmas of Black Manhood* (Curry, 2017), Black males are explained to be caricatures of thought and thinking because the characterological defect imposed by the white patriarchal society vacates the meanings Black men and boys can author for themselves about themselves. The Black is degraded by the imagination of others; those who imagine him have the power to rule him. The Black male is decimated by the projections of others. His aspirations are the fears others have of him, and his being is composed of the various monstrosities that occupy the minds of others. The Black male exists as a phantasmic threat – a shadow that haunts the existence of human others. This shadow can be the rapist, the taker of small children, the criminal, or simply a Black man. Because Black men are Not-Man, or not of mankind, he is thought to be a threat to all that is human. He is born from nihility – an absence of being and created endlessly through the projections of others.

Cooper argues that this psycho-social negation is built into the societal hierarchies and impacts how clinicians and scholars can discern the impact of anti-Black misandry.

According to Cooper, "Resilience is defined by the ability to be able to recover after experiencing trauma, assault, injury, or any other adverse experience and is a preferred approach than prevailing pathological models for understanding Black people." However, this notion of resilience is supposed to free autonomous individuals who exist as possible and positive entities in the world. The world can support their existence. For the Black male, who is negated for his presumed pathological nature, Cooper writes,

> Resilience does not provide a structural or systemic analysis. Consequently, structural violence (i.e., institutional decimation) in the form of anti-Black misandric aggression directed towards Black men is not examined but instead how well they can adjust, and cope is the focus.

The failure of our present theoretical orientation toward Black males sounds a clarion call for rethinking and innovation. How does one think of Black boys given the decimation of the Black male psychically and physically in the United States, what does he aim to become (Bowser, 1991)?

Yamonte Cooper's *Black Men and Racial Trauma* is an insightful contribution that further develops how Black Male Studies scholars think about the relationship between mental health, existential viability, and trauma. Cooper's research is daring and aims to decolonize the precepts of clinical practice toward Black men and boys. Unlike other theories of Black masculinity which focus primarily on the role that Black men and boys have in perpetrating violence (Curry, 2017, 2021b), Black Male Studies emphasizes the vulnerability Black men and boys have in the world committed to their negation and extermination for the benefit of others. The vulnerability of Black males in the United States and abroad, the "disadvantages that Black males endure compared with other groups; the erasure of Black males' actual lived experience from theory; and the violence and death Black males suffer in society" are not merely a sociological phenomenon (Curry, 2017, p. 29). It explains the process by which the degrading of Black men and boys makes him susceptible "to the will of others, how he has no resistance to the imposition of others' fears and anxieties on him" (Curry, 2017, p. 29). *Black Men and Racial Trauma* takes the vulnerability of the Black male to be its central problem. The conceptualization of Black men and boys as the foundation of how we theorize racism, resilience, sexual violence, and domestic abuse completely reorients how we come to think about the very idea of the victim and how racism as misandric aggression sustains the peculiar case of Black males in America. This book will be of tremendous service to our understanding of Black males in the years to come.

INTRODUCTION

The racial trauma that Black men experience is life altering and understudied.* Current articulations of racial trauma and Black men commonly provide superficial anecdotal soundbites that lack empiricism and depth, while some reinforce stereotypes about Black men. The racial trauma enterprise has grown exponentially over the past few years with articles and workshops, and trainings touting buzzwords such as *anti-racism, decolonizing*, and *healing*. Therefore, many professionals across disciplines are ill-equipped to be culturally responsive and appropriately serve Black men.

The impetus for this book is a culmination of the author's observations, research, and personal experiences. This included the author's experiences as a Black man in America and professional experience as a psychotherapist. The author has had his fair share of racial trauma that has ranged from experiences with the police to employment settings and other blocked opportunities. This book is about Black men and makes a distinction regarding the experiences of Black men that is empirically supported. The distinctive scope of the book details the systemic and structural racism and traumas that Black men are forced to navigate along with an emphasis on structural and clinical interventions.

Lethal violence and downward social mobility are primarily directed toward Black males. A national spotlight has been focused on anti-Black racism and state-sanctioned violence against Black men since the murder of Trayvon Martin a decade ago to the murder of George Floyd Jr. and Tyre Nichols. Although the media has intermittently focused on these horrific acts during the past decade, there has not been any specific and direct action in the form of public policy to ameliorate anti-Black misandric aggression and state-sanctioned violence against Black men.

The *New York Times* (2015) reported that there are 1.5 million Black men missing due to early death and hyperincarceration. Large numbers of Black men are missing from New York, Chicago, Philadelphia, Detroit, Memphis, Baltimore, Houston, Charlotte, Milwaukee, Dallas, Ferguson, N. Charleston, and the states of Georgia, Alabama, and Mississippi. Changes in incarceration over time were due to changes in policy and not changes in male behavior. Moreover, more than one out of every six Black men who would have been between the prime-age years of 25 and 54 years old has disappeared from daily life.[1]

Approximately 600,000 Black men are incarcerated, while approximately 900,000 are dead. According to the National Officer-Involved Homicide Database (NOIHD), 7,005 Black Americans were killed by police between the years 2000 and 2021 with 91 percent being Black men. Ninety-five percent of unarmed Black Americans killed by police between 2015–2022 were Black men. Approximately 96 percent of all Black children killed by police between 2015–2022 were Black boys. Even in the midst of the first year of the COVID pandemic, which was marked by social distancing, 241 Black Americans were shot and killed by police, whereas 239 of them were Black men. Police killings are preceding at the same pace as previous years, and no progress has been made in reducing deadly police violence in the

---

* Black is capitalized to recognize the struggle of Black Americans in the United States. Black and African American are used interchangeably throughout the text.

DOI: 10.4324/9781003430551-1

U.S. These figures are likely underestimates due to the systematic underreporting of police killings of Black Americans.[2]

The FBI 2020 Hate Crime Statistics indicated that approximately 62 percent of hate crimes were based on race/ethnicity/ancestry, 20 percent were based on sexual orientation, 13 percent were based on religion, approximately 3 percent were based on gender identity, 1 percent were based on disability, and approximately 1 percent were based on gender. Anti-Black bias was the largest category of race-based hate with 2,871 incidents (a 49 percent increase from 2019), which indicates that 56 percent of race-based hate crimes are motivated by anti-Black bias. Moreover, there were 517 anti-Hispanic (Latino/a) incidents and 279 anti-Asian incidents.[3]

Black men have lower incomes than white men in 99 percent of Census tracts and are the least likely of any group to experience upward mobility. English et al. (2014) found in their study that 89 percent of Black men reported experiencing racial discrimination. Black men report the highest rates of racial discrimination (e.g., job discrimination, police encounters, seeking employment, fair wages, getting a quality education, engaging with the health care system) than any group in the U.S. This includes racial discrimination and unfair treatment while shopping, while dining out, while at work, with the police, and while using public transportation. In addition, Black men report more experiences of racial discrimination and in more settings than women, including while seeking employment, working at their jobs, applying for bank loans, and interfacing with the justice system. A Gallup survey (2020) on Black adults and racial microaggressions found that Black men reported significantly higher rates of being feared, being treated with less courtesy, and mistrusted compared to Black women.[4]

This author attests that it is important to have a transdisciplinary approach in examining the racial trauma of Black men. Utilizing only a single discipline (e.g., psychology, counseling, social work, etc.) to address the racial trauma of Black men limits the articulation of racial trauma and is narrow in scope. The racial trauma of Black men is viewed from a clinical lens and a transdisciplinary approach that integrates psychology, counseling, sociology, history, political science, economics, education, demography, biology, neurobiology, business, law, philosophy, epidemiology, trauma studies, genocide studies, African American/ Black/Africana Studies, masculinity studies, gender studies, critical race theory (CRT), and decolonizing studies.

This volume provides a unified theory of racism (UTR), integrated model of racial trauma (IMRT), expanded frameworks of neo-slavery and digital Blackface, definition of Anti-Black racism, theory of plantation politics (anti-colonial theory), framework of race-based shame (RBS), theory of transgenerational trauma points (TTP), and theory of Black male negation (BMN). This definitive volume is the first of its kind to comprehensively center racial trauma and Black men. The current political milieu erroneously dictates that there should not be a focus on the experiences of Black males as they are positioned as an antagonism towards the experiences of other marginalized groups which can put anyone attempting to advocate for Black males in a precarious position.

Book chapters examine the manifestations of racial trauma in the lives of Black men followed by clinical implications. Chapter 1 defines various types of racism. Chapter 2 addresses racial discrimination and the relationship between racialized health disparities produced by anti-Black racism. Chapter 3 defines and discusses trauma and racial trauma. Chapter 4 examines the carceral state and Black men. Chapters 5 and 6 analyzes the economic deprivation of Black men. Chapters 7 and 8 examines the marginalization and vulnerability of Black men. Chapter 9 discusses the coping mechanisms of Black men and provides interventions.

This volume fills a critical and urgent void in the trauma studies field and emerging scholarship on racial trauma. This book is primarily directed towards therapists, but anyone who works with or cares for Black men will find it useful. This is an important contribution to the mental health field that provides clinicians (psychologists, marriage and family therapists, social workers, counselors, and psychiatrists) with the ability to begin to adequately recognize and articulate the racial trauma of Black men and provide responsive care and clinical interventions that inform treatment approaches. In addition, this book will be useful to Black people in general and other oppressed populations.

NOTES

1 Wolfers et al., 2015.
2 Wolfers et al., 2015; Fatal Encounters, n.d.
3 2020 FBI hate crimes statistics. (2021, November 17). https://www.justice.gov/crs/highlights/2020-hate-crimes-statistics; FBI Hate Crime Statistics, 2021; Equal Justice Initiative, 2021.
4 Chetty et al., 2018; Sidanius & Pratto, 1999; Sidanius & Veniegas, 2000; Lloyd, 2020.

CHAPTER 1

WHAT IS *RACISM*?

The term racism can have multiple meanings that produce confusion instead of clarity. This chapter defines various manifestations of racism. Racism is a term is that is used quite routinely in American society to describe a range of incidents and experiences. The term is frequently used in a binary and simplistic manner. What is regularly missing from the discourse is the range and manifestations along with the types of racism that is being discussed. Consequently, it is important that the many permutations of racism be defined to provide grounding and a reference point for the reader when examining the relationship between racism, racial trauma, and the experiences of Black men along with how the idea of race was constructed in the United States. Further, the history of racial hierarchy, stratification, and systemic racism in the U.S. continues to be endemic and ingrained in all aspects of life such as customs, laws, and traditions that permeate institutions and structures that create systems of education, employment, income and wealth, housing and neighborhoods, legal and judicial (criminal justice), and health and health care. These systems create barriers to equity and equality that profoundly impact the racially oppressed and subjugated with exposure to the many forms of racism. In addition, racism can be experienced vicariously. Therefore, it is imperative that this author defines the various constructs associated and also conflated with the term racism. The author has integrated multiple definitions of various forms of racism that are transdisciplinary in this chapter in an effort to provide a comprehensive unified theory of racism (UTR) that is multidimensional and includes race, prejudice, stereotypes, discrimination, oppression, white (white people), whiteness, white privilege, white supremacy, racism, individual racism, vicarious racism, scientific racism, cultural racism, traditional racism; modern/contemporary racism – color-blind racism/ideology, anti-Black racism, anti-Black misandry, symbolic racism, aversive racism; systemic racism – institutional racism, structural racism – structural violence; commodity racism (cultural appropriation) and digital Blackface, racial microaggressions, and implicit/unconscious bias that is grounded in social dominance theory (SDT) and the subordinate male target hypothesis (SMTH).[1]

DEFINITIONS

Race

Race is an unscientific sociopolitical construction in which people in the U.S. are classified by skin color, lineage, language, and physical features into grouped and ranked racial groups in the interests of maintaining racial hierarchies. Devoid of a scientific foundation, this false classification of people is not based on any real or accurate biological or scientific truth but biological fiction. Race is a political construction that historically has been weaponized for political self-interests in order to legitimize the dominance of white people over subjugated Black (African ancestry) and other non-white people. Racial group categories are utilized to distribute social rewards, economic resources, and access and opportunity. Chisom and Washington (1997) defined race as a false classification of human beings created by

DOI: 10.4324/9781003430551-2

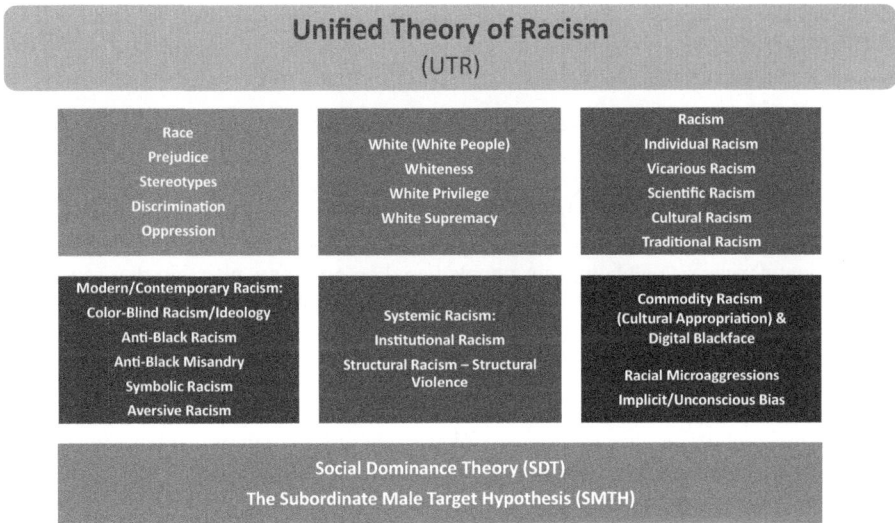

Figure 1.1 Unified Theory of Racism (UTR)

Europeans (whites) that assigns human worth and social status using "white" as the model of humanity and the height of human achievement for the purpose of establishing and maintaining power and privilege.[2]

Race is routinely associated with a group's culture. Culture is a system of meaning that includes values, norms, behaviors, language, and history that is passed generationally through socialization and participation in the group's organization and institutions. Routinely racial group membership refers to a person's social demographic and assumed cultural group.[3]

Prejudice

Operario and Fiske (2001) defined prejudice as negative attitudes directed towards a given out-group or individual based on out-group membership. Prejudice can operate as a pre-judgement or bias in favor of or directed against a person, a group, an event, an idea, or a thing. Action taken on a prejudgment is discrimination. Negative prejudgments are routinely referred to as a stereotype. Action taken based on a stereotype is routinely referred to as bigotry. What distinguishes prejudice from racism is that there is no power dynamic (e.g., structural power) implied or expressed by prejudice. Prejudice coupled with power (i.e., structural power) that affects or impacts people or a group is racism.[4]

Stereotypes

Stereotypes are defined as negatively constructed undesirable characteristics of a group that are either exaggerated or blatantly false and are utilized to justify the facilitation and implementation of oppressive and unfair acts such as discrimination and violence. This includes the belief that all people within a specific group possess the same traits or characteristics (Williams et al., 2012). Stereotypes can also include a positive assessment of a group that provides symbolic or material rewards for members of that group.

Discrimination

Discrimination is defined as the behavior that includes the inclusion or exclusion of someone based on their membership within a particular group. This includes the differential application of rules or regulations for people based on group membership that can have a negative impact on members of subordinate racial and ethnic groups.[5]

Oppression

Oppression is defined as an act or acts of violence that restricts a person's ability to evolve as a complete human being. Oppression includes individual or group attempts to exploit, block, and hinder an individual or group's pursuit of self-determination. Violence is deployed to achieve and maintain oppression and gradually permeates all aspects of the social order further impacting the lives of the oppressed. Over time, oppressive violence becomes normalized, implicit, and embedded in the institutional and psychological reality of society. Ultimately the violence of oppression develops permanence that consumes and dehumanizes the oppressed.[6]

White (White People)

The term white in reference to white people was created by Virginian white enslavers and colonial rulers in the 17th century. The purpose was to replace terms such as "Christian" and "Englishman" in order to distinguish European colonists from enslaved Africans and indigenous peoples. European colonial powers created white as a legal concept after Bacon's Rebellion of 1676 in which indentured servants of European descent and enslaved Africans united against the colonial elite. The legal distinction of white divided the servant class and enslaved Africans based on skin color and continent of origin. Therefore, the creation of "white" came with a granting of privileges while denying them to Africans with the justification of biological and social inferiority. Further, the invention of white people was a means for the ruling elites to retain power by providing a psychological wage linked to social gain for white workers. As a result, white workers were provided with a social status above enslaved Africans, which made it less likely that white workers would oppose the white power elite.[7]

Whiteness

Helms (2017) defined whiteness as the explicit and implicit socialization processes and practices, power structures, laws, privileges, and life experiences that support the white racial group over all others. This includes cultural and racial practices (e.g., customs, traditions), values, and attitudes that indicate what is considered normative with the ultimate effect of privileging white skin and naturalizing systems of white supremacy. Moreover, whiteness has been identified as a marker of racial, economic, and political privilege, a pervasive yet routinely invisible source of representational power, and an omnipresent state of being beyond racial identity. Further, whiteness has been conceptualized as property with appreciating value that is only available to those who are considered white by the legal, social, and cultural institutions of the U.S. Most definitions of whiteness center power, status, and identity associated with racial hierarchy. Schooley et al. (2019) defined whiteness as a multidimensional construct that encompasses racial attitudes, beliefs, behaviors, and experiences that are prevalent but not exclusive to white people as well as the privileged position white people embody in a racially hierarchical society. Whiteness is disseminated and repeatedly reproduced at individual, cultural, and institutional levels.[8]

White Privilege

McIntosh (1988, 1998) identifies two types of white privilege: (1) *unearned entitlements* and (2) *conferred dominance.* Unearned entitlements include life experiences that should be accessible to all people (e.g., feeling safe in public spaces, working in a place where people feel they belong, etc.) but are more accessible to white individuals resulting in unearned advantages. Unearned racial advantages result in a competitive edge that most white individuals are either unaware of or reluctant to acknowledge as well as relinquish. Conferred dominance grants white individuals power over other racial/cultural groups across generations. Conferred dominance is reflected in societal systems such as educational where Eurocentric-based curriculum validates white existence and the judicial system with the hypercriminalization/incarceration of Black people. This includes entertainment and sports where those who are in positions of power are white. White privilege is routinely unrecognizable to white individuals because acknowledging it means renouncing the U.S. perpetuated myth of meritocracy.[9]

Neville et al. (2001) identified white privilege as a multidimensional construct that operates on both a macrolevel and microlevel. The systemic nature of macrolevel white privilege manifests in the benefits, rights, and immunities afforded to white individuals in institutional settings in the U.S. This includes never having to defend being white as being white refers to behaving in ways that are culturally congruent with European American cultural values and expectations as opposed to Black individuals, who are frequently confronted to defend behaviors that are culturally congruent with the lived experiences of persons from their community. Microlevel white privilege includes individual and group-level advantages such as a sense of entitlement, social validation of whiteness, or white individuals being oblivious to the cultural norms, language, and customs of other groups without any resulting economic or social consequences.[10]

White privilege involves a historically based and institutionally perpetuated system that includes (1) treatment of and preferential prejudice for white people based solely on their skin color or ancestral origin from Europe, and (2) exemption from various forms of racial and national oppression based on skin color or ancestral origin from Africa, Asia, the Americas, and the Arab world. Harris and Ordona (1990) identified U.S. institutions and culture (e.g., economic, legal, military, political, educational, entertainment, familial, and religious) as privileging people from Europe over people from Africa, the Americas, Asia, and the Arab world. White supremacy as a system encompasses white privilege and racial oppression, which are correlated. Historical examples include white people being exempt from slavery, land theft, and genocide, which are identified as early forms of white privilege in the future U.S.[11]

White Supremacy

Welsing (1991) defined white supremacy as a behavioral power system of logic, thought, speech, action, emotional response, and perception that is consciously and unconsciously determined, where those who are classified as "white" are considered superior as well as their beliefs and value systems. White supremacy includes cultural, economic, ideological, military, political, psychological, religious, and social structures to sustain global conquest and domination. White supremacy has also been defined as a cultural, economic, and political system that supports white people's dominance over virtually all sectors of society and through which implicit and explicit ideas about white people's superiority are reproduced through everyday dynamics in a wide variety of institutional and social settings. Global white supremacy encompasses the following consistent three themes: (1) prevalent legal and extra-legal subordination of non-white groups; (2) promotion of white people's perspectives and interests across all areas of social life in both implicit (e.g., hypercriminalization/incarceration, gerrymandering) and explicit ways (e.g., alt-right, organized fascism); and (3) hostility toward individuals and social movements that are perceived as a threat to the assumed power and privilege of white people and the institutions they control. White supremacy permeates a range of contemporary social problems that include mental health, social justice, the murder and lynching of unarmed Black Americans by law enforcement, and the global war on terror. Colonial origins and the transatlantic slave trade form the foundation of white supremacy in the U.S. Lawrence and Keleher (2004) defined white supremacy as a historically based, institutionally perpetuated system of exploitation and oppression of continents, nations, and the darker races by white peoples and nations of the European continent with the intent to maintain and defend a system of wealth, power, and privilege.[12]

Racism

The term racism can be traced to the 1902 edition of the *Oxford English Dictionary* and is used to describe the U.S. policy toward Native Americans. The term began to become popularized as it was used as propaganda against anti-Semitism and racial eugenics targeted against Jews in Germany during the 1930s and the Second World War. The word racism was not formally used or accepted until the late 1960s even though the construct of racism had been lived, practiced, experienced for centuries, and understood by the subjugated. The word racism first appeared in the widely circulated Kerner Commission Report (1968) on civil unrest. The definition and application of the word racism has since varied. Eighteen definitions of racism from scholars representing the disciplines of sociology, anthropology, history, and social psychology were analyzed by Jones (1997). His analysis discovered that various accepted definitions over time reflect several different perspectives on racism. Definitions and conceptualizations of racism have established that racism is a complex set of rational and logical beliefs and attitudes that serve to justify the superiority of the dominant racial group while deemphasizing its systemic characteristics and sociohistorical context. Other definitions emphasize racism as attitudes and beliefs that deny minoritized groups of their dignity and access to resources. Moreover, some definitions focus on the role of racial group membership categories along with group-based self-interest and political processes. Further, other definitions recognize the systemic and structural component of racism and establish the sociohistorical context and the shifting nature of racism over time. Ahistorical conceptualizations of racism situate racism as a set of rational and logical beliefs or attitudes that are described by terms such as *nationalism, white nationalism, symbolic* racism, and *aversive* racism.[13]

Casas (2005) defined racism as beliefs that are reflected in behaviors that race is a biological entity and that other racial groups are intellectually, psychologically, and physically inferior. Bulhan (1985) defined racism as a form of oppression and violence that situates racial categories and systems of domination that identifies superior and inferior groups. These imagined differences are utilized in the justification for inequity, exclusion, or domination. Williams and Williams-Morris (2000) defined racism as an organized system that leads to the oppression of some human groups. Ranking and hierarchy determines a group's worth relative to other groups which leads to the development of negative beliefs and attitudes toward the deemed inferior *out-group*. These negative beliefs and attitudes form the justification for differential treatment by individuals and social institutions of out-group members. Clark et al. (1999) defined racism as beliefs, attitudes, institutional arrangements, and acts that tend to denigrate individuals or groups because of phenotypic characteristics. Jones and Carter (1996) defined racism as the transformation of racial prejudice into individual racism through the use of power directed against racial group(s) and their members, who are deemed as inferior by individuals, institutional members, and leaders. This is reflected in policy and procedures with the intentional and unintentional support and participation of the entire race and dominant culture. Gilmore (2007) defined racism as the state-sanctioned and extralegal production and exploitation of group-differentiated vulnerability to premature death. Curry (2017) defined racism as a complex nexus, a cognitive architecture used to invent, reimagine, and evolve the presumed political, social, economic, sexual, and psychological superiority of the white races in society, while materializing the imagined inferiority and hastening the death of inferior races. Therefore, racism is the manifestation of the social processes and concurrent logics that facilitate the death and dying of racially subjugated peoples. Grosfoguel (2016) defined racism as a hierarchy of superiority in relation to the human that has been politically, culturally, and economically constructed and reproduced for centuries by the institutions that encompass the capitalist/patriarchal Western-centric/Christian-centric modern/colonial world-system.

Individual Racism

Individual racism assumes the superiority of one's own racial group and rationalizes dominance and power of one group over another. This form of racism is typically targeted toward an individual and resides within individuals. Examples of individual racism include prejudice coupled with power, internalized oppression, and beliefs about racism influenced by the dominant culture.[14]

Vicarious Racism

Racism can be experienced vicariously through observing actions, nonverbal behavior, and the verbal statements of other people. These observations can reflect individual, cultural, and institutional racism. Vicarious racism includes the indirect exposure (e.g., hearing about or witnessing racist acts being committed) to prejudice and discrimination directed towards other members of one's racial group such as family members, close friends, and witnessing acts of racism either personally or through various media outlets (e.g., news, social media, etc.) that can cause distress as well as affect health. In addition, vicarious racism includes hearing about or seeing racism that is directed toward the entire racial group (e.g., public figures espousing racist rhetoric, racist social media posts, etc.).[15]

Scientific Racism

Scientific racism encompasses the logic of biological determinism in which the physical body signifies individual/group capacities and tendencies rather than social characteristics. Scholarship supporting scientific racism began to rise during the latter part of the 18th century with the writings of philosopher Voltaire, planter and jurist Edward Long, and physician Charles White of Manchester, England. In addition, philosophical underpinnings of scientific racism are traceable to the early work of hereditarians Charles Darwin and the publication of his book *The Origin of Species* (1859), which primarily focused on the biological evolution of animal species, but Social Darwinism was directed toward race and economics in the U.S., which ultimately supported American literature on the inferiority of African people that began to emerge in the 1840s and 1850s. This was followed by Herbert Spencer, who coined the phrase "survival of the fittest" and the belief in the principles of natural selection. The nation's first sociologist Graham Sumner and the nation's leading Social Darwinist believed that American slavery was a representation of the natural order of things. Some scholars in the 19th century began measuring heads and later other parts of the body in order to quantify differences among races with the stated intention of documenting race inequality. Towards the end of the 19th century there was a greater emphasis on the size and contents of the brain case, which led scientists to the next criterion of how race difference could be measured. This criterion was the development of tests that would measure the functions of the brain. The testing movement was led by Francis Galton and Alfred Binet. Galton was the father of the eugenics movement and believed heredity determined individual characteristics and eugenics was the answer to racially regenerate his native England. Galton developed a series of tests focusing on sensory and motor skill assessment in order to prove inherent differences between social classes in England. The first practical intelligence test was constructed in 1905 by Frenchmen Alfred Binet and Théophile Simon that would eventually become the Stanford-Binet Intelligence Scale and was one of the first to use the concept of the "intelligence quotient" (IQ). The modern fascination with testing was influenced by the social and human sciences to establish itself as a legitimate "science." The contemporary race and IQ studies of Arthur Jensen, Richard J. Herrnstein, and Charles Murray influence current discourse of scientific racism. Psychologist Arthur Jensen declared that Black Americans were intellectually inferior to whites. Herrnstein and Murray's book *The Bell Curve* (1994) repeat many of Jensen's assertions and appeals to the American public and policymakers to focus on genetics over environment as the central factor in the determination of human abilities. Intelligence tests became the principal means of scientists who were attempting to document and devise the narrative that there were significant differences between Black Americans and whites and establish Black inferiority and oppression which would be used as an instrument of genetic politics.[16]

Social Darwinism and the IQ testing movement enabled whites to justify long-standing ideological assumptions, policies, and oppressive behaviors. IQ tests became weapons of white supremacist ideology in a campaign of exploitation. This confirmed what had been believed ideologically that there was indeed a white racial hierarchy where whites were superior and Black Americans were inferior. In addition, by the early 20th century, Black Americans were considered a primitive people who could not be assimilated into a complex white civilization. Scientists speculated that Black Americans were doomed for extinction and analyzed census data and predicted the virtual extinction of Black Americans in the 20th century as they believed Black Americans were in the throes of a degenerative evolutionary process. They believed that Black Americans were prone to disease, vice, and crime and could not be helped by education or philanthropy. These late 19th and early 20th century anthropologists, ethnologists, and biologists were supported by the medical profession. This scientific racism reinforced the idea that Black Americans should be excluded from society as they were abstractions and one-dimensional figures. Scientific racism has routinely been used as a justification to propose, project, and enact racist social policies as well as provide a psychological and economic investment in the doctrine of Black inferiority.[17]

Cultural Racism

Jones and Carter (1996) defined cultural racism as the belief that the characteristics and values of one's racial group are superior to that of other racial groups. Cultural racism manifests in the assumed superiority of a language or dialect, standards of beauty, values, beliefs, worldviews, and cultural artifacts dominant in a society. It is passed on intergenerationally and encompasses white racial identity. Thus, it is embedded in all institutions and pervasive in all aspects of society. Consequently, power is exercised against a racial group deemed inferior by individuals and institutions with the intentional or unintentional support of the entire culture through the transformation of race prejudice or ethnocentrism with the ability to define social reality. Cultural racism's influence is mediated through institutional racism even though it is a precondition to individual racism. The intensity and frequency of individual acts of racism are regulated by cultural racism due to the extent that institutional racism has been deployed.[18]

Traditional Racism

Traditional racism refers to overt expressions of racial animosity and a belief in white racial superiority. It is the explicit belief that a group is biologically inferior in comparison to another group. Traditional racism includes negative beliefs about Black intelligence, ambition, honesty, and other stereotyped characteristics. This form of racism manifests in endorsement of direct and overt discriminatory practices and policies such as segregation.[19]

MODERN/CONTEMPORARY RACISM

Modern/contemporary racism are subtle forms of racism compared to the overt form of traditional racism. Modern racism is likely to be disguised and covert and has evolved from the traditional form of racism, which includes overt racial hatred and bigotry that is consciously and publicly displayed. Modern racism tends to be ambiguous and a nebulous form of racism that is more difficult to identify and acknowledge. Further, modern racism is thought to be more problematic, damaging, and injurious to Black people than traditional racism.[20]

Color-Blind Racism/Ideology

Color-blind racism/ideology endorses the belief amongst white individuals that consideration of race is no longer relevant in the U.S. Color-blind racism includes the denying, distorting, or minimizing race and racism. The endorsement of color-blind racism/ideology (e.g., "When I see people, I don't see color or race") provides whites with mechanisms of avoidance, delusions, cognitive dissonance, and dissociation in thinking and acknowledging that they are a member of a dominant racial or ethnic group. Bonilla-Silva (2001) defined color-blind racism as a complex array of shared beliefs or ideology that supports the racial structure in the U.S. It is a dominant racially based framework used to justify the racial status quo or to explain away racial inequalities in the U.S. by individuals, groups, and systems consciously or unconsciously. According to Bonilla-Silva (2001), there are four dominant types of color-blindness. These types include (1) abstract liberalism, which includes ideas such as race should not play a factor in college admissions or any other decision; (2) biological culture, which includes ideas that racism is due to cultural differences and not racism; (3) naturalization of racial matters includes ideas that racial hierarchy is a byproduct of natural tendencies toward in-group favoritism; and (4) minimization of racism includes the denial of structural racism.

According to Neville et al. (2013) color-blind racism includes two interrelated domains. These domains are color-evasion, which includes a denial of racial differences by emphasizing sameness and power-evasion, which includes the denial of racism by emphasizing equal opportunities. Those that endorse color-blindness still manage to racially discriminate, and their color-blind public policies still have racially discriminatory outcomes.[21]

Anti-Black Racism

This author defines anti-Black racism as the explicit and implicit socialization processes and practices, power structures, and laws that target, exploit, sanction, denigrate, demonize, and dispose of Black people. The function of anti-Black racism in the U.S. is to maintain subordination and racial hierarchy where descendants of slavery remain at the bottom of the racial hierarchy (e.g., incarceration, employment, education, income, wealth, housing and residential segregation, and health and health care) as a dispossessed undercaste, thus forming Black existence. In addition, social inequalities and violent events are utilized to manage the Black population in the U.S. Slavery and Jim/Jane Crow are two regimes that account for the bulk of U.S. history and were instrumental in the formation of anti-Black racism. As previously stated in the definition of *white (white people)*; anti-Black racism was forged in the U.S. when the Virginian white enslavers and colonial rulers in the 17th century created "white" as a racial designation in opposition to enslaved Africans following Bacon's Rebellion of 1676 in which indentured servants of European descent and enslaved Africans united against the colonial elite. The legal distinction of "white" divided the servant class and enslaved Africans based on skin color and continent of origin; slave versus free status. Therefore, the creation of "white" came with a granting of privileges while denying them to enslaved Africans with the justification of biological and social inferiority, which has been an impetus for hostility and violence leading to centuries of the death and dying of Black people in the U.S.[22]

Anti-Blackness includes various forms of captivity, terror, and subjection. Anti-Black racism is based on the historical narrative and construct that white people and Black people are essentially white and Black. Blackness is thought to contaminate the purity of whiteness. This includes the abstract imposition of darkness onto Black people and the mapping of moral codes and values (Manicheanism) of evil, sinfulness, impurity, dangerousness, and criminality onto Black bodies, thus fostering phobias. Moreover, Black people are considered inferior, and white people are considered superior. Which includes the belief that on an ontological level, Black Americans are not fully human, which has been calcified in law by the U.S. Supreme Court. Anti-Black racism is contingent upon the myth/doctrine of Black inferiority and the Black-white binary that encompasses racial hierarchy and stratification. These projections take explicit and implicit form and meaning ascribed to Black people in such a way that they become permanent affect charged associations supported by essentialist stereotypes and categorization that continually devalue Black lives. American and global media routinely perpetuate these projections and fears/anxieties/phobias (negrophobia) of Black people into form through the creation of symbolism and imagery. The effect is the criminalization of Blackness devoid of any specific action taken by the victim. Therefore, the mere presence of a Black person evokes hostility or incomprehensible violence as well as any indicator of "disobedience" or resistance to white order and oppression. Further legitimating a high tolerance for brutality, terrorism, perpetual warfare, and indifference toward the suffering of Black people.[23]

Anti-Black Misandry

Black men carry the burden of two stigmatized social identities in U.S. society as Black-Americans (anti-Black racism) and as a Black male (Black misandry). Anti-Black misandry is the hatred of Black men that includes stereotyping and marginality that Black men are forced to endure as they attempt to navigate through society. Smith et al. (2011) defined Black misandry as an exaggerated pathological aversion toward Black men that is produced and reinforced in societal, institutional, and individual ideologies and practices. In addition, Black misandry is an ideological pathology that is reinforced in scholarly ontologies, axiologies, and epistemologies where Black men are held in suspicion, marginalized, hated, rendered invisible, surveilled, or assigned to one or more socially prescribed stereotypical categories. Moreover, Black misandry describes how other groups position, conceptualize, define, redefine, and problematize Black males as subordinate, inferior, and criminal. Curry (2018) defined anti-Black misandry as the cumulative assertions of Black male inferiority due to problematic psychologies of deficiency and deviance or hyper-personality traits (e.g., hypersexuality or hypermasculinity) that provides the justification for criminalization, phobics (i.e., negrophobia), and the sanctioning of Black male life. These ideas encompass the group-based racial consciousness of white America and is part of the social structure and mythology of racism. Thus, exposure to the notions of Black male deviance and danger are commonplace in U.S. society. These stereotypes of Black males are held by whites (women and men), Black Americans (women and men), other ethnic groups, and LGBTQ+ groups. The hatred of Black men is routinely hidden by appeals to safety, civility, and democratic order as Black men are thought to be a phantasmic threat (i.e., boogeymen or living terrors) to America and the social order and is activated through extreme hypersurveillance, control, and death.[24]

Symbolic Racism

Symbolic racism is a form of modern racism that includes anti-Black affect and traditional American moral values that are embodied in the Protestant Ethic (e.g., self-reliance, individual achievement, and hard work). Symbolic racism emerged during the civil rights movement of the 1960s as a reaction to the end of legal segregation in the U.S. This form of racism is referred to as *symbolic* due to beliefs that are symbolic of an abstract system of learned moral values and ideals. It includes white Americans supporting the principles of equality for Black Americans but not supporting efforts to implement these principles (e.g., reparations). These anti-Black attitudes and feelings are embodied in the resistance to change racial status quo and caste based on moral feelings that Black Americans violate the traditional American values of individualism and self-reliance, the work ethic, obedience, and discipline. Further, symbolic racism is openly expressed by the following four themes and beliefs: (1) Blacks no longer encounter much prejudice or discrimination, (2) Blacks have failed to progress due to their unwillingness to work hard enough, (3) Blacks want too much too fast (equal rights), and (4) Blacks have received their fair share.[25]

Aversive Racism

Aversive racism is another form of modern racism that operates unconsciously in subtle and indirect ways. It is characterized by white individuals who publicly advocate egalitarian values but who hold views of racial superiority. Aversive racism includes ambivalence due to internal conflicts based on interactions and beliefs coupled with a sincere egalitarian value system (e.g., all humans are created equal under God) and unacknowledged negative affect and beliefs about Black Americans. Aversive racism encompasses feelings of antagonism and ambivalence about race and adherence to traditional American values. This form of racism is justified by American values and beliefs in equality. Therefore, the failure of minoritized groups to meet standards of conduct and social participation are routinely cited for their experiences. This places an emphasis on personal character rather than on systemic processes. An analysis of how the group in power defines what is acceptable and what is not is devoid from this discourse. Moreover, power dynamics that shapes values, behavior, and beliefs based on the group in power is largely ignored. Therefore, the group in power gets to determine when and if a group or its members fail to meet the standards of good character or appropriate behavior. As a result, a rational logic is applied to racism where one is able to maintain superiority without confrontation and accusations of racism.[26]

The psychological duality of aversive racism creates a state of cognitive dissonance in white individuals resulting in public advocacy for racial equality while privately harboring anxiety and fear of Black people. The dissonance further contributes to the avoidance of meaningful contact with Black people. Endorsement of egalitarian values coupled with the denial of negative and discriminatory attitudes toward Black Americans is a fundamental tenet of aversive racism. Therefore, explicit discrimination is only justifiable when it is based on factors other than race.[27]

Commodity Racism (Cultural Appropriation) and Digital Blackface

Chin (2015) defined commodity racism as the way in which race and commodities intersect and mutually inform one another (i.e., cultural appropriation). Commodity racism encompasses negrophilia, which is the fetishization of Black culture. Black bodies have historically been commodified in the U.S. beginning with slavery. Commodity racism represents a complex array of Black experiences (e.g., food, style of dress, vernacular, music, hair styles, digital Blackface, colloquialisms, Black death and dying, etc.) that are transformed into products/commodities from the ideological racial imaginings of whites and non-Black people that transfigures images of Black people into absurd decadent caricatures. These caricatures are routinely used in representational practices in popular culture. There is an inherent and perverted desire to embody and consume Blackness in order to inhabit it. This includes the reliance on the fetishization of Blackness and Black flesh. At face value it can appear as the celebration or appreciation of Black culture or people but is a mockery and form of parasitism that attempts to gain social or material capital/wealth through the absorption of Blackness that routinely is a grotesque or exaggerated version. Moreover, it takes form through racial stereotypes and minstrelsy in order to dehumanize and debase Black people through the commodification of racist tropes (e.g., Mammy, Saphire, Jezebel, Tom, Coon, Sambo, Buck, etc.) while defining Blackness. Embedding race into various media platforms and marketing techniques is a form of commodity racism. Commodity racism is a form of anti-Black racism and neocolonialism that markets white ideals of power and domination through images that idealize the oppression of Black people through commodity spectacle.[28]

Digital Blackface is a form of commodity racism. Minstrel Blackface in the U.S. has not ended but only emerged into more subtle forms of anti-Black racism through current technological mediums for mass consumption over the internet and mobile devices. Digital Blackface routinely is disseminated through GIFs, internet memes, and keyboard stickers (bitmojis) over social media platforms and text messages to share emotions and feelings of relatability. Black subjects are routinely mocked and used incessantly. White and non-Black people are able to anonymously claim a Black identity. Reaction GIFs are overwhelmingly Black subjects. Black bodies, art, and culture is exported for mass consumption while being reduced to a thing. Moreover, the circulation of digital Blackface contains memetic qualities that allow images of Black people to be commodified for mass entertainment in a perpetual feedback loop that reifies white identity while simultaneously dehumanizing Black people and normalizing/ritualizing anti-Blackness. Digital Blackface preserves legacies of anti-Black racism, which includes Black inferiority through repackaged minstrel Blackface that comprises cultural appropriation of language and expressions of Black people for entertainment while dismissing the lived experiences of Black people in the U.S. (e.g., police brutality, employment discrimination, wealth gap, hypercriminalization/incarceration, etc.). Historically, Blackface has served as a unifying tool of white people while promoting white supremacy and celebrating white power and American patriotism through symbolism. Whites who don't fit into mainstream whiteness are able to reassert their whiteness through Blackface while inhabiting the depraved Black thing. Digital Blackface reinforces and contributes to implicit biases against Black people.[29]

Racial Microaggressions

Pierce (1970) coined the term *microaggressions* to describe offensive mechanisms that are gratuitous incessant racial assaults upon the dignity and hope of Black people that are cumulative in nature. Racial microaggressions are routinely innocuous, automatic, and unconscious degradations that are steeped in the need to reaffirm and reassert feelings and ideas of white superiority. Included within the racial microaggressions framework are microassaults which are subtle and cumulative slights. Microaggressions can be experienced from individuals or a collective group. The cumulative nature of microaggressions can contribute to diminished mortality, augmented morbidity, and affect confidence and self-esteem. This leads to feelings of disconnection and helplessness. Racial microaggressions ensure that those who hold an inferior status are ignored, tyrannized, terrorized, and minimized. Moreover, racial microaggressions control space, time, energy, and mobility with subsequent feelings of degradation and the erosion of self-confidence and self-image.[30]

Pérez Huber and Solorzano (2015) defined racial microaggressions as everyday manifestations of racism that non-white people experience in their public and private lives. Racial microaggressions are a form of systemic racism that includes verbal (e.g., casual comments regarding appearance, language, or country of origin), nonverbal (e.g., body language), and visual (e.g., images in books/magazines, film, advertising) assaults that are directed towards the darker races in an automatic or unconscious fashion. The targets of racial microaggressions can experience a cumulative impact that takes a psychological and physiological toll. This includes self-doubt, anger, stress, racial battle fatigue, poor academic performance, poor health, etc. Racial microaggressions are undergirded by institutional racism that includes the formal and informal structural mechanisms of policies and processes that systematically subordinate, marginalize, and exclude non-white people. Therefore, racial microaggressions are everyday expressions of institutional racism through enactments of implicit biases against Black people. Racial microaggressions provide a framework for Black people to identify the pain caused by everyday racism without it being dismissed.

The "micro" in microaggression does not mean "minor," "less than," or "small" but it means "in the everyday." Racial microaggressions sometimes have debilitating consequences when experienced over a lifetime. The race-related stressors of racial microaggressions can contribute to high blood pressure, depression, anxiety, cardiovascular disease, and increased death rates among Black people.[31]

Sue et al. (2007) defined racial microaggressions as brief and common daily verbal, behavioral, or environmental indignities, whether intentional or unintentional, that communicate hostile, derogatory, or negative racial slights and insults toward Black people. Routinely there is a lack of awareness by the perpetrator of racial microaggressions that they have engaged in such communications when interacting with racial and ethnic people. Microaggressions from interactions are routinely unconsciously conveyed by subtle snubs or dismissive looks, gestures, and tones. The pervasiveness and automatic nature of microaggressions in interpersonal exchanges (e.g., daily conversations and interactions) contribute to them being dismissed and glossed over as being innocent and innocuous. Microaggressions may be environmental in nature, such as when a Black person is exposed to an office setting that unintentionally attacks their racial identity. Microaggressions are harmful to non-white people because they impair performance in a multitude of settings by depleting the psychic and spiritual energy of recipients and by creating inequities.[32]

Sue et al. (2007) expanded the racial microaggression framework by creating a taxonomy of racial microaggressions in everyday life that included three forms of racial microaggressions. These three forms of racial microaggressions include: **microassault**, **microinsult**, and **microinvalidation.** A **microassault** includes an explicit racial derogation that is primarily characterized by a verbal and nonverbal attack meant to hurt the intended victim through name-calling, avoidant behavior, or purposeful discriminatory actions. Examples include using racial epithets, deliberately serving a white patron before a Black person or displaying a swastika. Microassaults are a form of traditional racism conducted on an individual level. They are likely to be conscious and deliberate and routinely expressed in limited or private situations that provide the perpetrator some degree of anonymity. A **microinsult** includes interaction that conveys rudeness and insensitivity and demeans a person's racial heritage or identity. Microinsults are routinely unconscious (perpetrator) subtle snubs that convey a hidden insulting message to the non-white person. Examples include a white employer telling a prospective Black candidate that the most qualified person should get the job regardless of race or when a non-white employee is asked how they got their job. Further, microinsults can occur nonverbally when a Black person's presence is not acknowledged or ignored, which conveys the message that their very being and presence or contributions hold no value or are unimportant. **Microinvalidations** include communication that excludes, negates, or nullifies the psychological thoughts, feelings, or experiences of a Black person. Examples include the perpetrator telling Black people that they don't see color or that we are all a part of the human race.[33]

Sue et al. (2007) identified nine categories of microaggressions with distinct themes. The categories fall under microinsults and microinvalidations, and they include the following: (1) alien in one's own land that sends a message that you are not American or that you are a foreigner; (2) ascription of intelligence, which includes assigning intelligence to a Black person based on their race and sends the message that Black people are generally not as intelligent as whites; (3) color-blindness include statements that indicate a white person is avoiding acknowledging race, which sends messages that deny a non-white person's racialized and ethnic experiences or that they should assimilate and acculturate to the dominant culture; (4) criminality/assumption of criminal status includes the presumption that a Black person is dangerous, criminal, or deviant on the basis of their race, which sends the message that a Black person is a criminal, going to steal, poor, don't belong, and they are dangerous; (5) denial of individual racism is made in a statement by whites when denying their racial biases, which sends the message that they are immune to racism because they have Black friends or that they experience sex/gender oppression that is no different than racism; (6) myth of meritocracy include statements that assert race does not play a role in life successes, which sends the message that Black people are given unfair benefits because of race or are lazy and incompetent and need to work harder; (7) pathologizing cultural values and communication styles with the notion that the values and communication styles of the dominant white culture is ideal, which sends the message to assimilate into the dominant culture or leave your cultural baggage behind; (8) second-class status/citizen occurs when a white person is provided with preferential treatment as a consumer over a Black person, which sends the message that non-white people are servants to whites and don't occupy a high-status position, whites are more valued as customers, or you don't belong and are a lesser being; and (9) assumption of inferior status includes the presumption that a Black person is uneducated, poor, or a menial worker, which includes "credentials" and "social class" that characterize the nature of this assumption and sends the message that Black Americans are uneducated, poor, and occupy low-status positions.[34]

Racial microaggressions create psychological dilemmas that lead to an increase in levels of anger, mistrust, and self-esteem and are routinely ambiguous and invisible to the perpetrator as well as the recipient. White individuals frequently perpetuate racial microaggressions who routinely don't consciously recognize the racist origins or implications of their actions. Therefore, microaggressions tend to be subtle, indirect, and unintentional; are typically present when other explanations can be offered for prejudicial behavior as opposed to explicit prejudice; and can routinely occur when whites adhere to color-blind ideology (microinvalidation) and claim to not notice differences or that "color" was not involved in various actions. Routinely racial microaggressions result in a negative racial climate where the victim is left with self-doubt, frustration, isolation, and depression. Microaggressions are an invisible and unconscious reflection of white supremacy that assails the racial reality of Black Americans; are manifested at individual, institutional, and cultural levels; create psychological distress in Black people; and produce education, employment, and healthcare disparities in Black communities.[35]

Implicit/Unconscious Bias

Implicit bias is defined as the pervasive and robust attitudes or stereotypes that affect our understanding, actions, and decisions in an unconscious manner. These biases are activated involuntarily and without an individual's awareness or intentional control and include both favorable and unfavorable evaluations. Implicit biases are not accessible through introspection and reside deep in the unconscious and are different from explicit biases that individuals may choose to conceal for the purpose of social and political correctness. The implicit associations that people harbor cause them to have feelings and attitudes about other people based on race, ethnicity, age, and appearance that affect behavior. These associations develop over the course of a lifetime beginning at a very early age through exposure to direct and indirect messages as well as in-group preferences. The media and news programming contribute to implicit associations as well. Moreover, exposure to commonly held attitudes about social groups permeate the unconscious of individuals without their active consent through media exposure and by the passive observation of who occupies valued roles and devalued roles in society. According to De Castillo (2018), the implicit bias model avoids a central aspect of unconscious racial prejudice which includes the underlying motivations and incentives for harboring racist attitudes and beliefs that activate psychological resistances (i.e., active ignorance and persistent defensiveness) to awareness or changing prejudices.[36]

Everyone possesses implicit biases, even those with avowed impartiality such as court judges, and implicit bias has been documented in children. Implicit and explicit biases are related but distinct mental constructs that may influence each other and are not mutually exclusive. Implicit attitudes may predict and influence behavior more than self-reported explicit attitudes. It is important to consider implicit and explicit attitudes in order to understand prejudice-related responses. Implicit associations do not necessarily align with declared beliefs or even reflect explicitly endorsed stances as they are held outside of conscious awareness. Implicit biases tend to favor one's in-group but can be held against one's in-group and is routinely an automatic and unconscious process.[37]

The Black/White Implicit Association Test (IAT) analyzes the speed at which participants categorize white and Black faces with positive (e.g., happiness, joy, etc.) and negative (e.g., terrible, angry, etc.) words. The racial group that is most quickly associated with positive terms indicates a positive implicit bias towards that group. Most Americans (approximately 70 percent) regardless of race exhibit a pro-white/anti-Black bias on the Implicit Association Test. This includes Asian and Latino/a respondents who indicate a pro-white bias at levels comparable to white respondents as well as children as young as six years old. Further, close to half of Black respondents display a pro-white/anti-Black bias on the Implicit Association Test.[38]

Research has demonstrated that there is a clear implicit anti-Black bias against Black Americans. Pediatricians are more likely to prescribe painkillers for white patients as opposed to Black patients; people with "Black-sounding" names (e.g., Jamal and Lakisha) are 50 percent less likely to get called for a job than people with "white-sounding" names, Black boys as young as 10 years old are viewed as older and less innocent than their peers among a sample of police officers in large urban areas, college students demonstrated implicit racial bias against Black students, and research participants (college students and police officers) are more likely to "shoot" if the target is Black than white.[39]

SYSTEMIC RACISM

Feagin (2013) defined systemic racism as a complex array of recurring exploitive, discriminatory, and other oppressive practices targeting non-white people; the institutional economic and other social resource inequalities that includes racial hierarchy and the dominant white racial frame that was created to justify and ensure white privilege and dominance over the darker races. Systemic racism encompasses institutional and structural racism.

Institutional Racism

Institutions are comprised of individuals and characterizes the cumulative experiences of individuals over time, which produces the represented culture and creates the ability of institutions to operate independently from individual influence. The blueprint and architecture of the organization of institutional racism is provided by cultural racism. The objectives of institutional racism are white dominance, and the criterion of success is white privilege. Gross and unequal outcomes in social systems and organizations such as in education, health, occupation, and politics reflect institutional racism. Further, policies and practices within organizations and institutions that contribute to discrimination for a group of people that continually leads to adverse outcomes and racial inequality is representative of institutional racism. Moreover, institutional racism occurs within and between institutions and is discriminatory treatment, unfair policies, inequitable opportunities, and impacts that are based on race and produced and perpetuated by institutions such as schools, mass media, etc. Institutional power is exercised when individuals within institutions act in ways that advantage and disadvantage people based on race. An example would be a police officer who treats someone with racial bias, thus engaging in institutional racism because they are representing a law enforcement institution. Institutions thrive on racist cultural scripts of white supremacy and Black inferiority and is continued within and across generations which reinforces cultural racism. In addition, individual expressions of racism are preceded and preconditioned by institutional racism.[40]

Structural Racism

Structural racism includes a social system of stratification that limits a group's access to opportunity from social, educational, economic, and political participation. From a sociological perspective, this includes a denial of primary structural assimilation, which translates into a lack of proximal relationships of a close personal nature with people from groups in positions of power and authority that ultimately operates as systemic barriers that limit access to power. Moreover, this comprises social structures at all levels of society that manifests in ethnic prejudices as shared group beliefs and in discriminatory actions by individuals of the dominant group. This includes discourses, organization, or relationships within and among groups, institutions, classes, or other social formations. Lawrence and Keleher (2004) defined structural racism in the U.S. as the normalization and legitimization of a range of dynamics that include historical, cultural, institutional, and interpersonal that consistently advantage whites while producing cumulative and chronic adverse outcomes for Black people. Egede and Walker (2020) defined structural racism as the ways in which societies foster discrimination through mutually reinforcing inequitable systems. Interconnected systems that embed inequities in laws and policies are created by discriminatory practices in one sector that reinforce parallel practices in other sectors. Structural racism encompasses mutually reinforcing practices that sanction discriminatory beliefs, stereotypes, and unequal distribution of resources through education, employment, housing, credit markets, health care, and the justice system. Further, it is a system of racial hierarchy and inequity that is supported by white supremacy and includes the preferential treatment, privilege, and power of white people at the expense of Black people, Native American, Latino/a, Asian, Pacific Islander, Arab, and other racially oppressed groups.[41]

Structural racism incorporates the entire system of white supremacy and is dispersed and inculcated in all aspects of society including history, culture, politics, economics, and the social fabric of the U.S. Structural racism encompasses three foundational areas of American society. These areas are (1) history, which routinely is a distorted revisionist version that is implicit providing the foundation to white supremacy; (2) culture, which is an omnipresent fixture of American life that provides the normalization and replication of racism; and (3) interconnected institutions and policies that provide the fundamental relationships and rules across American society, which exercise legitimacy and reinforcements to maintain and perpetuate racism. Moreover, it has been argued that structural racism is the most profound and pervasive form of racism as all other forms of racism emerge from structural racism. Inequalities in power, access, opportunities, treatment, and policy impacts and outcomes whether intentional or nonintentional are key indicators of structural racism. Structural racism involves the reinforcing effects of multiple institutions and cultural norms, past and present, that continually produce new, and reproduce old forms of racism therefore making it difficult to locate in a particular institution.[42]

Structural violence is a power system that is an aspect of structural racism. According to Lee (2016), structural violence is a form of violence where social structures or social institutions harm people by preventing them from meeting their basic needs. Structural violence often includes racial, sex, health, and economic disparities and is frequently a subtle and less visible form of violence but greater in scope and implication. Societies place limitations (e.g., political, economic, religious, cultural, and legal institutions of authority) on groups of people that prevent them from reaching an optimal quality of life where they can thrive. The structural violence is embedded within social structures and manifested through institutional practices and normalized as ordinary life difficulties or hardships. Societies form and organize the institutions that creates structures, and the violence causes deprivation, injury, and death.

SOCIAL DOMINANCE THEORY (SDT) AND THE SUBORDINATE MALE TARGET HYPOTHESIS (SMTH)

Social dominance theory (SDT) indicates that all human societies tend to be structured as systems of group-based social hierarchies. Routinely, one or a small number of dominant hegemonic groups are at the top and one or a number of subordinate groups are at the bottom of the hierarchical social structure. The dominant group possess a disproportionate large share of *positive social value* (e.g., political authority and power, good and plentiful food, splendid homes, the best available health care, wealth, and high social status, etc.), which includes all the material and symbolic rewards for which people strive. Subordinate groups possess a disproportionate large share of *negative social value* (e.g., low power and social status, high-risk and low-status occupations, relatively poor health care, poor food, modest or miserable homes, and severe negative sanctions such as prison and death sentences). SDT attempts to identify the various mechanisms that produce and maintain group-based social hierarchy. Group-based hierarchy refers to the social power, prestige, and privilege that an individual acquired by virtue of their membership in a socially constructed group such as race, religion, clan, tribe, lineage, linguistic/ethnic group, or social class. An individual's social status, influence, and power are a function of their group membership and not simply due to their abilities or characteristics. SDT posits that there are three distinctly different stratification systems. These stratification systems are an age system where adults and middle-age people have disproportionate social power over children and younger adults; a sex/gender system where males have disproportionate social and political power compared to females (patriarchy); and an arbitrary-set system that is filled with socially constructed and highly salient groups based on characteristics such as race, caste, social class, clan, ethnicity, estate, nation, religious sect, regional grouping, or any other socially relevant group distinction that is constructed from the human imagination. The arbitrary-set system is associated with the greatest degree of violence, brutality, and oppression and routinely far exceeds the other two systems in terms of intensity and scope.[43]

SDT encompasses three primary assumptions that are foundational: (1) age and sex/gender-based hierarchies routinely exists within all social systems and arbitrary-set systems of social hierarchy will consistently emerge within social systems producing sustainable economic surplus; (2) most forms of group conflict and oppression (e.g., racism, ethnocentrism, sexism, nationalism, classicism, regionalism) are different manifestations of human predisposition to form group-based social hierarchies; (3) human social systems (societies) are subject to the counterbalancing influences of *hierarchy-enhancing* (HE) forces that produce and maintain higher levels of group-based social inequality and *hierarchy-attenuating* (HA) forces that produce greater levels of group-based social equality. HE and HA both include legitimizing ideologies and social institutions. Social ideologies include beliefs, myths, and religious doctrines that are utilized to justify and defend group-based social inequality. HE social institutions advantage dominant groups through the allocation of social resources while disadvantaging subordinate groups. HE social institutions include internal security forces, the criminal justice system, and large corporations. HA social institutions include human and civil rights organizations, charities, and legal aid groups focused on the poor and indigent. Group-based hierarchy is motivated by three proximal processes of *aggregated individual discrimination*, *aggregated institutional discrimination*, and *behavioral asymmetry*. These proximal processes are in part regulated by legitimizing myths. The level of endorsement, desire, and support of group-based social hierarchy is related to the extent that an individual endorses legitimizing myths. The generalized orientation toward group-based social hierarchy is referred to as *social dominance orientation* (SDO). SDO includes the degree to which individuals desire and support group-based hierarchy and the domination of groups deemed "inferior" by "superior" groups. High status groups typically are higher in SDO than low status groups. SDO correlates with numerous sociopolitical attitudes that are relevant to intergroup inequality and domination that predicts endorsement of racism, sexism, nationalism, cultural elitism, political-economic conservatism, belief in meritocracy, pro-military attitudes, punitive legal policies, and rejection of social welfare policies. Aggregated individual discrimination refers to simple, daily, and inconspicuous individual acts of discrimination by an individual against another. Aggregated institutional discrimination refers to the rules, procedures, and actions of social institutions. These social institutions include private or public institutions including courts, lending institutions, hospitals, retail outlets, and schools. Aggregated institutional discrimination can be identified within institutions based on institutional decisions that result in disproportionate allocation of positive or negative social value across the social status hierarchy regardless of whether institutional discrimination is conscious/unconscious or deliberate/unintended. Moreover, institutions assist in the maintenance of the integrity of social hierarchy through the deployment of systematic terror (e.g., violence or threats of violence disproportionately directed against subordinates).[44]

Behavioral asymmetry is a mechanism that produces and maintains group-based hierarchy. Behavioral asymmetry includes the differences in behavioral repertoires of individuals belonging to groups across different levels of the social power continuum. The group-based hierarchical relationships within the social system (society) reinforce these behavioral differences while the behavioral differences contribute to group-based hierarchy. Behavioral asymmetry is also affected by socialization patterns, stereotypes, legitimizing ideologies, psychological biases, and systematic terror. Therefore, the constrained agency of the subordinates maintains group-based hierarchies and are routinely cooperative with group-based domination. This passive and active cooperation with their own oppression provides systems of group-based hierarchy with resiliency, robustness, and stability. Therefore, social hierarchy is not solely maintained by the oppressive behavior of dominants but also by the deferential and compliant behavior of subordinates. There are four varieties of behavioral asymmetry: *asymmetrical in-group bias, out-group favoritism* or *deference, self-debilitation,* and *ideological asymmetry.* Behavioral asymmetry illustrates the cooperative nature of intergroup oppression and group-based social hierarchies that are coordinated and collaborative activities of both dominants and subordinates. Legitimizing myths (LMs) are ideological instruments that affects group-based hierarchy. LMs consists of consensually shared ideologies that include stereotypes, attributions, cosmologies, predominant values or discourses, shared representations, etc. that provide moral and intellectual justification for the distribution of social value through social practices while providing explanations for why things are how they are and suggesting how people and institutions should behave. LMs routinely have the appearance of being true due to being consensually and closely associated with the structure of society. LMs can be identified by two independent characteristics of either functional type or potency.[45]

The **Subordinate Male Target Hypothesis** (**SMTH**) of SDT posits with supporting research that out-group males rather than out-group females are the primary targets of arbitrary-set discrimination. Women from both arbitrary-set in-groups and out-groups will be exposed to sex/gender discrimination and the dynamics of patriarchy (paternalism/control), while arbitrary-set out-group females will suffer from the effects of arbitrary-set discrimination generally due to their close associations (e.g., husbands, sons, fathers, brothers, and lovers) with arbitrary-set out-group males but are not the primary targets of arbitrary-set discrimination. The explanation provided is that arbitrary-set discrimination is primarily a form of intrasexual competition that is perpetrated by in-group males and directed against out-group males. Moreover, this arbitrary-set discrimination against out-group males has a ferocity that can be interpreted as a form of low-level warfare meant to harm, destroy, or debilitate. Evidence across various domains include encounters with police and the criminal justice system (e.g., incarceration and death penalty), labor market (employment and salary), housing, educational outcomes, banking and financial sectors, and retail sales sectors of society support the SMTH.[46]

ORIGINS OF ANTI-BLACK RACISM

The most significant sociodemographic distinction in the U.S. is race. Kendi (2016) identified the book *The Chronicle of the Discovery and Conquest of Guinea* as the beginning of a recorded history of anti-Black racism. This book was published in 1453 and written by Gomes Eanes de Zurara, who was commissioned by Portugal's King Afonso V. The book was a biography on the life and slave-trading of King Afonso V's uncle Prince Henry and was the first European book on Africans in the modern era. Zurara was a commander in Prince Henry's Military Order of Christ, who obscured Prince Henry's economic decision to exclusively participate in African slave trading. Zurara's book reflected Prince Henry's racist policies regarding African slave-trading. The Portuguese were the first Europeans to bring enslaved Africans back to Europe. These slave-trading ventures were framed by Zurara as missionary expeditions, and African captives were framed as barbarians and beasts who not only needed religious but also civil salvation. Enslavement was presented as an improvement over their free state in Africa. The Portuguese became the primary resource of knowledge on the unknown continent of Africa and African people for slave-traders and enslavers in Spain, Holland, France, and England.[47]

The word *race* first appeared in Frenchman Jacques de Brézé's 1481 poem *The Hunt*, which refers to hunting dogs. The term *race* was eventually expanded to include humans over the next century, where it was used to primarily identify, differentiate, and animalize African people. The term *race* made its debut in a dictionary in 1606, where French diplomat Jean Nicot included a definition that referenced the *descent* of a man, horse, or dog being from a "good or bad race," which was utilized by the British to collapse Native Americans and multiethnic Africans into the same racial groups. In 1758, Swedish taxonomist and botanist Carl von Linne (Linnaeus) coined the term *Homo sapiens* (Humans) and was the first to position humans in a taxonomy of animals in his book *Systema Naturae*. Humans were divided into four groups on the basis of physical and psychological impressions. In 1775, German anthropologist and anatomist Johann Blumenbach used the word *race* to classify humans into five divisions of Caucasian, Mongolian, Ethiopian, American, and Malay. He coined the term *Caucasian* as he believed that the Caucasus region of Asia Minor created "the most beautiful race of men." Race categorization continues today even though phenotypic and biochemical variations do not correlate simply with genotypic differences. The use of the word *race* has remained largely unchanged in common and medical texts, and racial taxons are still widely used in medical teaching, practice, and research despite evidence that race is biological fiction. The medicalization of race groupings is legitimatized by the use of race groupings in medical literature and practice as acceptable descriptive labels that are fundamental to the proper diagnosis and treatment of disease in humans.[48]

In what was to become the United States, there was a labor shortage in the British North American Colonies that would eventually become the United States. The items grown in the colonies were labor intensive and included tobacco, cotton, wheat, and corn. There were approximately 250,000 indentured servants in the British North American colonies during the colonial era. In addition, religious nonconformists, convicts, and kidnap victims were sent to the colonies as well. But there was still an insufficient supply of labor to meet the demand in the colonies. At the time, race was not yet the major social division, which was to occur years later.[49]

In 1664, young British aristocrat Nathaniel Bacon settled in Jamestown, Virginia. As a recent arrival, he was excluded from Governor William Berkeley's inner circle and the subsequent advantages, which included social networks that would have allowed him to participate in the lucrative fur trade. Bacon was frustrated by this exclusion and recognized the discontentment of various groups in the Virginia colony. Bacon formed a coalition of two disparate groups that consisted of a group of aristocrats and a group of farmers, former indentured servants, indentured servants, and enslaved Africans. The group of aristocrats had been excluded from the elite circles of social networks which affected their ability to generate greater wealth. The group of farmers, former indentured servants, indentured servants, and enslaved Africans desired to create a more egalitarian society. Their complaint was that the colonial government failed to adequately provide for their well-being. This included complaints of being over-taxed and the government failing to clear indigenous land for their usage and failing to protect them from attacks by Native Americans as well as complaints from former indentured servants that they had not received land that was promised to them concluding their servitude. In addition, indentured servants and enslaved Africans experienced harsh treatment in the Virginia colony. Therefore, government under Berkeley's rule was regarded as cliquish, corrupt, and ineffective. Bacon was able to generate support from these disaffected groups in his effort to overthrow Berkeley's government with the intention of creating a new social order in the Virginia colony. Bacon's Rebellion took place in 1676, and Governor Berkeley was unable to quell the rebellion. Jamestown was raided by Bacon's supporters, and the governor's mansion was burned down to the ground, forcing Berkeley to flee. Troops were sent by King Charles II as a result of Berkeley's inability to subdue the uprising. The rebellion came to an end as a result of the additional firepower and Bacon's death from dysentery.[50]

Bacon's Rebellion failed to overthrow the Virginia colonial government but forged class solidarity between indentured servants and former indentured servants and enslaved Africans. This posed a serious threat to the ruling elite that could happen again and potentially overthrow the ruling elite. Therefore, race was used as a wedge between Black and white workers in order to maintain power. Whites were offered social advantages that were denied to Black Americans, and Black Americans were made slaves for life. This severed the bond of solidarity between the two groups. Poor landless whites were promised and able to obtain property, own firearms, become plantation overseers, and have the right to vote, while Black Americans were enslaved for life and relegated to the status of property and a permanent racial undercaste. Their undercaste status included the denial of employment opportunities, education, political rights, access to courts, ownership of property, and residential locations. The ruling elite were able to buy the support of working-class whites by offering them benefits with the illusion that they were partners in the political system, thus allowing them to identify with the ruling-class whites who were oppressing them. The effect was the prevention of a spreading class consciousness among the lower class that was multiracial and could potentially spark mass uprisings. The planters wanted to avoid class conflict among white people by switching from white servants to an enslaved Black labor force that would never become free or control firearms. Further, this practice was codified with the passage of the Virginia Slave Codes of 1705. The Virginia Slave Codes prohibited Black Americans from owning firearms and gave white enslavers the right to kill slaves with impunity.[51]

The aftermath of Bacon's Rebellion created a modern system of racial stratification (slavocracy) in the U.S. that maintains social and racial inequality and ultimately prevented a more equitable society which represented a deepening of past praxis. Therefore, a racial paradigm was created that affects the way people of different races in the U.S. related to each other. This included making Black Americans a permanent undercaste open to gratuitous violence who were excluded from having political agency while providing immigrants and poor whites who shared white skin with a minimum political participation under the illusion that they were partners with the elite in the governing process and shared a connection through whiteness. Further providing an ideological basis to resolve conflict between propertied and unpropertied whites and produced racial solidarity among whites regardless of class differences as they were able to partake in white privilege and create an identity that was in opposition to Black Americans who were lower on the social scale (racial under-caste) while identifying and supporting the policies of the upper class. The term "white" began to replace "Christian" and "Englishman," which continued through the 21st century. Whiteness (white) transcended ethnicity followed by religious boundaries that had been at the center of religious conflict that devastated Europe. Moreover, whiteness created a mutual interest in exploiting Black Americans. Slavery for Black Americans led to greater freedom for poor whites where the labor force was systematically changed from the indentured servitude of whites to the lifelong generational bondage of Black Americans as well as propertyless whites not only obtaining literal property but their whiteness being a form of property and currency. Consequently, more than 17,000 congressmen enslaved Black Americans. Freedom became synonymous with whiteness, where in order to be American one had to be free, and to be free, one had to be white. Black Americans were not viewed as true Americans because they were not white and therefore not free and did not have the right to vote. The invention of race has been the most efficient mechanism of social domination. The relative dominance of Euro-Americans over Black Americans has remained unchanged since the European occupation of the New World more than 400 years ago, thus maintaining a system of racial stratification and hierarchy through white supremacy even in the face of intense efforts to eliminate anti-Black racism from U.S. life.[52]

NOTES

1 Carter, 2007.
2 Carter, 2007; Western States Center, 2003; Carter & Pieterse, 2005; Marger, 2003.
3 Marger, 2003; Carter, 2007.
4 Lawrence & Keleher, 2004.
5 Williams et al., 2012; Feagin, 1991.
6 Freire, 1970; Fanon, 1952, 1963; Bulhan, 1985.
7 Adair & Howell, 1988; Allen, 1994; Du Bois, 1935; Roediger, 1991; Buck, 2001.
8 Giroux, 1997; Harris, 1993; Lipsitz, 1998; Moreton-Robinson, 2005; Schooley et al., 2019; Dyer, 1997; Matias, 2016; Twine & Gallagher, 2008.
9 Utsey et al., 2008.
10 Utsey et al., 2008.
11 Lawrence & Keleher, 2004.
12 Fuller, 1969; Ansley, 1997; Khair, 2016; Puar, 2007; Reddy, 2011; Bell, 1992.
13 Howard, 2016; Blaut, 1992; Carter, 2007; Kerner Commission, 1968; Feagin et al., 1995; Ani, 1994; Goldberg, 1990.
14 Jones, 1997; Lawrence & Keleher, 2004.
15 Harrell, 2000; Heard-Garris et al., 2018; Chae et al., 2021.
16 Hickey, 2006; Smedley & Smedley, 2005; Dennis, 1995; Brandt, 1978; Fredrickson, 1971.
17 Hickey, 2006; Smedley & Smedley, 2005; Dennis, 1995; Brandt, 1978; Fredrickson, 1971.
18 Bowser, 2017; Belgrave & Allison, 2018; Jones, 1972; Essed, 1991.
19 Allport, 1954; Belgrave & Allison, 2018; McConahay, 1986.
20 Sue et al., 2007; Sue, 2003.
21 Bonilla-Silva, 2006; Neville et al., 2006.

22 Gordon, 1995; Adair & Howell, 1988; Curry, 2020.
23 Gordon, 1995; Deliovsky & Kitossa, 2013; Phillips & Pon, 2018; Fanon, 1952.
24 Smith et al., 2007; Smith, 2010.
25 Kinder & Sears, 1981; McConahay, 1982; Bowser, 2017; Henry & Sears, 2008.
26 Gaertner & Dovidio, 1986, Dovidio & Gaertner, 1998; Carter, 2007; Jones, 1997.
27 Dovidio & Gaertner, 1998; Gaertner & Dovidio, 2000.
28 White, 2011; Borgman, 2019; McClintock, 1994.
29 White, 2011; Wong, 2019; Byrne, 2016.
30 Pierce, 1970, 1974, 1988, 1995.
31 Pérez Huber & Solorzano, 2015; Franklin et al., 2014.
32 Franklin, 2004; Sue, 2004.
33 Sue et al., 2007; Helms, 1992.
34 Sue et al., 2007.
35 Sue et al., 2007, 2008; Constantine et al., 2008.
36 Lawrence, 1995; Blair, 2002; Beattie, 2013; Kang et al., 2012; Castelli et al., 2009;
    Kang, 2012; Rudman, 2004a, 2004b; Dunham et al., 2008; Dasgupta, 2013.
37 Rachlinski et al., 2009; Baron & Banaji, 2006; Newheiser & Olson, 2012; Rutland et al.,
    2005; Dasgupta, 2013; Kang, 2009; Wilson et al., 2000; Kang et al., 2012; Bargh &
    Chartrand, 1999; Ziegert & Hanges, 2005; Son Hing et al., 2008; Graham & Lowery,
    2004; Greenwald & Krieger, 2006; Reskin, 2005.
38 Dovidio et al., 2002; Greenwald et al., 1998, 2009; Nosek, 2005; McConnell & Liebold,
    2001; Nosek et al., 2002; Rachlinski et al., 2009; Baron & Banaji, 2006; Newheiser &
    Olson, 2012; Rutland et al., 2005.
39 Sabin & Greenwald, 2012; Sadler et al., 2012.
40 Bowser, 2017; Carter, 2007; Belgrave & Allison, 2018; Lawrence & Keleher, 2004.
41 Carter, 2007; Marger, 2003; Van Dijk, 1987; Bailey et al., 2017; Paradies et al., 2015.
42 Lawrence & Keleher, 2004.
43 Sidanius & Pratto, 1999, 2012.
44 Sidanius & Pratto, 1999, 2012; Sidanius et al., 1994, 2000; Pratto et al., 1994; Schmitt
    & Wirth, 2009.
45 Sidanius & Pratto, 1999, 2012.
46 Sidanius & Pratto, 1999; Sidanius & Veniegas, 2000.
47 Kendi, 2016; Zurara et al., 1896; Thomas, 1997; Russell, 2000.
48 Kendi, 2016; Takaki, 1993; Witzig, 1996; Blumenbach & Bendyshe, 1865; Cavalli-
    Sforza et al., 1994.
49 Tatum, 2017; Williams, 1994.
50 Tatum, 2017; Kendi, 2016.
51 Tatum, 2017; Encyclopedia of Virginia, n.d.; Willhelm, 1986.
52 Tatum, 2017; Horne, 2018; Wilderson, 2017; Bell, 1988; Acebo, 2012; Quijano, 2000;
    Sidanius & Pratto, 1999; Gans, 1999; Weil et al., 2022.

CHAPTER 2

RACIAL DISCRIMINATION AND HEALTH

There has been very minimal research done to better understand the health effects of racial trauma. This chapter examines the biopsychosocial health effects of racial trauma along with specific historical events that have contributed to the trauma of Black men. Racial Battle Fatigue (RBF), weathering, telomeres, epigenetics, mortality, trauma, COVID-19, depression, health care, the Tuskegee Experiment, and schizophrenia are all examined in relation to the racial trauma and the health impacts on Black men. The relationship between racialized health disparities and unequal social and economic conditions produced by anti-Black racism has been documented by Du Bois (1899) as early as the late 19th century. The director of the Centers for Disease Control and Prevention (CDC) declared racism a serious public health threat. The assault on Black life is correlated with racial public health inequalities. A Black person dies prematurely every seven minutes, which equates to more than 200 Black Americans a day due to racial discrimination. Black Americans report higher rates of racial discrimination than any other group in the U.S. In addition, Black Americans have been the primary targets of continuous racial discrimination for one of the lengthiest periods in the entire history of the human race. The four centuries of sustained oppression is longer than any other group with the exception of indigenous groups in several colonized areas. The permanence of racism in American society has been pervasive in Black life with deleterious health effects. Racism is a potent psychosocial stressor that includes both social ostracism and blocked economic opportunity. In addition, racism is a form of structural violence as it produces socially unjust conditions that predispose Black communities to disability and death (e.g., chattel slavery, mortgage redlining, white terrorism (lynching), political gerrymandering, lack of Medicaid expansion, employment discrimination, and health care provider bias). This reality is normalized/ritualized and reproduced within the practices and policies of long-standing public and private institutions.[1]

Racial discrimination takes place in various domains and everyday experiences, creating an additional layer of stress to those who are subjected to it. Racial discrimination is the behavioral component of racism and is a risk factor for poor health outcomes that can range from restricted access to health care, exposure to environmental stressors that negatively impact physical and mental health.[2]

Environmental adversity contributes to PTSD, major depression, alcoholism, substance use disorders, and nonspecific distress. Institutional racism is reflected in policies and procedures that produce a lack of access to housing, neighborhood and educational quality, employment opportunities, and other desirable societal resources, thus shaping socioeconomic status (SES) and opportunities. Economic status and health are negatively affected by cultural racism that is reflected at the societal and individual level through a policy environment that is hostile to egalitarian policies, thus triggering stigma, negative stereotypes, and discrimination that are pathogenic and foster health-damaging psychological responses (e.g., internalized oppression, stereotype threat, John Henryism, etc.).[3]

Racial discrimination is routinely divided into two main types: major discriminatory events and day-to-day discrimination events (i.e., racial microaggressions or everyday racism). Physiological reactions to racial discrimination may include changes in eating patterns, sleep, blood pressure, and increased alcohol use as well as other substances. Emotional

DOI: 10.4324/9781003430551-3

responses to racial discrimination may include depression, anxiety, hopelessness, helplessness, despair, and social isolation. Cognitive reactions to racial discrimination may involve
attempts to explain or make sense of the cause of the experience, the meaning attributed
to the experience in relation to an individual's self-esteem, and future coping strategies and
interactions with others. Therefore, racial discrimination is experienced as a potent psychosocial stressor that can lead to adverse changes in health status and altered behavioral
patterns that can increase health risks.[4]

Racially stigmatized groups in the U.S. have worse health than whites. The poorer
health of racialized/minoritized populations include higher rates of mortality, earlier onset
of disease, greater severity and progression of disease, and higher levels of comorbidity and
impairment. Racialized populations tend to have both lower levels of access to medical care
and receive poor quality care. These disparities are persistent over time and are evident at
every level of income and education even though income and education reduce these disparities. Racism operates through multiple intervening mechanisms to fundamentally affect
health as well as altering and transforming other social factors that can exacerbate the negative effects of other risk factors for health. Stressors created by racism such as racial discrimination and historical trauma are intervening pathways that can affect the levels, clustering,
and impact of stressors such as unemployment, neighborhood violence, or residential and
occupational environments that cause physical and chemical exposure. Racial health disparities have routinely been viewed as genetic, biological, or intractable and deeply embedded
cultural values and behaviors. But research indicates that institutional and cultural racism
are the significant contributors to initiating and sustaining racial inequalities that combine
in a broad range of societal outcomes to create inequalities in health.[5]

Most racial incidents take place at work or school and are recurring. Perceived discrimination (e.g., subjective belief that one was passed over for a job promotion due to ethnicity or
race) can be just as negatively impactful as being victimized by objective discrimination (e.g.,
being called a racial slur). Everyday racism also identified as racial microaggressions encompasses subtle and unconscious forms of discrimination that is experienced daily and refers to
familiar practices that reflect systematic and institutional bias in daily attitudes and behaviors. This includes familiar and recurrent patterns of being devalued in various ways and
across different contexts. The stress from everyday racism has a cumulative effect on mental and physical health. Black Americans have consistently reported higher levels of racial
discrimination than any other racial or ethnic group. Moreover, Black men report experiences of racial discrimination more frequently than Black women. Klonoff and Landrine
(2000) found dark-skinned Black Americans were more likely to experience frequent racial
discrimination than their light-skinned counterparts, while Borrell et al. (2006) found that
Black men reported higher rates of discrimination associated with darker skin color. But
they found a moderate association between skin color and racial discrimination and posited
that Black Americans may be seen and treated as Black by the majority in the U.S. regardless of their tone or shade. Moreover, Klonoff et al. (1999) found that racial discrimination
significantly contributed to the psychiatric symptoms of Black Americans. The impact of
racial discrimination on symptomology was significantly above and beyond contextual factors such as age, sex, education, social class, and generic stressors. Depression, anxiety, and
anger about racism are the most common problems presented in psychotherapy by Black
Americans. Racial discrimination is linked to higher levels of depression and PTSD among
Black Americans. Raced-based discrimination is associated with significantly higher odds
of the lifetime endorsement of Generalized Anxiety Disorder (GAD), and everyday racial
discrimination is associated with Social Anxiety Disorder (SAD) among Black Americans.

In addition, racial discrimination is attributed to an increase in somatization as well as intrusion and avoidance symptoms among Black Americans.[6]

Racial discrimination is associated with elevated blood pressure, greater hypertension prevalence, artery calcification, visceral fat, heart disease, inflammation (C-reactive protein/CRP), neuroendocrine risk markers (glucocorticoids and pro-inflammatory cytokines), and poor sleep. Sims et al. (2012) found smoking to be positively correlated with everyday discrimination as well as BMI, dietary fiber, and sodium intake. Further, racial discrimination is a stressor that contributes to the psychological distress impacting Black parental and intimate relationships. Racial discrimination is associated with preterm and low-birthweight deliveries as well as uterine myomas (fibroids) and breast cancer. Moreover, the majority of racial discrimination against Black Americans occurs in semi-public and public settings. This includes daily public harassment that can be expressed as verbal and non-verbal hostility. Everyday discrimination on the job that is experienced as minor, pervasive mistreatment and unfairness is associated with impaired physical well-being among Black Americans.[7]

BLACK MEN

Black men carry the burden of two negative social identities that include being Black (anti-Black racism) and a Black male (anti-Black misandry). Black men are subjected to unique and specific anti-Black male misandry that contributes to worsening health. Racial discrimination is a persistent noxious environmental stressor for Black men. Black men report the highest rates of racial discrimination (e.g., job discrimination, police encounters, seeking employment, fair wages, getting a quality education, engaging with the healthcare system) than any group in the U.S. This includes racial discrimination and unfair treatment while shopping, while dining out, while at work, with the police, and while using public transportation. In addition, Black men report more experiences of racial discrimination and in more settings than women (e.g., while seeking employment, working at their jobs, applying for bank loans, and interfacing with the justice system). A Gallup survey (2020) on Black adults and racial microaggressions found that Black men reported significantly higher rates of being feared, being treated with less courtesy, and mistrusted compared to Black women. English et al. (2014) discovered in their study that 89 percent of Black men reported experiencing racial discrimination. This sex/gendered racism comes at an emotional, physiological, and psychological cost. Black men experience greater unemployment and underemployment, earn less, are more likely to be victims of homicide, and have high rates of incarceration and criminal victimization. The *New York Times* (2015) reported that 1.5 million Black men are missing due to early deaths and hyperincarceration. Further, more than one out of every six Black men have disappeared from daily life who today should be between 25 and 54 years old.[8]

The level of violence that Black males are exposed to is comparable to what is witnessed in active warzones. Homicide is the most common cause of death for Black men ages 15 to 34. Data collected by the Justice Department between 1996 and 2007 found that young Black men were the most likely to be robbed every year more than any other demographic in the U.S. as well as the most likely to be victimized by overall violence. Moreover, they are frequently exposed to and are the victims of stabbings, shootings, and other acts of violence within the urban communities they grow up in more than any other racial group. Further, Black men are the most vulnerable racial-sex group for almost every health condition that medical researchers monitor in the U.S. This includes higher risk for hypertension and major cardiovascular events such as cardiac death, myocardial infarction, stroke, heart failure, and respiratory disease.

Black men and boys have the lowest life expectancy and highest mortality rates in the U.S., and in 1990, it was reported that the Black male in Harlem had less of a chance of reaching age 65 than the average male resident of Bangladesh, which at that time was one of the poorest countries in the world. The life expectancy of Black men in the U.S. experienced an unprecedented drop every year from 1984 to 1989. From birth there are approximately the same number of Black boys as girls, but this begins to change during teenage years with the number of Black males declining throughout the twenties, peaking in the thirties, and then remaining persistent throughout the rest of adulthood. The life expectancy gap between Black males (lowest group) and Asian females (highest group) in 2001 was nearly 21 years. The overall life expectancy of Black men is now recorded to be approximately 70 years, but it was reported that Black men lost three years of life expectancy in the year 2020 due to COVID-19.[9]

Racial discrimination and the internalization of negative group attitudes are both risk factors for cardiovascular disease among Black Americans. High levels of racial discrimination and implicit anti-Black bias have been correlated with hypertension among Black men. Bennett et al. (2004) found that Black men who had been exposed to an ambiguous scenario compared to an overtly racist scenario experienced more negative affect reactivity. Routinely ambiguous racial discrimination presents itself as everyday racism. Chae et al. (2010) found a positive association between cardiovascular disease among Black men who endorsed negative beliefs about Black Americans, which also moderated the effect of racial discrimination. Black men who reported racial discrimination and disagreed with negative beliefs about Black Americans were at higher risk of cardiovascular disease. However, the risk of cardiovascular disease was greatest among Black men who endorsed negative beliefs about Black Americans and who reported not experiencing racial discrimination. Further, the combination of internalizing negative beliefs about Black Americans and the absence of the reporting of racial discrimination are attributed to poor cardiovascular health. Black men experience unique social stressors and psychological challenges that may contribute to greater risk for developing cardiovascular disease. This includes racial profiling and racial discrimination in domains such as employment, housing, education, and health care. These stressful life experiences may manifest through psychological and behavioral reactions to stress by engagement of the stress response that indirectly impacts cardiovascular health via its impact on biological systems.[10]

Racial Battle Fatigue (RBF)

Smith (2010) developed the Racial Battle Fatigue (RBF) framework to describe the physiological and psychological strain (i.e., race-based stressors) experienced by Black male college students due to attempts at coping with exposure to racial microaggressions (i.e., anti-Black misandric micro/aggressions) at historically white institutions (HWIs). RBF is an interdisciplinary theoretical framework that includes the increase in psychosocial stressors and subsequent psychological, physiological, and behavioral/emotional responses to resisting racial microaggressions in mundane extreme environmental stress (MEES). The psychological responses include frustration, defensiveness, apathy, irritability, sudden changes in mood, shock, anger, disappointment, resentment, anxiety, worry, disbelief, disappointment, helplessness, hopelessness, and fear. The physiological responses include headaches, backache, "butterflies," grinding teeth, clenched jaws, chest pain, shortness of breath, pounding heart, high blood pressure, muscle aches, indigestion, gastric distress, constipation or diarrhea, increased perspiration, intestinal problems, hives, rashes, sleep disturbance, fatigue, insomnia, and frequent illness. The behavioral/emotional responses include stereotype threat, "John Henryism," or prolonged high-effort coping with difficult psychological stressors, increased commitment to spirituality, overeating or loss of appetite, impatience, argumentative, procrastination, increased use of alcohol or drugs, increased smoking, withdrawal or isolation from others, self-doubt, neglect of responsibility, poor school or job performance, and changes in close family relationships.[11]

The following provides a description of MEES. Mundane (M) represents how race-related and societal stress is ubiquitous and routinely taken for granted. Extreme (E) characterizes the excessive influence on the physiological, psychological, emotional, and cognitive reactions. Environmental (E) signifies the historical and institutional ideology that informs the policy practices, behaviors, culture, and custom of the dominant environment. Stress (S) indicates that the combination of these elements is distressful and ultimately consumes valuable time and energy that could be invested in more creative, educative, professional, and humanitarian pursuits. Racism and racial microaggressions are psycho-pollutants in the social environment that contribute to the overall race-related stress of Black men and women. RBF provides a conceptual link between the experience of racial discrimination and GAD.[12]

Weathering

Weathering refers to the early health deterioration that Black Americans experience as a result of the cumulative impact of repeated experience with social or economic adversity and political marginalization that cannot be explained by racial differences in poverty. Health can be profoundly impacted on the physiological level as a consequence of high-effort coping with acute and chronic stressors. The overexposure to the primary stress hormone cortisol can flood the bloodstream and wear the body down (e.g., insulin resistance leading to diabetes) where the immune system becomes compromised, and sickness, disease, and aging (weathering) becomes prevalent. Black Americans experience earlier deterioration of health than whites. The inherent stress of living in a racist society that stigmatizes and disadvantages Black men may cause disproportionate physiological deterioration that may manifest the morbidity and mortality that would be typical in a significantly older white individual. The weathering process begins to accelerate in young adulthood and through middle age with a marked increase between the ages of 35 and 64 years. The poorer health that Black Americans experience at earlier ages accumulates and produces greater racial inequality in health with ages through middle adulthood. Weathering encompasses multiple biological systems (e.g., cardiovascular, metabolic, immune, etc.) and includes impacts on them that might not yet clinically register. Turney et al. (2022) found that brain aging was most prominent among Black adults than white and Latino/a adults, which they attributed to weathering.[13]

Telomeres

Racial discrimination contributes to racial disparities in the onset and progression of aging-related diseases via the chronic activation of the physiologic stress response over time. The burden placed on biological systems as a result of chronic psychosocial stress contributes to physiological weathering and premature declines in health, which are indexed by health indicators including biomarkers that reflect elevated disease risk, and one of these measures that reflects this process is telomere length. Telomeres are repetitive sequences of DNA that cap the ends of chromosomes and are pivotal in supporting chromosomal stability and protecting against DNA degradation. Telomere attrition occurs during cell replication, which results in shorter length on average over time and is associated with chronological aging. Psychosocial and physiologic stressors can accelerate telomere shortening. Further, telomere length has been posited as a biological marker of replicative history and a cumulative indicator of cellular level "wear and tear." Leukocyte telomere length (LTL) is a marker of immune system aging as well as general systemic aging and earlier mortality. In addition, LTL is associated with several aging-related health outcomes that include cardiovascular diseases, diabetes, metabolic syndrome, osteoporosis and osteoarthritis, dementia, Alzheimer's disease, cognitive decline, and earlier mortality.[14]

Racial discrimination has been associated with LTL shortening in Black Americans. Racial discrimination in multiple settings is a source of social adversity that can result in biological tolls. Chae et al. (2014) found that racial discrimination was associated with shorter LTL among Black men who had anti-Black bias. They posit that Black men with an implicit anti-Black bias may be compromised in their ability to manage or cope with stress that arises from racial discrimination. Internalizing an anti-Black bias in concert with external anti-Black racial discrimination may threaten both self- and group-identity that combine to create detrimental consequences for telomeric aging. Therefore, multiple levels of racism that includes interpersonal racial discrimination and the internalization of negative racial bias jointly operate to accelerate the biological aging of Black men.[15]

Epigenetics

Epigenetics are the heritable changes in chromatin and gene expression without alterations in the DNA sequence. Therefore, the genotype of an organism remains intact while the outward expression (phenotype) is altered. The three major types of mechanisms that encompass epigenetics are non-coding RNAs (ncRNAs), histone modifications (e.g., acetylation), and DNA methylation. The epigenetic mechanism of DNA methylation involves direct chemical modification of DNA. Gene regulation through DNA methylation is sensitive to environmental input and life experiences. Yehuda et al. (2016) found methylation in Jewish Holocaust survivors as well as in their offspring. Perroud et al. (2014) discovered methylation in both female survivors of the Tutsi genocide and their offspring. Both findings indicate the possibility of environmental influences in the transmission of parental trauma with epigenetic alterations found in both the exposed parent and their offspring. Moreover, potential insight is provided into how severe psychophysiological trauma can have transgenerational effects. This includes the transgenerational epigenetic priming of the physiological response to extreme stress in the offspring of highly traumatized individuals, thus increasing their risk of psychopathology. In addition, these findings support the possibility that Black Americans have experienced transgenerational epigenetic alterations as a result of transgenerational trauma points [Walk of Sorrow, Middle Passage, enslavement, Second Middle Passage, and various forms of neo-slavery that includes Black codes and convict leasing, Jim/Jane Crow, lynching, the Great Migration (Third Passage), the crack epidemic, the war on drugs, and hypercriminalization/incarceration] that makes them vulnerable to health disparities.[16]

Mortality

Chae et al. (2015) found a correlation between Google searches containing the "N-word" [nigger(s)] and Black mortality rates of Black Americans age 25 and over. Their research reviewed area racism, which was the proportion of Google searches of the "N-word" in 196 designated market areas (DMAs/media market) out of 210. These searches were concentrated in the rural Northeast and South of the U.S. In addition, residence in the Midwest and South compared to the Northeast were associated with a greater mortality rate. There was no significant difference in Black mortality rates when comparing residence in the West and Northeast. They found that area racism was significantly correlated with an increase in all-cause Black mortality rates that were the equivalent of 30,000 deaths annually nationwide. Cause-specific Black mortality rates revealed associations with heart disease, cancer, stroke, and diabetes. Black men had greater mortality rates than Black women. Their findings indicate that area racism that was indexed by the proportion of Google searches containing the "N-word" is significantly associated with the all-cause Black mortality rate as well as the Black-white disparities in mortality.

Trauma

Exposure to traumatic events is highest among Black Americans and specifically Black men. Black Americans have an elevated risk for PTSD due to racial discrimination, race-related verbal assaults, and racial stigmatization. The current configuration of PTSD fails to consider and account for the daily and recurring dangerous exposure that Black males experience. The PTSD framework fails to capture the extent of the injuries sustained by Black males exposed to racial trauma (e.g., the violence of anti-Black misandry and its many permutations), which exceeds the limited scope of the diagnostic criteria established for a PTSD diagnosis. Research on Black men and trauma indicates that approximately 62 percent had directly experienced a traumatic event in their lifetime, 72 percent witnessed a traumatic event, and 59 percent had learned of a traumatic event involving a friend or family member. The research of Smith Lee and Robinson (2019) found that Black males (aged 18–24 years old) in Baltimore (MD) disclosed witnessing (e.g., witnessing police beat up and injure older Black men) and experiencing (e.g., racial profiling, harassment, physical injury, threats, and verbal aggression) police violence that began in childhood and continued into emerging adulthood, which met the *DSM-5* criteria for trauma exposure and embodied theoretical conceptualizations of racial trauma. The police violence progressed from primarily witnessing police violence in childhood to directly experiencing harassment, verbal abuse, and physical injury from police officers during adolescence and emerging adulthood.[17]

The exposures to police violence informed Black males' appraisals and understandings of their vulnerability (Black male vulnerability to physical, psychological, social, economic, or legal harm) to police violence (i.e., racial profiling, injury, and death) across the life course. In addition, some of the participants disclosed losing loved ones to police killings, which activated hypervigilance and grief. The participants were challenged to navigate morbidity, mortality, and traumatic loss as a function of community violence while concomitantly challenged to navigate the chronic risk of exposures to violence and premature death due to police encounters. Sibrava et al. (2019) found that the reported frequency of experiences with discrimination significantly predict a PTSD diagnosis in Black Americans. Moreover, Black Americans have higher levels of violent victimization. Black Americans are more than twice as likely to be unarmed when killed during encounters with the police than white people. Police brutality is conduct that is taken in bad faith with the intent to dehumanize and degrade its target, which includes excessive use of physical violence. Police brutality is a social determinant of health and a public health epidemic.[18]

Alang et al. (2017) include the five interconnected mechanisms through which police brutality is linked to excess morbidity among Black Americans at both individual and community levels: (1) the increase of population-specific mortality rates as a result of fatal injuries; (2) an increase in morbidity as a result of adverse physiological responses; (3) race-based stress caused by racist public reactions; (4) the financial strain of arrests, incarcerations, legal, medical, and funeral bills; and (5) systemic disempowerment from integrated oppressive structures.

Police killings of Black men saw a massive spike beginning in the late 1960s. Among all groups, Black men and boys face the highest lifetime risk of being killed by police. Over the life course, approximately 96 per 100,000 Black men will be killed compared to 5 Black women. Police violence is one of the leading causes of death for young Black men and the only group that legal intervention is a leading cause of death. Police kill more than 300 Black Americans each year in the U.S. with at least a quarter of those killed unarmed. Ninety-two percent of unarmed Black Americans killed by police between 2013 and 2016 were Black men. Ninety-five percent of unarmed Black Americans killed by police between 2015 and 2022 were Black men. Approximately 96 percent of all Black children killed by police between 2015–2022 were Black boys. In the year 2020, 241 Black Americans were shot and killed by police, and 239 of them were Black men even in the midst of a COVID year that was marked by social distancing (this figure does not include George Floyd as he was not killed by shooting). According to the National Officer-Involved Homicide Database (NOIHD), 7,005 Black Americans were killed by police between the years 2000 and 2021. Ninety-one percent were Black males, 8 percent Black females, and approximately 1 percent were trans identified. Seventy-six percent of Black children killed by police during this time were Black males. Moreover, approximately 83 percent of unarmed Black Americans killed during this time were Black males.[19]

Police killings are preceding at the same pace as previous years, and no progress has been made in reducing deadly police violence in the U.S. These figures are likely underestimates due to the systematic underreporting of police killings of Black Americans. Further, very little public information is available regarding the prevalence of nonlethal police violence that results in injury or disability. Arseniev-Koehler et al. (2021) reviewed legal intervention-related deaths of males (4,981) from law enforcement and coroner text summaries (2003–2017) that were drawn from the U.S. National Violent Death Reporting System (NVDRS). They found that Black male decedents were younger, and their deaths were less likely to include public health worker (PHW) coded mental health or substance use histories, weapon use, or positive toxicology for alcohol or psychoactive drugs compared to white male decedents. Therefore, themes of physical aggression or escalation were more likely to be attributed to white men, while Black men had a lower threat profile. Arseniev-Koehler et al. (2021) indicated that the greater risk that Black males pose that warrants their deaths in greater numbers remains undetermined. DeAngelis (2021) found that Black victims of police killings had 60 percent lower odds of exhibiting signs of mental illness, 23 percent lower odds of being armed, and 28 percent of higher odds of fleeing in comparison to whites. Therefore, the threshold for being perceived as dangerous and related lethal police violence is higher for white civilians. Bor et al. (2018) discovered that Black Americans who were exposed to one or more police killings of unarmed Black Americans in their state of residence was associated with an increase in poor mental health days with respondents on average experiencing four days of poor mental health. Each additional killing of an unarmed Black person was associated with up to 0.14 additional poor mental health days. They estimated that police killings of unarmed Black Americans could contribute to 1.7 additional mental health days per year or 55 million excess mental health days per year among Black adults in the U.S. Police killings can cause heightened perceptions of threat and vulnerability, lack of fairness, confirm racial caste, beliefs about one's own value or worth, activation of prior traumas, and identification with the deceased.[20]

It has been determined that police killings of unarmed Black Americans have adverse effects on the mental health of Black adults in the general population. In addition, researchers have found elevated or heightened depressive symptoms among Black mothers in Baltimore (MD) following Freddie Gray's death while in police custody as well as pregnant Black women in Atlanta (GA) as a result of anticipation of negative encounters between Black youth and police. High rates of PTSD and depression were found in Ferguson (MO) after Michael Brown's death. It has been reported that Philando Castile was pulled over 49 times in 13 years. Aggressive policing practices (e.g., stop-and-frisk, threats of violence, or harshly addressed with racial insults) have been associated with trauma and anxiety among Black men and predicted a higher prevalence of PTSD among Black males than Latino males. Reviewing police killings of Black Americans as well as distressing news directed towards Black Americans are related to poor mental health outcomes.[21]

Police killings of Black Americans are recorded for public scrutiny and consumption. Lipscomb et al. (2019) found that Black males who heard, read, or viewed the fatal shooting of Stephon Clark by police officers of the Sacramento Police Department reported posttraumatic stress-related symptoms (fear, hypervigilance, and flashbacks). Three significant themes emerged from their research, which included emotional reactions of anger and sadness; psychophysiological symptoms of hypervigilance, avoidance, and dissociation; and the targeting of Black males (i.e., targeting of Black male bodies; Black male vulnerability). The research of Motley et al. (2020) on young Black males (ages 18 to 25) with a history of involvement in the criminal justice system and exposure to community-based violence (CBV) revealed that viewing a video of police violence was significantly associated with an increase in feeling sad, angry, and fearful. Staggers-Hakim (2016) discovered that Black adolescent males exposed by the media to nationally publicized cases of police killings indicated a fear of police and significant concern for their personal safety and mortality while in the proximity of police officers. Tynes et al. (2019) found an association between exposure to traumatic events online (TEO) and PTSD symptoms among Black adolescents. It was posited that the viewing of viral videos of police killings of Black Americans may increase rumination about the event. Media exposure keeps the acute stressor active and alive in a person's mind. Moreover, disparaging messages and images based on race can cause individuals and communities to self-identify with the individuals directly affected by such trauma as well as perceiving a potential threat based on racial/ethnic group membership. In addition, individuals may be keenly aware that the individuals in the video could easily have been them, thus decreasing their sense of control over what happens to them leaving them with a sense of helplessness. Viral videos are a constant reminder of the devaluing of Black lives and Black Americans' low social position (racial undercaste). The message sent to Black communities and Black men specifically through the witnessing or experiencing harassment, routine unwarranted searches, and deaths that go unpunished is that their bodies are police property, disposable, and underserving of dignity and justice. Therefore, Black males' direct and indirect exposures to police violence and police killings in Black communities is a severe form of not only generalized trauma but racial trauma.[22]

COVID-19 (Coronavirus 2019)

The severe negative health impact of COVID-19 on Black Americans is primarily due to structural racism and the resulting location of Black Americans to various viral exposures. Syndemic theory provides a framework of interacting, co-present, or sequential diseases, and the social environment factors that promote and enhance the negative effects of disease inter-action. Syndemic theory encompasses the adverse interactions between diseases and health conditions of all types, such as infections, chronic non-communicable diseases, mental health problems, behavioral conditions, toxic exposure, and malnutrition are likely to emerge under conditions of health inequality caused by poverty, stigmatization, stress, and structural vio-lence. Social conditions contribute to the formation, clustering, and spread of disease, which creates conditions that are either exacerbated or have a bidirectional relationship with increas-ing susceptibility and reduced immune function which contributes to disease progression.[23]

COVID-19 is a pandemic/plague that has disproportionately affected Black Americans. Black Americans made up 30 percent of COVID-19 cases in 14 states in which racial data was available and nationwide represented a third of hospitalized COVID-19 patients even though they made up 13 percent of the population. Black men are the most likely among Black Ameri-cans and white Americans to die of COVID-19. One of the nation's hotspots was Chicago where Black Americans made up 42 percent of the cases and 60 percent of the deaths from the virus.[24]

The multiple historical and present-day factors have created the syndemic conditions that Black Americans have experienced and exacerbated death and dying as a result of the lethal force of COVID-19. Black Americans are overrepresented in "essential" service or font-line industries that include low-wage and little autonomy in healthcare sectors such as home health aides, nursing home staff, hospital janitorial, food service and delivery, laun-dry, childcare, travel industry, postal service, transportation sectors, and other sectors that have suffered the largest job losses during the pandemic, thus creating high unemployment rates with a loss of available health insurance. Many of these low-wage jobs do not provide adequate health insurance, if provided at all, including sick leave, childcare, or other bene-fits that protect higher wage workers from COVID-19 exposures. Therefore, their employ-ment may interfere with their ability to stay home and social distance and placing them at high exposure risk to viral transmission. Stay-at-home orders and social distancing carry an assumption of socioeconomic privilege, such as the ability to work from home and transition from in-person communications to online platforms and remote working.[25]

Further, the surrounding environment that many Black Americans find themselves in magnifies risk. Black Americans live in hypersegregated communities where they are con-centrated in cities in the industrial Midwest and South. Segregation is a mechanism of struc-tural racism that determines a large portion of the life trajectory of Black Americans such as the availability and types of employment, place of residence, and the conditions that they are subjected to live and die through which drive infection risk. Hypersegregation not only refers to where one lives but includes how broader inequity is shaped from housing, edu-cation, employment, etc. Approximately, one-third of all Black metropolitan residents live in a hypersegregated location. This includes living in densely populated areas and crowded settings such as public housing and multigenerational housing units where the ability to practice social distancing is significantly limited and even impossible as well as having to rely on public transportation. In addition, Black Americans were not only dying because they could not access care but were being refused care and were not being tested or treated by hospitals and emergency clinicians when they displayed symptoms (all are examples of benign indifference). Therefore, Black men lost three years of life expectancy, and Black women lost more than two years of life expectancy in the year 2020 due to COVID-19.[26]

Long-standing public and private institutions normalize and reproduce this reality through practices and policies. Examples are exemplified through the history of chattel slavery, mortgage redlining, white terrorism (lynching), political gerrymandering, lack of Medicaid expansion, employment discrimination, and healthcare provider bias. Americans are not at equal risk; thus COVID-19 is a racialized disease. Anti-Black racism is institutionalized throughout the American political system that actively produces racial health inequities that are not random nor passive. Black Americans are forced to exist within a society as a substantially more vulnerable population (racial undercaste) than the white majority due to the formation of racial hierarchy and the constitutive racial discrimination. Systemic racism is a dynamic functioning epidemic that has converged with the COVID-19 pandemic/plague to accelerate exposure, disease, and mortality among Black Americans. Therefore, the impact of social and political decisions outweighs individual choices as these decisions have a historical and present-day context. Moreover, research from Skinner-Dorkenoo et al. (2022) revealed that whites who perceived COVID-19 racial disparities to be greater reported reduced fear of contracting COVID-19, empathy for vulnerable populations, and support for COVID-19 safety precautions. This indicated that publicizing racial health disparities potentially reduces support for policies among whites that would protect public health and reduce disparities.[27]

Depression

Depression is one of the most common mental disorders that affects an estimated 17 million people in the U.S. each year and the leading cause of disability within the U.S. Major depression is a psychiatric disorder that is extremely prevalent and debilitating in the U.S. and worldwide. The average onset is the mid-20s even though major depressive disorders can begin at any age. Consistent depressive symptoms over two weeks or more may indicate a depressive diagnosis. Moreover, depression is a leading cause of worldwide disability and the second leading contributor to the global burden of disease. Black Americans may suffer from more severe forms of depression than other racial or ethnic groups. Psychosocial coping, economic status/income, and racial discrimination are major factors that contribute to depression and depressive symptoms in Black men. Moreover, racial discrimination is a catalyst for depressive symptomology among Black men.[28]

Lifetime prevalence of everyday discrimination has been directly associated with depressive symptoms among Black men. Exposure to racial discrimination has been found to precede depressive symptomology. Moreover, self-esteem has been found to be a mediator between everyday discrimination and depressive symptoms among Black men. Hudson et al. (2012) examined whether exposure to racial discrimination among Black Americans would attenuate the positive effects of increased levels of socioeconomic position (SEP). They found that Black men compared to women were significantly more likely to report incidents of both major (acute, i.e., racial discrimination that could potentially block social mobility) and everyday discrimination (chronic; routine racial discrimination, i.e., racial microaggressions). Further, racial discrimination was associated with an increased risk of depression among Black men who possessed greater levels of education and income. The interaction between education and major discrimination were associated with greater odds of depression among Black men. In addition, they found interactions between income and both everyday discrimination and major discrimination. Thus, racial discrimination toward Black men potentially diminished the effects of increased socioeconomic position.[29]

In addition, Britt-Spells et al. (2018) and Hoggard et al. (2019) found a positive association between perceived racial discrimination and depressive symptoms, somatic complaints, and interpersonal problems among Black men. The research of Goodwill et al. (2021)

revealed that race-based everyday discrimination was significantly associated with increased rates of depressive symptoms and suicide ideation. Racial discrimination diminishes mastery and self-efficacy, increases hopelessness, and prevents Black men from assuming important or idealized male roles such as provider and protector. The threat or prevention of Black men from assuming these roles can compromise the realization of their potential and hinder their individual growth and life fulfillment (i.e., social mobility), thus exacerbating depressive symptomology. [30]

Health Care

Modern medicine in the U.S. has historical roots in scientific racism and eugenics movements. Scientific racism reified the concept of race as a biological and later genetic attribute through culturally influenced scientific theory and inquiry. The eugenics movement formed in the U.S. in the early 20th century which led to laws prohibiting "miscegenation" and the forced sterilization of undesirable races with the intention of creating a better and more intelligent white nation. Scientific arguments were weaponized under the guise of neutrality and objectivity by well-respected medical doctors who cast Black Americans as innately diseased and dehumanized their suffering. The father of American psychiatry, Dr. Benjamin Rush, believed that Black skin was the result of a mild form of leprosy that he referred to as "negritude." In 1851, his onetime apprentice, Southern physician Samuel Cartwright, created "drapetomania" as a mental illness that caused enslaved Black Americans to escape their confinement (referred to as "absconding from service") and recommended whippings as the remedy that would ensure submission. Cartwright also created the disease "dysaesthesia aethiopica" for enslaved Black Americans that was characterized by reduced intellectual ability, laziness, and partial insensitivity of the skin. In addition, the father of modern gynecology physician J. Marion Sims repeatedly operated on enslaved Black women without anesthesia or consent. Medical schools across the U.S. bought the bodies of deceased enslaved Black Americans from southern white enslavers for dissection and research, which offered white enslavers a profitable way to make Black bodies disappear if needed due to murder from inflicted punishments. Enslaved Black Americans' bodies were a commodity in life as well as death.[31]

Today, bias, prejudice, and stereotyping contribute to widespread difference in health care by race and ethnicity. Black Americans receive poorer care than white patients, and this unequal treatment is partly based on enduring racist cultural beliefs and practices. Hoffman et al. (2016) found half of white medical students and residents held unfounded beliefs about intrinsic biological differences between Black and white people. This included false beliefs and assessments that Black patients' pain was less severe than white patients as well as inappropriate treatment decisions for Black patients. Moreover, segregated Black communities are routinely under/non-resourced (e.g., fewer clinicians, etc.) because of systematic disinvestment in public and private sectors within these communities. Thus, making it difficult to recruit experienced and well-credentialed primary care providers and specialists, which ultimately affects access and utilization. Black communities have become medical training grounds and a source of profit which reinforces the modern American medical racial caste system. The limited and substandard care that Black Americans are forced to endure is ensured by medical schools, healthcare providers, insurers, health systems, legislators, and employers. This inequitable treatment is accepted and normalized through the historical belief that Black Americans are intrinsically disease-prone and implicitly/explicitly not deserving of high-quality care. The construct of race as biological difference exemplifies and contributes to a broader system of structural racism.[32]

The Tuskegee Experiment

The medical communities' beliefs about Black Americans in the early 20th century was formed by mythology concerning sex, sexuality, and disease while discounting the socioeconomic conditions that affected Black health and mortality. The U.S. Public Health Service (PHS) initiated its Study of Syphilis in the Untreated Negro Male routinely referred to as *Tuskegee Syphilis Study* in 1932. Free medical care was promised to approximately 600 sick, extremely poor sharecroppers in Macon County, Alabama. The PHS claimed the study was designed to study the progression of syphilis in Black men. Scientists had long made claims that the venereal disease manifested differently in Black Americans than in whites. PHS scientists decided to document this, locating a pool of infected Black men and withholding treatment from them while charting the progression of symptoms and disorders.[33]

The subjects/victims were lied to by PHS and were convinced that they were being treated, not studied. The physician-researchers autopsied the men when they died to trace the precise ravages of the disease in their bodies. The PHS expected to validate its racist belief that syphilis operated differently in Black bodies than whites. It was thought that syphilis caused the worst damage to the neurological systems and brains of whites, while the worst damage was to the cardiovascular systems of Black Americans, thus sparing their primitive and "underdeveloped" brains. The sharecroppers of Macon County were plagued by poor nutrition, a lack of decent housing, and rampant infectious disease that ranged from malaria to tuberculosis to syphilis. Treatment could eradicate syphilis, but 99 percent of the cases in Black Americans had never been treated. Syphilis is caused by the bacterial organism *Treponema pallidum* and can be acquired through sexual activity or congenitally from an infected mother. The initial stage of sexually transmitted syphilis includes a chancre which is a hard and painless sore that appears on the genitals or other point of entry that is followed by flulike symptoms. Untreated, syphilis enters into a long latent stage before the emergence of an assortment of skin growths, running sores, gumma, bone decay, and heart damage. The final tertiary stage may cause profound neurological damage, including blindness, insanity (paresis), paralysis, and death several decades later.[34]

Black Americans were thought of by PHS doctors as resistant to health measures, intellectually inferior, impetuous, degenerate, most importantly motivated by uncontrollable frighteningly powerful sexual drives (hypersexual). Their medical speculation contributed to the image of Black Americans as sexually promiscuous and infected with syphilis. Their belief was that sexual irresponsibility condemned Black Americans to chronic syphilitic infection and referred to Black Americans as "a notoriously syphilis-soaked race" (Washington, 2006, p. 160). It was theorized by Dr. Frank Lydston that Black Americans were more likely than white men to spread venereal disease, and Dr. S. S. Hindman estimated that the national prevalence rate of syphilis among Black Americans was at 95 percent, which was based on his imagination and not evidence. Moreover, 61 percent of the true syphilis cases in Macon County were congenital nonvenereal syphilis and were not contracted through sexual activity. This fact was consistently ignored in publications and investigations by medical researchers who persistently characterized syphilis in Black Americans due to sexual degeneracy. Further, the Wassermann test for syphilis was notoriously nonspecific, and not all the men who tested positive for syphilis really had the disease as men who suffered from related illnesses such as yaws also tested positive.[35]

Yaws is a common nonvenereal infectious disease that is endemic to West Africa and is caused by the subspecies of the *treponema pallidum* bacterium that causes syphilis. Yaws was prevalent in the South in 1932, particularly among Black Americans due to impoverished conditions such as malnourishment, exposure to the elements, being shoeless, and frequent injuries that broke the skin (e.g., daily injuries as a result of picking cotton), which made them vulnerable to infections by pathogens that caused yaws. PHS doctors routinely defended their failure of treatment by insisting that Black Americans with syphilis would never voluntarily seek treatment even though they enticed Black men with their services as a treatment program and not an experiment. The PHS doctors were aware that most of these men had never seen a doctor and being cared by one who claimed to be devoted to restoring their health was a godsend to the sick and forgotten Black Americans of Macon County. Therefore, PHS announced that they would perform a day of free health assessments and screening tests in Macon County. Tests were conducted by the physicians who told the men that they were being treated for the nebulous disorder "bad blood," which referred to a wide range of symptoms such as anemia, muscle aches, general malaise, parasitic infections, gonorrhea, syphilis, and other venereal diseases. The "treatment" of those suspected of having syphilis consisted of vitamins, ineffectual doses of arsenic, aspirin, and a useless mercury salve. Aspirin was thought to be a miracle drug for these overworked and sickly men who were amazed by its ability to assuage their omnipresent aches and pains. But mercury was ineffectual in treating syphilis and caused devastating side effects, including injury to the nervous system, profound mental deficits, hair and tooth loss, kidney and heart disease, and lung injury. The state-of-the-art treatment of arsenic compounds such as arsphenamine and neoarsphenamine (i.e., Salvarsan or Compound 606) for syphilis was withheld.[36]

The first clinics enabled doctors to identify syphilitics and 399 Black men with syphilis were selected as subjects to observe. PHS regarded these men as living cadavers who were more valuable to American medicine dead than alive. They were intently monitored, and most did not receive treatment for 40 years (1932–1972). PHS performed autopsies and regularly published the results in medical journals as the men began to die. Study results were even shared in 1936 during an American Medical Association (AMA) meeting where many white physicians were informed of the study's details. Black physicians were largely barred from AMA membership during this time.[37]

It was revealed in the 1936 report that 84 percent of the infected men showed signs of illness. The death rate of the infected a decade later was twice that of the control subjects. Nearly one-third of the autopsied men by 1955 had died directly of syphilis, and many of the survivors were suffering from its deadliest complications. Moreover, 40 wives were infected, and at least 19 children were born with syphilitic birth defects. The PHS awarded a certificate of appreciation signed by the surgeon general replete with a gold seal in 1958 that included $25 (a dollar for each year of the study). The new cure of penicillin for syphilis was nationally dispensed by PHS clinics in 1943, but the Surgeon General Thomas Parran opted for the continued experimentation of Black men of Macon County instead of providing them with the cure and sought to prevent them from receiving treatment. Physical examinations and autopsies revealed by 1969 that as many as 100 of the men had died of syphilis and syphilis-related complications, and others had died of syphilis-related heart disease and a CDC committee during this time decided that the study should continue. In 1972, a whistleblower revealed the story to a journalist friend, and eventually the story was revealed to the Associated Press, and the government convened an ad hoc panel to investigate. During this time, 74 of the test subjects were still alive. The Tuskegee researchers regarded these Black men as less than human. It has been posited that these men provided fresh supplies of blood products that contained the syphilis bacterium to develop new, more reliable, and profitable tests for syphilis 20 years before scientists learned to culture cells and grow pathogens such as the syphilis bacterium in a laboratory. This assertion is supported by the routine blood tests and spinal taps of these Black men. Tuskegee has become the iconic symbol of racialized medical abuse and has contributed to a general sense of distrust of physicians, medical industry, and healthcare systems. The Tuskegee Syphilis Study is not an aberration but part of a centuries-old pattern of experimental abuse, pain, and humiliation at the hands of physicians that Black Americans have integrated into their rich oral tradition of remembering. Therefore, Black distrust is not an overreaction but a perfectly understandable reaction to American medicine's persistent experimental and medicalized abuse of Black Americans.[38]

Schizophrenia

Prior to the 1960s, schizophrenia was associated with white middle-class housewives based on official descriptors that emphasized the generally calm nature of such persons. Studies in the 1960s by the National Institute of Mental Health (NIMH) found that Black Americans had a 65 percent higher rate of schizophrenia than whites. A series of studies in 1973 in the *Archives of General Psychiatry* found that Black patients were significantly more likely than white patients to receive a schizophrenia diagnosis and significantly less likely than white patients to receive other mental health diagnoses such as depression or bipolar disorder (affective disorders). A host of articles from leading psychiatric and medical journals throughout the 1980s and 1990s demonstrated that doctors diagnosed the paranoid subtype of schizophrenia in Black men five to seven times more often than in white men as well as more frequently than in any other ethnic racialized/minoritized groups.[39]

Schizophrenia sustained a change beginning in the 1960s due to American assumptions of race, sex, and temperament. Schizophrenia suddenly began to be described as an illness manifested not by white feminine docility but rage according to many leading medical and popular sources. Leading psychiatric journals published a growing number of research articles that claimed that schizophrenia was a condition that also afflicted Black men ("Negro men") and the Black forms of the illness were manifested through volatility and aggression. Many psychiatric authors conflated the schizophrenic symptoms of Black patients with their perceived schizophrenia of civil rights protests. This perception was ascribed particularly to those civil rights protests that were organized by Black Power, Black Panthers, Nation of Islam, or other activist groups. Psychiatrists Walter Bromberg and Frank Simon in a 1968 article in the *Archives of General Psychiatry* described schizophrenia as a "protest psychosis" where Black men had developed "hostile and aggressive" feelings and "delusional anti-whiteness" because of listening to the words of Malcolm X, joining the Black Muslims, or affiliating with groups that espoused militant resistance to white society. Black men required psychiatric intervention because their symptoms threatened not only their own sanity but the social order of white America according to Bromberg and Simon.[40]

Pharmaceutical companies began to advertise pharmaceutical treatments that depicted similar themes for schizophrenia in the 1960s and 1970s. Advertisements in leading psychiatric journals for antipsychotic medication Haldol showed angry Black men with clenched Black power fists and an urban background with messaging that chemical management was required for their symptoms of social belligerence. Moreover, mainstream white newspapers began in the 1960s and 1970s to describe schizophrenia as a condition of angry Black masculinity, including warnings of crazed Black schizophrenic killers on the loose. The confluence of social and medical forces changed schizophrenia's rhetorical transformation from an illness of white feminine docility to one of Black male hostility. These forces included biased actions by individual doctors, researchers, and drug advertisers and at structural levels. The structural levels included the shifting language associated with the official psychiatric definition of schizophrenia. In the 1960s, the frame changed, and in 1968, the second edition of the *Diagnostic and Statistical Manual* (*DSM*) was published during a political climate that was marked by profound protests and social unrest. The *DSM* recast the paranoid subtype of schizophrenia as a disorder of masculinized belligerence. This language was consistently used in an increasing number of research articles from the 1960s and 1970s and asserted that schizophrenia was a condition that also afflicted Black men ("Negro men") and that the Black form of this illness was more hostile and aggressive than it was for whites. The schizophrenia diagnosis was even applied to Black men who had not had direct involvement in the civil rights movement and became part of structural attempts to control and contain Black men. Consequently, Black men are more likely to be described by healthcare professionals as being hostile or violent and receive higher dosages of antipsychotic medications than do white male psychiatric patients. Racial bias and overt racism were written into diagnostic language that are now invisible and are perpetuated by institutional racism. Schizophrenia literally and figuratively became a Black disease of Black men.[41]

CLINICAL IMPLICATIONS

The health effects of racial trauma are understudied. The biopsychosocial health effects of racial trauma along with specific historical events have contributed to the trauma of Black men. Racial trauma and its health impacts on Black men can be examined through RBF, weathering, telomeres, epigenetics, mortality, trauma, COVID-19, depression, health care, the Tuskegee Experiment, and schizophrenia. Trauma, RBF, depression, the overdiagnosis of schizophrenia, and the lack of trustworthy health care are issues raised in this chapter that are within the scope of clinical practice. Trauma will be addressed in Chapter 3. RBF overlaps with the symptoms of GAD (General Anxiety Disorder) and SAD (Social Anxiety Disorder) that are associated with race-based discrimination and racial microaggressions/everyday discrimination. GAD symptoms include excessive anxiety and worry (e.g., regarding various events and situations), difficulty controlling worry, irritability, concentration problems, muscle tension, feeling wound up, tense, or restless, fatigue, and difficulty with sleep. SAD is the most common anxiety disorder and is defined by an intense and unreasonable fear of social and performance situations, which causes distress and impaired functioning in some life domains. SAD impacts social and vocational functioning and reduces subjective quality of life. SAD is thought to develop due to internal representations of the self that are based on how one believes they are perceived by others (i.e., viewed negatively/social-evaluative threat cues), which culminates in anxiety about their abilities in social situations. The relationship between awareness of racism and cultural mistrust may be associated with social anxiety symptoms.[42]

Two decades worth of research on Black men and depression indicates that the major factors that contribute to depression and depressive symptoms are psychosocial coping, economic status/income, and racism/discrimination (anti-Black misandric micro/aggressions). Assari et al. (2018) found that Black males of a higher socioeconomic status (SES) were at an increased risk of having a major depressive episode (MDE). Self-esteem among Black men has been found to mediate the relationship between everyday discrimination and depression, and greater perceived discrimination is associated with greater depressive symptoms, while race-based everyday discrimination is the only type of discrimination that is significantly associated with increased rates of both depressive symptoms and suicide/death ideation. Racial discrimination has not only been positively associated with depressed affect but also somatic complaints and interpersonal problems. Culturally expressed Major Depressive Disorder (MDD) symptoms among Black men include irritable mood, increased hostility, increased agitation, internalized anger, decreased observed mood, anxiety symptoms, decreased appetite, insomnia, and psychomotor agitation or retardation. Issues that affect the presentation of MDD among Black men are higher levels of cultural distrust, increased guardedness, increased self-consciousness, increased hypochondriasis, increased physical symptoms, increased somatization, increased physical disability, and increased somatic symptom severity. Lastly, clinicians should be aware that Black men and Black Americans have historically been overdiagnosed with schizophrenia and underdiagnosed with affective disorders.[43]

NOTES

1 CDC, 2021; Williams, 2021; Chou et al., 2012; Feagin, 2004, 2010; Feagin & Bennefield, 2014; Williams & Mohammed, 2013; Chae et al., 2014; Poteat et al., 2020; Massey & Denton, 1993; Durst, 2018; Farmer et al., 2006; Soto et al., 2011; Yetman, 1985; Dohrenwend, 2000; Krieger, 2000; Brondolo et al., 2008; Thompson, 1996, 2002; Graetz et al., 2022; Carter & Forsyth, 2010; Essed, 1991; Forman et al., 1997; Kessler et al., 1999; Sellers & Shelton, 2003; Banks et al., 2006; Soto et al., 2011; Siegel et al., 2014; Broman et al., 2000; Landrine & Klonoff, 1996; Klonoff & Landrine, 1999; Deitch et al., 2003; Krieger & Sidney, 1996; Murry et al., 2001; Lewis et al., 2011, 2006, 2009, 2010, 2013; Williams & Neighbors, 2001; Mays et al., 2007; Mustillo et al., 2004; Deitch et al., 2003; Brondolo et al., 2008; Wise et al., 2007; Taylor et al., 2007.

2 CDC, 2021; Williams, 2021; Chou et al., 2012; Feagin, 2004, 2010; Feagin & Bennefield, 2014; Williams & Mohammed, 2013; Chae et al., 2014; Poteat et al., 2020; Massey & Denton, 1993; Durst, 2018; Farmer et al., 2006; Soto et al., 2011; Yetman, 1985; Dohrenwend, 2000; Krieger, 2000; Brondolo et al., 2008; Thompson, 1996, 2002; Graetz et al., 2022; Carter & Forsyth, 2010; Essed, 1991; Forman et al., 1997; Kessler et al., 1999; Sellers & Shelton, 2003; Banks et al., 2006; Soto et al., 2011; Siegel et al., 2014; Broman et al., 2000; Landrine & Klonoff, 1996; Klonoff & Landrine, 1999; Deitch et al., 2003; Krieger & Sidney, 1996; Murry et al., 2001; Lewis et al., 2011, 2006, 2009, 2010, 2013; Williams & Neighbors, 2001; Mays et al., 2007; Mustillo et al., 2004; Deitch et al., 2003; Brondolo et al., 2008; Wise et al., 2007; Taylor et al., 2007.

3 CDC, 2021; Williams, 2021; Chou et al., 2012; Feagin, 2004, 2010; Feagin & Bennefield, 2014; Williams & Mohammed, 2013; Chae et al., 2014; Poteat et al., 2020; Massey & Denton, 1993; Durst, 2018; Farmer et al., 2006; Soto et al., 2011; Yetman, 1985; Dohrenwend, 2000; Krieger, 2000; Brondolo et al., 2008; Thompson, 1996, 2002; Graetz et al., 2022; Carter & Forsyth, 2010; Essed, 1991; Forman et al., 1997; Kessler et al., 1999; Sellers & Shelton, 2003; Banks et al., 2006; Soto et al., 2011; Siegel et al., 2014; Broman et al., 2000; Landrine & Klonoff, 1996; Klonoff & Landrine, 1999; Deitch et al., 2003; Krieger & Sidney, 1996; Murry et al., 2001; Lewis et al., 2011, 2006, 2009, 2010, 2013; Williams & Neighbors, 2001; Mays et al., 2007; Mustillo et al., 2004; Deitch et al., 2003; Brondolo et al., 2008; Wise et al., 2007; Taylor et al., 2007.

4 CDC, 2021; Williams, 2021; Chou et al., 2012; Feagin, 2004, 2010; Feagin & Bennefield, 2014; Williams & Mohammed, 2013; Chae et al., 2014; Poteat et al., 2020; Massey & Denton, 1993; Durst, 2018; Farmer et al., 2006; Soto et al., 2011; Yetman, 1985; Dohrenwend, 2000; Krieger, 2000; Brondolo et al., 2008; Thompson, 1996, 2002; Graetz et al., 2022; Carter & Forsyth, 2010; Essed, 1991; Forman et al., 1997; Kessler et al., 1999; Sellers & Shelton, 2003; Banks et al., 2006; Soto et al., 2011; Siegel et al., 2014; Broman et al., 2000; Landrine & Klonoff, 1996; Klonoff & Landrine, 1999; Deitch et al., 2003; Chou et al., 2012; Krieger & Sidney, 1996; Murry et al., 2001; Lewis et al., 2011, 2006, 2009, 2010, 2013; Williams & Neighbors, 2001; Mays et al., 2007; Mustillo et al., 2004; Deitch et al., 2003; Brondolo et al., 2008; Wise et al., 2007; Taylor et al., 2007.

5 CDC, 2021; Williams, 2021; Chou et al., 2012; Feagin, 2004, 2010; Feagin & Bennefield, 2014; Williams & Mohammed, 2013; Chae et al., 2014; Poteat et al., 2020; Massey & Denton, 1993; Durst, 2018; Farmer et al., 2006; Soto et al., 2011; Yetman, 1985; Dohrenwend, 2000;

Krieger, 2000; Brondolo et al., 2008; Thompson, 1996, 2002; Graetz et al., 2022; Carter & Forsyth, 2010; Essed, 1991; Forman et al., 1997; Kessler et al., 1999; Sellers & Shelton, 2003; Banks et al., 2006; Soto et al., 2011; Siegel et al., 2014; Broman et al., 2000; Landrine & Klonoff, 1996; Klonoff & Landrine, 1999; Deitch et al., 2003; Chou et al., 2012; Krieger & Sidney, 1996; Murry et al., 2001; Lewis et al., 2011, 2006, 2009, 2010, 2013; Williams & Neighbors, 2001; Mays et al., 2007; Mustillo et al., 2004; Deitch et al., 2003; Brondolo et al., 2008; Wise et al., 2007; Taylor et al., 2007.

6 CDC, 2021; Williams, 2021; Chou et al., 2012; Feagin, 2004, 2010; Feagin & Bennefield, 2014; Williams & Mohammed, 2013; Chae et al., 2014; Poteat et al., 2020; Massey & Denton, 1993; Durst, 2018; Farmer et al., 2006; Soto et al., 2011; Yetman, 1985; Dohrenwend, 2000; Krieger, 2000; Brondolo et al., 2008; Thompson, 1996, 2002; Graetz et al., 2022; Carter & Forsyth, 2010; Essed, 1991; Forman et al., 1997; Kessler et al., 1999; Sellers & Shelton, 2003; Banks et al., 2006; Soto et al., 2011; Siegel et al., 2014; Broman et al., 2000; Landrine & Klonoff, 1996; Klonoff & Landrine, 1999; Deitch et al., 2003; Chou et al., 2012; Krieger & Sidney, 1996; Murry et al., 2001; Lewis et al., 2011, 2006, 2009, 2010, 2013; Williams & Neighbors, 2001; Mays et al., 2007; Mustillo et al., 2004; Deitch et al., 2003; Brondolo et al., 2008; Wise et al., 2007; Taylor et al., 2007.

7 CDC, 2021; Williams, 2021; Chou et al., 2012; Feagin, 2004, 2010; Feagin & Bennefield, 2014; Williams & Mohammed, 2013; Chae et al., 2014; Poteat et al., 2020; Massey & Denton, 1993; Durst, 2018; Farmer et al., 2006; Soto et al., 2011; Yetman, 1985; Dohrenwend, 2000; Krieger, 2000; Brondolo et al., 2008; Thompson, 1996, 2002; Graetz et al., 2022; Carter & Forsyth, 2010; Essed, 1991; Forman et al., 1997; Kessler et al., 1999; Sellers & Shelton, 2003; Banks et al., 2006; Soto et al., 2011; Siegel et al., 2014; Broman et al., 2000; Landrine & Klonoff, 1996; Klonoff & Landrine, 1999; Deitch et al., 2003; Chou et al., 2012; Krieger & Sidney, 1996; Murry et al., 2001; Lewis et al., 2011, 2006, 2009, 2010, 2013; Williams & Neighbors, 2001; Mays et al., 2007; Mustillo et al., 2004; Deitch et al., 2003; Brondolo et al., 2008; Wise et al., 2007; Taylor et al., 2007.

8 Smith et al., 2007; Gary, 1995; Wolfers et al., 2015; McCord & Freeman, 1990; Bond & Herman, 2016; Klonoff & Landrine, 1999, 2000; Borrell et al., 2006; Smith et al., 2011; Burd-Sharps et al., 2008; Santhanam, 2021; Forman et al., 1997; Chou et al., 2012; Chae et al., 2014; Clark et al., 1999; Pieterse & Carter, 2007; Gallup, 1997; Lloyd, 2020; Sidanius et al., 2018; Banks et al., 2006; Krieger & Sidney, 1996; Klaus & Maston, 2008; Sellers & Shelton, 2003; English et al., 2014; Heron, 2009; Lauderdale et al., 2006; Mouzon et al., 2020; Singletary, 2020; Britt-Spells et al., 2018; Broman et al., 2000; Broman, 1996; Weitzer & Tuch, 1999; Welch et al., 2001; Hausmann et al., 2008; Taylor & Turner, 2002; Barnes et al., 2004; Brown, 2001; Din-Dzietham et al., 2004; Herring et al., 1998; Ifatunji & Forman, 2006; Sigelman & Welch, 1991; Ifatunji & Harnois, 2016; Hudson et al., 2012.

9 Smith et al., 2007; Gary, 1995; Wolfers et al., 2015; McCord & Freeman, 1990; Bond & Herman, 2016; Klonoff & Landrine, 1999, 2000; Borrell et al., 2006; Smith et al., 2011; Burd-Sharps et al., 2008; Santhanam, 2021; Forman et al., 1997; Chou et al., 2012; Chae et al., 2014; Clark et al., 1999; Pieterse & Carter, 2007; Gallup, 1997; Lloyd, 2020; Sidanius et al., 2018; Banks et al., 2006; Krieger & Sidney, 1996; Klaus & Maston, 2008; Sellers & Shelton, 2003; English et al., 2014; Heron, 2009; Lauderdale et al., 2006; Mouzon et al., 2020; Singletary, 2020; Britt-Spells et al., 2018; Broman et al., 2000; Broman, 1996; Weitzer & Tuch, 1999; Welch et al., 2001; Hausmann et al., 2008; Taylor & Turner, 2002; Barnes et al., 2004; Brown, 2001; Din-Dzietham et al., 2004; Herring et al., 1998; Ifatunji & Forman, 2006; Sigelman & Welch, 1991; Ifatunji & Harnois, 2016; Hudson et al., 2012.

10 Smith et al., 2007; Gary, 1995; Wolfers et al., 2015; McCord & Freeman, 1990; Bond & Herman, 2016; Klonoff & Landrine, 1999, 2000; Borrell et al., 2006; Smith et al., 2011;

Burd-Sharps et al., 2008; Santhanam, 2021; Forman et al., 1997; Chou et al., 2012; Chae et al., 2014; Clark et al., 1999; Pieterse & Carter, 2007; Gallup, 1997; Lloyd, 2020; Sidanius et al., 2018; Banks et al., 2006; Krieger & Sidney, 1996; Klaus & Maston, 2008; Sellers & Shelton, 2003; English et al., 2014; Heron, 2009; Lauderdale et al., 2006; Mouzon et al., 2020; Singletary, 2020; Britt-Spells et al., 2018; Broman et al., 2000; Broman, 1996; Weitzer & Tuch, 1999; Welch et al., 2001; Hausmann et al., 2008; Taylor & Turner, 2002; Barnes et al., 2004; Brown, 2001; Din-Dzietham et al., 2004; Herring et al., 1998; Ifatunji & Forman, 2006; Sigelman & Welch, 1991; Ifatunji & Harnois, 2016; Hudson et al., 2012.

11 Smith et al., 2011; Pierce, 1974, 1975a, 1975b, 1995; Soto et al., 2011.

12 Smith et al., 2011; Pierce, 1974, 1975a, 1975b, 1995; Soto et al., 2011.

13 Geronimus et al., 2006.

14 Chae et al., 2011; Williams & Mohammed, 2013; Chae et al., 2014, 2020; Geronimus et al., 2006, 2010; Harris & Schorpp, 2018; McEwen & Stellar, 1993; McEwen, 1998; Buxton et al., 2014; Mason et al., 2011; Riethman, 2008; Aviv, 2006; Müezzinler et al., 2013; Cherkas et al., 2006; Epel et al., 2004, 2006; Simon et al., 2006; Monaghan, 2010; Blackburn et al., 2015.

15 Chae et al., 2020; Massey et al., 2018; Needham et al., 2014; Park et al., 2015.

16 Dupont et al., 2009; Huang et al., 2014; Moore et al., 2013.

17 Norris, 1992; Breslau, 2001; Motley & Banks, 2018; Roberts et al., 2011; Loo, 1994; Loo et al., 2005; Edwards et al., 2018, 2019; Ellis et al., 2008; Yimgang et al., 2017; Jackson et al., 2017; Holman et al., 2014, 2020; Galovski, 2016; Geller et al., 2014; Schmader et al., 2015; Alang et al., 2017; Bandes, 1999; Krieger et al., 2015; Hartfield et al., 2018; Heard-Garris et al., 2021; Washington Post, 2022; Swaine et al., 2015; Singletary, 2020.

18 Norris, 1992; Breslau, 2001; Motley & Banks, 2018; Roberts et al., 2011; Loo, 1994; Loo et al., 2005; Edwards et al., 2018, 2019; Ellis et al., 2008; Yimgang et al., 2017; Jackson et al., 2017; Holman et al., 2014, 2020; Galovski, 2016; Geller et al., 2014; Schmader et al., 2015; Alang et al., 2017; Bandes, 1999; Krieger et al., 2015; Hartfield et al., 2018; Heard-Garris et al., 2021; Washington Post, 2022; Swaine et al., 2015; Singletary, 2020.

19 Norris, 1992; Breslau, 2001; Motley & Banks, 2018; Roberts et al., 2011; Loo, 1994; Loo et al., 2005; Edwards et al., 2018, 2019; Ellis et al., 2008; Yimgang et al., 2017; Jackson et al., 2017; Holman et al., 2014, 2020; Galovski, 2016; Geller et al., 2014; Schmader et al., 2015; Alang et al., 2017; Bandes, 1999; Krieger et al., 2015; Hartfield et al., 2018; Heard-Garris et al., 2021; Washington Post, 2022; Swaine et al., 2015; Singletary, 2020.

20 Norris, 1992; Breslau, 2001; Motley & Banks, 2018; Roberts et al., 2011; Loo, 1994; Loo et al., 2005; Edwards et al., 2018, 2019; Ellis et al., 2008; Yimgang et al., 2017; Jackson et al., 2017; Holman et al., 2014, 2020; Galovski, 2016; Geller et al., 2014; Schmader et al., 2015; Alang et al., 2017; Bandes, 1999; Krieger et al., 2015; Hartfield et al., 2018; Heard-Garris et al., 2021; Washington Post, 2022; Swaine et al., 2015; Singletary, 2020.

21 Norris, 1992; Breslau, 2001; Motley & Banks, 2018; Roberts et al., 2011; Loo, 1994; Loo et al., 2005; Edwards et al., 2018, 2019; Ellis et al., 2008; Yimgang et al., 2017; Jackson et al., 2017; Holman et al., 2014, 2020; Galovski, 2016; Geller et al., 2014; Schmader et al., 2015; Alang et al., 2017; Bandes, 1999; Krieger et al., 2015; Hartfield et al., 2018; Heard-Garris et al., 2021; Washington Post, 2022; Swaine et al., 2015; Singletary, 2020.

22 Norris, 1992; Breslau, 2001; Motley & Banks, 2018; Roberts et al., 2011; Loo, 1994; Loo et al., 2005; Edwards et al., 2018, 2019; Ellis et al., 2008; Yimgang et al., 2017; Jackson et al., 2017; Holman et al., 2014, 2020; Galovski, 2016; Geller et al., 2014; Schmader et al., 2015; Alang et al., 2017; Bandes, 1999; Krieger et al., 2015; Hartfield et al., 2018; Heard-Garris et al., 2021; Washington Post, 2022; Swaine et al., 2015; Singletary, 2020.

23 Singer et al., 2017.

24 Azar et al., 2020; Poteat et al., 2020; BLS, 2019; Farmer et al., 2006; Massey & Denton, 1993; Durst, 2018; Ajilore & Thames, 2020; CDC, 2021; Andrasfay & Goldman, 2021; Bechteler et al., 2020; Santhanam, 2021; Richardson et al., 2021; Curry, 2020; Eligon & Burch, 2020; Egede & Walker, 2020.

25 Azar et al., 2020; Poteat et al., 2020; BLS, 2019; Farmer et al., 2006; Massey & Denton, 1993; Durst, 2018; Ajilore & Thames, 2020; CDC, 2021; Andrasfay & Goldman, 2021; Bechteler et al., 2020; Santhanam, 2021; Richardson et al., 2021; Curry, 2020; Eligon & Burch, 2020; Egede & Walker, 2020.

26 Azar et al., 2020; Poteat et al., 2020; BLS, 2019; Farmer et al., 2006; Massey & Denton, 1993; Durst, 2018; Ajilore & Thames, 2020; CDC, 2021; Andrasfay & Goldman, 2021; Bechteler et al., 2020; Santhanam, 2021; Richardson et al., 2021; Curry, 2020; Eligon & Burch, 2020; Egede & Walker, 2020.

27 Azar et al., 2020; Poteat et al., 2020; BLS, 2019; Farmer et al., 2006; Massey & Denton, 1993; Durst, 2018; Ajilore & Thames, 2020; CDC, 2021; Andrasfay & Goldman, 2021; Bechteler et al., 2020; Santhanam, 2021; Richardson et al., 2021; Curry, 2020; Eligon & Burch, 2020; Egede & Walker, 2020.

28 Kessler et al., 2003; Kessler & Üstün, 2004; Williams et al., 2007; Üstün et al., 2004; Mereish et al., 2016; Watkins et al., 2006; English et al., 2014; Gee et al., 2012; Hammond et al., 2016; Polanco-Roman & Miranda, 2013; Ward & Mengesha, 2013.

29 Kessler et al., 2003; Kessler & Üstün, 2004; Williams et al., 2007; Üstün et al., 2004; Mereish et al., 2016; Watkins et al., 2006; English et al., 2014; Gee et al., 2012; Hammond et al., 2016; Polanco-Roman & Miranda, 2013; Ward & Mengesha, 2013.

30 Kessler et al., 2003; Kessler & Üstün, 2004; Williams et al., 2007; Üstün et al., 2004; Mereish et al., 2016; Watkins et al., 2006; English et al., 2014; Gee et al., 2012; Hammond et al., 2016; Polanco-Roman & Miranda, 2013; Ward & Mengesha, 2013.

31 Bailey et al., 2021, 2017; Warner, 2021; Jackson et al., 2005; Willoughby, 2018; Smedley et al., 2003; Jones-Rogers, 2019; Agency for Healthcare Research and Quality, 2018; Bynum, 2000.

32 Bailey et al., 2021, 2017; Warner, 2021; Jackson et al., 2005; Willoughby, 2018; Smedley et al., 2003; Jones-Rogers, 2019; Agency for Healthcare Research and Quality, 2018; Bynum, 2000.

33 Brandt, 1978; Washington, 2006; Jones, 1981.

34 Brandt, 1978; Washington, 2006; Jones, 1981.

35 Brandt, 1978; Washington, 2006; Jones, 1981.

36 Brandt, 1978; Washington, 2006; Jones, 1981.

37 Brandt, 1978; Washington, 2006; Jones, 1981.

38 Brandt, 1978; Washington, 2006; Jones, 1981.

39 Metzl, 2010; Baker & Bell, 1999; Mukherjee et al., 1983; Pavkov et al., 1989; Bromberg & Simon, 1968; Brody, 1961; American Psychiatric Association, 1968; Segal et al., 1996.

40 Metzl, 2010; Baker & Bell, 1999; Mukherjee et al., 1983; Pavkov et al., 1989; Bromberg & Simon, 1968; Brody, 1961; American Psychiatric Association, 1968; Segal et al., 1996.

41 Metzl, 2010; Baker & Bell, 1999; Mukherjee et al., 1983; Pavkov et al., 1989; Bromberg & Simon, 1968; Brody, 1961; American Psychiatric Association, 1968; Segal et al., 1996.

42 Soto et al., 2011; Levine et al., 2014; Watkins et al., 2006; Mereish et al., 2016; Britt-Spells et al., 2018; Goodwill et al., 2021; Hoggard et al., 2019; Walton & Shepard Payne, 2016; Baker & Bell, 1999; Metzl, 2013.

43 Soto et al., 2011; Levine et al., 2014; Watkins et al., 2006; Mereish et al., 2016; Britt-Spells et al., 2018; Goodwill et al., 2021; Hoggard et al., 2019; Walton & Shepard Payne, 2016; Baker & Bell, 1999; Metzl, 2013.

CHAPTER 3

RACIAL TRAUMA

The phenomenon of racial trauma is understudied and ill-defined. This chapter defines trauma and racial trauma. It is important that trauma and racial trauma be defined to provide a foundational reference point for the reader. This includes reviewing Acute Stress Disorder (ASD), posttraumatic stress disorder (PTSD), Big "T" and Little "t" trauma, complex trauma, Complex PTSD (CPTSD), racial trauma, stress, traumatic stress, raced-based traumatic stress (RBTS), cultural trauma, historical trauma, and introducing the integrated model of racial trauma (IMRT) and transgenerational trauma points (TTP). Routinely the word *trauma* is used to describe anything that is stressful or troublesome. But everything upsetting is not trauma. The term *trauma* and *racial trauma* are commonly used terms that lack clear coherent operational definitions. The terms have become catch-all phrases that are now a part of the pop culture lexicon. Although it is important that engagement in discussions related to trauma and racial trauma are being highlighted, it is also problematic as the discussions are not grounded in a working definition and theory. This chapter attempts to provide operational definitions and racial trauma theory that clinicians can apply in practice.

Trauma is the Greek word for "wound." According to the Merriam-Webster dictionary (n.d.), the definition of trauma is as follows:

1. An injury (such as a wound) to living tissue caused by an extrinsic agent; a disordered psychic or behavioral state resulting from severe mental or emotional stress or physical injury; an emotional upset.
2. An agent, force, or mechanism that causes trauma.

Therefore, this author's definition of trauma is a wound that affects how a person or community organizes themselves and makes sense of the world. This self or communal organization is created and enforced by oppressive, violent, or threatening incidents perpetuated by individuals or systems that can be historical or present day in nature or both. This wound (trauma) is experienced emotionally, physically, psychologically, spiritually, and systemically. The wound leaves an individual or community feeling untethered and unsafe without a sense of well-being or value. Therefore, a distorted false belief about the self is internalized and continually reinforced by a societal negative feedback loop. To ward off the imposed distorted false belief, individuals and communities experience intrusion, avoidance, and hyperarousal with negative changes in mood and cognitions.

Trauma is not a diagnosis, it is an experience or stressor and the subsequent reactions. Diagnosis can result from an unprocessed traumatic experience. The *DSM-5* is used to diagnose clusters of symptoms to name psychological disorders that may arise.

ACUTE STRESS DISORDER (ASD)

The acute stress disorder (ASD) diagnosis first appeared in the *DSM-4*. This diagnostic category was created to recognize and codify intrusive, avoidant (particularly dissociative), and

DOI: 10.4324/9781003430551-4

hyperarousal-related psychological reactions to an acute stressor that occur relatively immediately after the traumatic event has transpired. ASD also serves the function of identifying
those who may eventually progress onto PTSD. The relevant symptoms must last for at least
three days but not exceed four weeks in duration in the *DSM-5*.[1]

ASD shares numerous similarities with PTSD with the exception that it is diagnosed
more acutely and does not include a requirement that any given symptom cluster be represented in the client's distress. Instead, it is only necessary that a total of nine or more
symptoms be present. An ASD diagnosis does not equate to an automatic progression onto
PTSD. Further, it has been argued that there is insufficient evidence for the existence of
ASD as a disorder separate from early PTSD. Nonetheless, ASD is a useful diagnosis for
those suffering from severe symptoms immediately after accidents, major disasters, mass
trauma, or interpersonal victimization. (Briere & Scott, 2014).

POSTTRAUMATIC STRESS DISORDER (PTSD)

Herman (1992) identified the many symptoms of posttraumatic stress disorder falling into
three main categories. These categories are *hyperarousal, intrusion,* and *constriction.* Hyperarousal includes the persistent expectation of danger, while intrusion includes the permanent imprint of the traumatic moment, and constriction includes the numbing response
of surrender. Since Herman's publication (1992), PTSD now includes avoidance and constriction, which is now described as negative alterations in mood and cognitions. Therefore, PTSD symptomology now includes the four main categories of intrusion, avoidance,
hyperarousal, and negative alterations in mood and cognitions following exposure to a traumatic event. Symptoms of intrusion includes reexperiencing of the traumatic event, that can
involve images, flashbacks (dissociative reactions), and dreams. Avoidance includes efforts
to avoid memories, thoughts, feelings, and physical stimuli related to the traumatic event.
Hyperarousal includes difficulties with sleeping or concentrating, irritability, hypervigilance,
reckless behavior, and an intensified startle response. Alterations in mood and cognition can
occur that may include a consistent negative emotional state and disconnection from others.
This includes guilt, shame, and mistrust.[2]

During the late 19th century and in the early 20th century, trauma was recognized in
psychiatric and mental health diagnostic systems. Stress-related trauma was recognized as
the result of combat (shell shock) or railway accidents in civilian life. During the American
Civil War, terms such as "soldier's heart" or "nostalgia" were used to describe traumatic stress
reactions. Research in the social and physical sciences revealed that stress, which resulted in
trauma, had distinct psychological, social, and physiological components. Research in the
biological sciences discovered that exposure to certain events caused a response that produced distinct physiological and psychological changes. These physiological and psychological changes to extreme stress reactions resulted in an increase in adrenaline and decrease in
endorphin production, which resulted in increased muscle tension and greater sensitivity to
pain. In addition, this manifested in psychological symptoms to the reaction as well. Further,
traumatic events stimulated the release of cortisol and catecholamine potentially resulting
in an integrated traumatic memory that becomes clinically expressed through intrusive rec-
ollections, flashbacks (dissociative reactions), and repetitive nightmares, which potentially
facilitates conditioned emotional responses. Thus, a positive feedback loop is created when
the traumatic memory is vividly recalled in which cortisol, epinephrine, and norepinephrine
are released, further strengthening the memory.[3]

PTSD has been the foundation utilized for understanding trauma in mental health practice and research. Further, PTSD as a diagnostic condition in the history of the *DSM* has created more controversy about boundaries of the condition, symptomatological profile, central assumptions, clinical utility, and prevalence with the exception of dissociative identity disorder (DID). PTSD was originally classified as an anxiety disorder within the *DSM*. This view was supported by the pronounced fear and classical conditioning believed to be central among survivors and treatment approaches that aimed to extinguish such fear-based responses. Therefore, Zoellner et al. (2011) warned that reclassifying PTSD would create the incorrect assumption among clinicians and researchers that fear and anxiety are not central to understanding PTSD. However, other researchers advocated for the creation of a trauma-related disorders diagnostic category where the traumatic event and not the symptoms designate such disorders. Therefore, the traumatic event is the foundation for the diagnosis that encompasses the intensely heterogenous nature and symptomatic presentation of the disorder.[4]

PTSD was initially defined in the *DSM-3* due to the political pressure placed on the mental health field to acknowledge the observed psychological effects of war as well as concentration camp survivors. The PTSD diagnosis was recommended to recognize that persistent psychological reactions to horrific events were a representation of an illness that required care and treatment. The *DSM-3* included a minimum of 4 out of a possible 12 symptoms from three symptom criteria. The *DSM* expanded the potential symptoms in later iterations from 12 to 17 because of criticism that it narrowly focused on Vietnam veterans and Jewish Holocaust survivors but not any other events such as natural disasters. In addition, the definition of a traumatic event was expanded to include experiencing, witnessing, or being otherwise confronted with any event that involves actual or threatened physical harm to self or others along with some symptoms switching criteria. With the *DSM-5*, the definition of trauma became more explicit. Now the *DSM-5* includes 20 PTSD symptoms and yields over 600,000 possible symptom combinations with an extension of the traditional fear response focus to encompass other affective responses. A formal diagnosis of PTSD requires a minimum of 8 out of 20 possible symptoms where symptoms cause significant distress or impairment. PTSD is changing and heterogeneous and so is client presentation. But raced-based traumatic stress is not included under the PTSD diagnosis even though Black persons display PTSD symptomology as a result of racist experiences.[5]

PTSD is the most recognized trauma-specific diagnosis in the *DSM-5*. Further, PTSD is a diagnosable disorder following a traumatic event, and after one month of symptoms from each of the four clusters of *intrusion, hyperarousal, avoidance,* and *negative alterations in mood and cognitions. Intrusive* symptoms include reexperiencing of the traumatic event in the form of nightmares, flashbacks (dissociative reactions), and intrusive thoughts or memories of the trauma as well as the subsequent distress and physiological reactivity upon exposure to stimuli that is a reminder of the event. Therefore, traumatic experiences are unforgettable, outside of an individual's ordinary experience, and not integrated into a person's meaning systems. Attempts to process and integrate the trauma result in intrusive memories, rumination, and perseveration.[6]

Hyperarousal refers to hyperreactivity and the chronic overstimulation of the nervous system where a person is constantly on alert for danger. This may present as "jumpiness," which is a lowered startle threshold, as well as irritability, sleep disturbance, self-destructive behavior, and attention and concentration difficulties. Increases in heart rate, blood pressure, and skin conductance in response to sounds, images, and thoughts that resemble the trauma are part of hyperarousal symptomology. These symptoms can get paired with neutral stimuli as well. Anger control problems are routinely comorbid with PTSD with chronic irritability and anger being problematic. Moreover, psychosomatic complaints and physical problems such as headaches, hypertension, back pain, and gastrointestinal difficulties can occur as a result of hyperarousal.[7]

Avoidance compensates for intrusion and hyperarousal. Symptoms may be cognitive, such as avoiding or suppressing upsetting thoughts, feelings, or memories or behavior such as avoiding activities, people, places, or conversations that may trigger memories of the stressor. Avoidance includes "shutting down," dissociating, suppressing feelings and memories of the trauma, avoiding situations that are reminders of the trauma, utilizing maladaptive behaviors such as substance abuse and self-injury. *Negative alterations in mood and cognitions* include numbing, which may involve diminished interest, detachment, amnesia, as well as persistent negative beliefs and emotional states. A hallmark of PTSD is numbing, which is also linked to depressive shutting down. Avoidant and hyperarousal symptoms are typically more enduring, while the reexperiencing symptoms are routinely the first to fade over time. Avoidance can serve an adaptive function in the short-term but can prevent processing and integration of trauma while perpetuating trauma symptoms in the long-term. In addition, there are several prevalent associated features of PTSD following interpersonal victimization that include cognitive distortions, personality disorder-like difficulties in areas such as relatedness and affect regulation.[8]

Trauma can cause cognitive disruptions where a person's sense of self, others, and reality is shattered. The view of self and the world involves basic assumptions about invulnerability, personal safety, others as mostly trustworthy, and a just world. These assumptions are incompatible and disrupted when trauma is introduced. The exposure to trauma results in hypervigilance, self-blame, survivor guilt, distrust, and alienation. PTSD is associated with increased rates of major depressive disorder, substance-related disorders, panic disorder, agoraphobia, obsessive-compulsive disorder, generalized anxiety disorder, social phobia, bipolar disorder, and borderline personality disorder. These disorders can precede, follow, or co-occur with PTSD. It is important to note that the following classifications of types of traumas (e.g., big "T" and little "t," complex trauma, and complex PTSD) are debated and not uniformly accepted among trauma experts.[9]

BIG "T" AND LITTLE "T" TRAUMA

Big "T" and little "t" trauma was coined by Shapiro (2001) to distinguish between a major traumatic event and mundane traumatic event. Big "T" trauma is a major traumatic event with imminent danger and harm, overwhelming, immobilizing, such as sex assault, rape, abuse, tsunami, earthquake, car crash, fire, etc. Big "T" trauma routinely refers to experiences that cause PTSD and impacts victims in terms of how they behave, think, and feel about themselves and their vulnerability to symptomology. Routinely overlooked but no less significant than big "T" trauma is little "t" trauma. Little "t" trauma is the various day-to-day or periodic happenings that can have a cumulative effect and cause distress, anxiety, guilt, fear, and shame that did not receive a repair and affect our ability to cope. Examples of little "t" trauma include interpersonal conflict, infidelity, divorce, abrupt or extended displacement, legal trouble, and financial worries or difficulty. The accumulation of small "t" trauma over a short period of time can lead to an increase in distress and emotional functioning. Although the distress from small "t" trauma is not considered life or bodily integrity threatening, it can leave a person feeling helpless.[10]

COMPLEX TRAUMA

Although not listed in the *DSM-5*, the field of trauma studies has adopted the term *complex trauma* that describes the experience of multiple, chronic, and prolonged, developmentally adverse traumatic events, most often of an interpersonal nature (e.g., sexual or physical abuse, war, community violence, etc.) and early life onset that is adequately reflected in the diagnostic formulation of PTSD. Initially, Herman (1992) coined the term *disorders of extreme stress not otherwise specified (DESNOS)* to describe the array of symptomology that accompanies what has recently been identified as complex PTSD. Therefore, trauma is categorized into two types. Type I trauma includes exposure to a single, unexpected disturbing event (e.g., car or industrial accident, a natural disaster, or a single assault) that causes fear, horror, or feelings of helplessness that ultimately become conditioned behavioral and biological responses to reminders of the trauma. The exposure and responses are associated with the symptoms of PTSD. Type II is routinely referred to as complex trauma and pertains to prolonged, repeated exposure to extremely disturbing events (e.g., social or political violence through war or torture, domestic violence as a victim or witness, or child abuse) that includes a constellation of disturbances known as complex PTSD and can include the symptomology of PTSD, dissociation, anxiety, depression, and somatic complaints as well as maladaptive behaviors such as substance abuse and self-harm, and personality pathology. Research demonstrates that exposure to multiple traumatic events is more common than exposure to a single traumatic event. In children, this type of trauma is routinely experienced in the form of abuse or neglect from caregivers or other known individuals. Complex trauma during childhood includes physical, sexual, or emotional abuse as well as physical and emotional neglect. PTSD from exposure to a single traumatic event is relatively rare compared to cases with exposure to multiple trauma.[11]

Diagnostic categories are routinely deployed for research and treatment of mental illness. These categories are intended for clinicians and researchers to be able to identify those who have a disorder based on a clear set of symptoms and symptom categories. The *DSM-5* framework attempts to define symptom requirements for illness in order for researchers and clinicians to be able to identify predictors and correlates of specific mental illnesses. Therefore, clinicians and researchers can develop and apply more targeted treatments. Unfortunately, many of the diagnostic classifications are not simple or specific. People with the same diagnosis can have distinctly different symptom presentations. Thus, the *DSM-5* diagnoses and treatment tools are questionable. Further, there are limitations with the *DSM-5* diagnoses as the field of trauma psychology is in its infancy in recognizing and understanding trauma spectrum disorders. Therefore, beyond the *DSM-5*, the causes and manifestations of trauma can vary. Further, the hypothalamic pituitary adrenal (HPA) axis is our central stress response system that often is a potential objective indicator of PTSD when the return to normal levels of arousal are disrupted. Subjective indicators of trauma and PTSD are an individual's overwhelmed coping mechanisms.[12]

COMPLEX PTSD (CPTSD)

Herman (1992) first used the term *complex PTSD* to describe a syndrome experienced by survivors of repeated, prolonged trauma that involved alterations in affect regulation, consciousness, self-perception, and relationships to the perpetrator as well as others. In 2019, the World Health Organization (WHO) formally issued the latest revision to the International Classification of Diseases (ICD-11) with significant changes to the PTSD diagnosis. PTSD was replaced by two diagnoses of PTSD and CPTSD. PTSD requirements include evidence of the re-experiencing of traumatic events in the present, deliberate avoidance, and a current sense of threat and functional impairment. CPTSD includes the same requirements in addition to evidence of disturbances in self-organization (DSO) that consists of affect dysregulation, negative self-concept, and disturbance in relationships. Affective dysregulation may present as hyperactivation where intense emotions cannot be readily moderated or hypoactivation where there is an absence of normal feeling states or both. Negative self-concept may present as feelings of worthlessness or being a failure. The disturbances in relationships may present as detachment and withdrawal from others. Evidence of impairment in important life roles must accompany the symptoms. The enduring changes to one's self-organization typically result from exposure to sustained or multiple traumas from which escape is difficult or impossible. The ICD-11 situates CPTSD as a separate diagnosis from PTSD in which a person can be diagnosed with one or the other but not both. But CPTSD must include the same evidence of re-experiencing in the present, avoidance, and a sense of threat. Therefore, both diagnoses share an explicit focus on specific identifiable traumatic events that are prominent in consciousness. Moreover, chronic or repeated trauma is a risk factor but not a requirement for CPTSD.[13]

SYMPTOM DEVELOPMENT

It has been hypothesized that traumatic experiences are encoded in memory as a multi-modal network of information or fear structure. The encoded information includes the neurobiological, cognitive, affective, and stimulus response of the traumatic experience. Any reminders or stimuli resembling the traumatic event can activate the entire network or fear structure. Classical conditioning is learning that occurs through association of an environmental stimulus and a naturally occurring stimulus, and it is thought to account for the development of chronic PTSD. Operant conditioning is learning that occurs through rewards and punishments for behavior and is thought to account for maintenance of disturbance such as avoiding trauma feelings and memories that can be a negative reinforcer. Reminders of trauma are not the only precursor to PTSD reactions, but neutral stimuli such as loud noises can activate a trauma response, indicating a loss of stimulus discrimination.[14]

Research studies indicate that trauma memories tend to be implicit, behavioral, and somatic. Moreover, trauma memories tend to be vague, overgeneralized, fragmented, incomplete, and associated with disorganized personal narratives. Further, it is theorized that traumatic experiences are encoded primarily in right-brain experiential (nonverbal) memory in the form of emotions, images, and bodily sensations but are not processed on a symbolic or verbal level and are not integrated with other life experiences. Neuroimaging studies of individuals recalling trauma memories indicate increased sensory processing, particularly of visual information accompanied by decreased verbal processing. This research supports clinical observations of low verbal processing and high sensory experiencing by trauma survivors.[15]

RACIAL TRAUMA

Racial Trauma

According to Lebron et al. (2015), the trauma of racism includes kidnapping from Africa, chattel slavery, socially sanctioned rape, Jim/Jane Crow and segregation, lynching, de facto and legal discrimination, marginalization, oppression, employment discrimination, poverty, social alienation, hate crimes, demonization of non-white cultures, discriminatory child welfare practices, hypercriminalization/incarceration, racially biased justice systems, mandatory sentencing, inhumane treatment within societal institutions, unethical medical experiments on Black people, forced sterilization of Black women, the school-to-prison pipeline, inferior schools and education, the achievement gap, the sequestering of Black students in special education programs, racial housing segregation, inhumane housing conditions, and discriminatory policing.

This author provides an integrated and comprehensive theory of racial trauma. The integrated model of racial trauma (IMRT) includes cultural trauma, historical trauma, and race-based traumatic stress (RBTS) theories. Carter's (2007) theory of RBTS provides a foundation and guide to meet narrow psychological and diagnostic standards. Much of the scholarship on racism has tended to focus on the social, economic, and political impacts of racism. Less is understood about the impacts of racism psychologically and the reactions of those who are targeted. Most discussions regarding the psychological harm due to racism tend to be general and global in reference to racism as a form of oppression and violence.

Racism and trauma share common features as both can be experienced directly or vicariously. In addition, racism can cause trauma, and this author posits that anti-Black racism is a form of trauma where Black Americans are often victimized. Black Americans have suffered from cultural, historical, and transgenerational traumas as a result of slavery, anti-Black racism, and discrimination. The trauma of racism refers to the chronic and cumulative negative impact of racism in the lives of Black Americans. This includes the damaging effects of ongoing societal and group racial microaggressions, internalized oppression, overt forms of racism, discrimination, and oppression in the lives of Black Americans. Therefore, it is problematic to refer to many of these experiences as *posttraumatic* as they often are perpetual and not a specific, time-limited event except for historical trauma [e.g., transgenerational trauma points (TTP)].

The PTSD framework fails to account for the daily and recurring dangerous exposure that Black males experience and capture the extent of the injuries sustained by their exposure to racial trauma (e.g., the violence of anti-Black misandry and its many permutations). Chronic and unresolved racial trauma can cause severe emotional pain and distress that overwhelms a person's and community's ability to cope resulting in feelings of powerlessness. The cumulative effect of racial trauma is transgenerational and has created societal vulnerabilities for Black Americans. Racial trauma can be directly or vicariously experienced and is significantly associated with increased psychiatric and physical symptoms among Black Americans. Not everyone who experiences racist incidents will be traumatized, but some people develop posttrauma symptoms in response to racist incidents. But direct experiences with racism are associated with higher levels of anxiety, guilt/shame, and hypervigilance.[16]

Racism is an abuse of human rights and a form of torture and terrorism and a submission-dominance dynamic. Torture is the deliberate and the systematic infliction of physical and mental suffering with the intent of forcing people to conform. Terrorism is actual or threatened violence to obtain attention, thus reinforcing a submission-dominance dynamic or to reestablish the power of the terrorists and their importance or cause. Submission and dominance are maintained through the monopolization of the victim's perception. Thus, the victim's space, time, energy, and mobility must be yielded to the oppressor. Racism, torture, and terrorism require the dehumanization and degradation of the victim. This includes daily insults and aggressions that most Black Americans are subjected to, which are routinely referred to as racial microinsults and microaggressions. They are offensive mechanisms that function to keep Black Americans in an inferior, dependent, and helpless role. These mechanisms (nonverbal and kinetic) produce feelings of degradation and are situated to control space, time, energy, and mobility; thus they are potentially debilitating to Black Americans.[17]

Racist incidents are a form of victimization that produces trauma symptomology. Race-based physical and verbal assaults and threats to a person's livelihood affect's their sense of self and well-being. These numerous threats to a person's emotional and psychological well-being can suddenly occur or be systemic in nature, intentional or nonintentional, vague, and ambiguous, or direct and specific, and can be perpetuated by a person (individual racism), institution (institutional racism), or cultural power and oppression (cultural racism). Racist incidents are a form of violence and emotional abuse and thus traumatic. Racism is motivated by power or the desire to impose a sense of dominance over someone who is less powerful. Power and domination are sustained by communicating and convincing others that the victim or target of oppression is unworthy, lazy, or deserving of differential or abusive treatment. Those targeted and victimized live with fear and are socially isolated with no awareness of when the next violation is to occur. This contributes to anxiety and hyperarousal due to the violence and emotional abuse of racism. Headaches, body pains and aches, trouble sleeping, and difficulty remembering may manifest in Black Americans subjected to these experiences. In addition, they may experience self-blame, confusion, shame, or guilt. The perpetrators of racism routinely fail to assume responsibility, do not experience social or legal repercussions for their actions, and the victim's role as well as their character becomes the social and legal focus in causing the assault. The incident is not viewed as racist or a violation of a Black person's rights and is routinely dismissed or minimized if they are viewed as "arrogant," stepped out of their societally prescribed place, attempted to get more than they deserved, is seen as overly sensitive, or has a criminal record.[18]

Stress and trauma are interchangeable terms to describe the biological, psychological, and social interaction of external events (stressors). The appraisal of an event as either positive, unwanted, negative, or taxing that requires one to adapt or cope in some way is described as stress. A more severe form of stress that overwhelms a person's ability to cope is trauma. What is missing from the discourse are the specific aspects of racism that are connected to emotional and psychological harm in consideration of an individual's response pattern and coping with these adverse experiences. Racism causes psychological harm from the stress or trauma that is experienced. These encounters occur through individuals, institutional, and cultural forms of racism, thus impacting psychological and physical health. Racism as a stressor that can harm or injure its targets is routinely not recognized.[19]

Racial discrimination has been correlated with clinical depression, anxiety, PTSD, or personality disorders as a result of major stress. Racial trauma should be treated as the result of a situational event(s) that produced emotional pain rather than treating the reactions as a mental disorder such as PTSD. Reliance on mental disorders or diagnoses is a dispositional approach that holds those victimized by racism responsible for situational factors outside their control. These experiences should be conceptualized as an *injury* which accurately depicts the external violations and assaults that emanate from racism or race-based encounters and experiences. Moreover, psychological injury indicates that the person who was injured had their rights violated. A nonpathological stance includes the conceptualization of an injury that encompasses reactions to specific forms of racism that are external and situational that have the capacity to affect mental health rather than a mental disorder.[20]

For racial trauma to be identified, the type of racism event(s) of either *racial discrimination, racial harassment,* or *discriminatory harassment* must be experienced as negative (emotionally painful), sudden, and uncontrollable (helplessness). In addition, aspects of the traumatic reactions of intrusion, avoidance, or hyperarousal should be experienced. The trauma reactions may be manifested cognitively, behaviorally, emotionally (affect), somatically, relationally, and spiritually as a result of the greater presence of intrusion and avoidance, which contribute to greater levels of hyperarousal. Cognitive effects potentially include difficulty concentrating, remembering, and focusing. Behaviorally, those targeted and victimized may begin to self-medicate through substance abuse or other forms of self-harm. Affective effects potentially include numbness, depression, anxiety, grief, and anger. Somatic complaints potentially include migraines, nausea, and body aches. Distrust of dominant group members or distrust of members of the same racial group because of internalized oppression may manifest relationally. Spiritually, those targeted and victimized may question their faith in God, humanity, or both. Other manifestations potentially include external locus of control, dissociation, and a sense of a foreshortened future or hopelessness. The trauma reactions may also manifest as anxiety, anger, rage, depression, low self-esteem, shame, and guilt. Racial trauma may be clustered or cumulative racist encounters that may be triggered by a "last straw" event. Stress may not become traumatic until a threshold is reached due to a trigger or last straw after a series of emotional wounds and blows. Traumatic experiences are painful, and the person experiencing the trauma relives the event (last straw) in multiple ways and attempts to psychologically avoid the memory (avoidance) and the resulting pain. This is characterized by a pervasive feeling of vulnerability that is representative of a wound that will not heal. The reactions from the intrusion that causes an open wound are anger, depression, general anxiety, irritability, hostility, poor social and interpersonal relationships, lack of trust, self-blame, or multiple combinations of these reactions.[21]

Denial is a coping mechanism in response to a lifetime of racism. Denial can be a sign that an event(s) was traumatic when it becomes memory loss. A person can become numb emotionally in order to avoid feeling the pain and impact of the constant or sudden assaultive indignities or sense of self. Moreover, a person may dissociate to a place where they cannot be reached or touched by the pain of racism. Avoidance reactions may include depression, aggression, low self-esteem, racial identity confusion, complicated interpersonal relationships, shame, and guilt. Those targeted and victimized might blame themselves for their circumstances without any awareness of the role of racism, or they might be aware of the presence of racism and how it has impacted them but feel helpless.[22]

Psychological trauma (psychology) describes a *wound* within the psyche of an individual, while cultural trauma (sociology) refers to a collective experience (i.e., *wound*) of a group. Cultural trauma is an invasive and overwhelming event (i.e., extreme violence) that undermines or overwhelms a significant aspect of or the entirety of a culture. Culture encompasses the patterns of elements (i.e., values, norms, beliefs, ideologies, knowledge, etc.) that structures a group's meaning-system. Therefore, a cultural trauma is a rupture in the group's meaning system and can threaten collective identity, where dramatic loss of identity and meaning occurs. Both psychological and cultural trauma describe a crisis in meaning and identity but are distinctly different in that a psychological trauma occurs in an individual's psyche, and cultural trauma is a social process. Psychological trauma is contextual, while cultural trauma is historically produced through social phenomenon. Moreover, negative affect/emotions (e.g., fear, sadness, anger, and shame) are fundamental to a cultural trauma where a precognitive emotional response to an event is elicited. The emotional response disrupts social life and activates the impacted group to assign meaning to the event. Therefore, cultural trauma includes a dual process of an emotional experience and an interpretive reaction. An event might cause shock and horror amongst a group along with strong emotions that cause the group to make meaning of the event that potentially transforms the group's collective identity.[23]

Collective memory is a historical narrative of the making of a group's collective identity. A group is unified through time and space by collective memory, which provides a collective story (i.e., narrative frame). Collective memory is fundamental for the endurance of a group as it diachronically connects past and present and synchronically connects group and individual. Trauma can be encapsulated within the collective memory (e.g., cultural trauma-slavery, Jim/Jane Crow, resistance, etc.) that forms the identity of a group (e.g., Black American). The history of slavery in the U.S. forms Black American collective identity in the face of ongoing anti-Black racism. It becomes a cultural process where the formation of a collective identity and the construction of collective memory/history is linked to trauma. The trauma refers to an event(s) that has left wounds for later generations. A collective identity is forged through meaning-making and the remembrance of the trauma. A collective identity is reconstituted or reconfigured to repair a tear or rupture in the social fabric of that group. Reconciling present/future needs includes the process of reinterpreting the past. Historical trauma includes the collective, spiritual, psychological, emotional, and cognitive distress perpetuated intergenerationally due to multiple denigrating experiences beginning with the slave trade/slavery and continuing with various forms of anti-Black racism and discrimination that extends to the present day.[24]

Black Americans have endured more than 300 years of captivity (e.g., enslavement and Jim/Jane Crow) in the U.S., ethnic cleansing through eugenics, and forced acculturation. Historical trauma theory encompasses three theoretical frameworks in social epidemiology. This includes psychosocial theory that connects disease to both physical and psychological stress that is caused by the social environment. Psychosocial stressors create susceptibility to disease and operate as a direct pathogenic mechanism affecting biological systems in the body. The second theoretical framework is political/economic theory, which incorporates the political, economic, and structural determinants of health and disease, including power relations of dominance and racial inequality. The third theoretical framework is social/ecological systems theory, which identifies the multidimensional dynamics and interdependence of present/past, proximate/distal, and life course factors that are correlated with disease causation.[25]

Four distinct assumptions underpin historical trauma theory: (1) a dominant and subjugating population deliberately and systematically inflicts mass trauma upon a target population; (2) trauma continues over an extended period of time and is not limited to a single event; (3) a universal experience of trauma is created as a result of traumatic events reverberating throughout the population; and (4) the population is derailed from its natural projected historical course due to the magnitude of the trauma experience resulting in a legacy of physical, psychological, social, and economic disparities that persists across generations. The constructs of the theory include the historical trauma experience, the historical trauma response, and the intergenerational transmission of historical trauma. Physiological, environmental, and social pathways serve as the conduit for the psychological and emotional consequences of the trauma experience that is transmitted to subsequent generations with the effect of an intergenerational cycle of trauma response.[26]

Historical trauma originates with a dominant group subjugating a population. The successful subjugation requires at least four elements: (1) overwhelming physical and psychological violence, (2) segregation or displacement, (3) economic deprivation, and (4) cultural dispossession. The dominant group enforces subjugation through various mechanisms including military force, police force, war, bio-warfare, national policies, genocide, ethnic

cleansing, incarceration, colonialism, slavery, as well as laws that prohibit freedom of movement, economic development, and cultural expression. These legacies remain in the form
of racism, discrimination, and social and economic disadvantage even when the overt legitimization of subjugation may have been rescinded. The targeted population is affected from
physical and psychological trauma through the universal experience of subjugation.[27]

Psychological and emotional responses stem from experiencing violence, severe stress,
pervasive hardship, and chronic grief as a result of loss. This may manifest in PTSD, depression, anxiety, self-destructive behaviors, shame, anger/rage, complex bereavement, as well as
physical disease. Maladaptive behaviors and related social problems can result in substance
abuse, physical/sexual abuse, and suicide. Vicarious trauma can occur through collective
memory, storytelling, and oral tradition. Moreover, traumatic events can become embedded in the collective social memories of the population. Ancestral knowledge of historical
trauma is reinforced through racial discrimination and everyday racism (i.e., racial microaggressions). The cumulative effects of historical trauma result in poor health outcomes across
generations. Cultural and historical trauma theories support the author's ***transgenerational trauma points*** (TTP) theory that includes the traumatic historical events of the
Walk of Sorrow, Middle Passage, enslavement, Second Middle Passage, and various forms
of neo-slavery that includes Black codes and convict leasing, Jim/Jane Crow, lynching, the
Great Migration (Third Passage), the crack epidemic, the war on drugs, and hypercriminal-
ization/incarceration. These historical tragedies are indexed within this theory and have
had devasting and lasting consequences that reverberate today. TTP theory does not support
a pathologizing claim that Black Americans are suffering from intergenerational psychological disorders (e.g., psychological dysfunction) or biological inferiority (e.g., genetic defects)
due to cultural and historical traumas but rather highlights how cultural and historical traumas not only inform identity through collective memory but impacts present-day health
outcomes that can be connected to specific events. Thus, Black Americans are positioned as
a vulnerable population.[28]

Stress

Stress is an emotional, physical, and behavioral response to an event(s) that is assessed as
positive or unwanted. The initial assessment is followed by a second assessment that focuses
on action to cope and adapt to the event. Further, stress reactions intensify if mechanisms of
coping or adaptation fail. A person's personal characteristics and predispositions correlates
with the extent to which a person is affected by stress. The stress response can be adaptive but

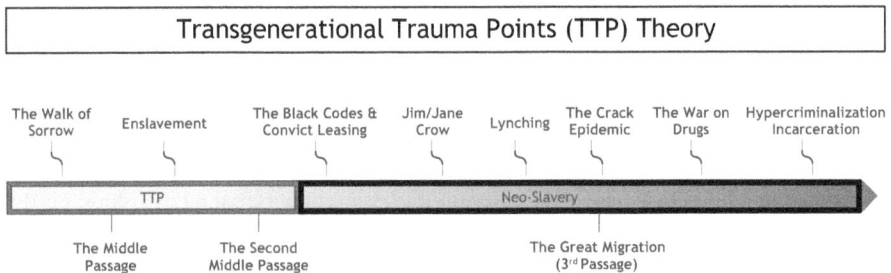

Figure 3.1 Transgenerational Trauma Points (TTP) Theory

harmful as well, affecting mental and physical health. The stress response becomes harmful during prolonged periods or if the stress produces trauma. Therefore, health outcomes are impacted negatively as a result of exposure to stress.[29]

Stress increases when events are ambiguous, negative, unpredictable, and uncontrollable. Stress tends to be greater if there are problems and conflicts with central roles such as personal relationships, work, and parenting. Moreover, negative life events in personal relationships tend to be stronger predictors of depression. Stress reactions occur regardless of whether the stressor is objective, such as a sudden death or accident, or subjective, such as perception of discrimination, as both independently predict psychological and health effects. Some people exposed to stressful situations or events are able to adapt and cope effectively, while others may not be able to adapt and cope effectively when exposed to stressful situations or events. People suffer negative psychological and physical consequences because of long-term and chronic stress.[30]

People can adapt to or experience strain as a result of ongoing stressful events. For some people, it is difficult to adapt to highly stressful situations. Physiological changes resulting from long-term stressful situations may continue and impact psychological well-being even after psychological adaptation to long-term strain from prolonged stress has occurred. Stress is problematic not only because it is a difficult experience but because of the persistent long-term effects and overall cumulative damage.[31]

The reactions to stressful life events routinely result in depression and anxiety. Stressful life events include unemployment, discrimination, poverty, sudden death, marriage, war zone combat, assault, accidents, natural and technological disasters, etc. More severe stress reactions such as posttraumatic stress due to exposure to a life-threatening event is a significantly different area of scholarship than the study of life event stress and psychological health. Therefore, life event stress focuses on major and everyday events such as marriage, moving, or work-related activities, while posttraumatic stress focuses on less common events that are more extraordinary and severe. Both forms of stress are critically different by the level of severity of the event and the reaction that creates the stress or trauma.[32]

Stress has been consistently characterized as an emotional, physical, and behavioral response to an event that is appraised as positive or unwanted. A secondary assessment follows the initial appraisal that focuses on action to cope and adaptation to the event. Cognitive appraisal moderates the environmental stimulus (potential stressor) and either increases or mitigates a person's response (psychophysiological) to the stimulus. Stress affects both mental and physical health, and stress and reactions intensify if coping or adaptation fails. A stress response can be simultaneously adaptive and harmful. It becomes harmful when the stress response is prolonged or produces trauma. Social structures must be considered in comprehending stress and stress reactions. Social structures or systems of social stratification that includes race, sex, and socioeconomic status are routinely related to where a person is situated within that structure and has a direct correlation with stressful experiences. Stress is a fundamental construct in RBTS that can be conceptualized as an emotional trauma brought on by the stress of racism. Moreover, ambiguous, negative, and uncontrollable experiences increase stress. Problems and conflicts with central roles in one's life such as personal relationships, work, and parenting add to the weight of stress. Stronger predictors of depression tend to be connected to negative life events in personal relationships. Further, people suffer negative psychological and physical consequences under conditions of long-term and chronic stress. People experiencing chronic stress can adapt or experience strain, but it is difficult for some people to adapt to these events that are highly stressful. Moreover, physiological changes can result from prolonged stress even after psychological adaptation, but the physiological changes can eventually impact psychological well-being.[33]

Person-environment transactions involving race contribute to life stress. Racism is embedded and experienced within interpersonal, collective, cultural-symbolic, and socio-political contexts as sources of stress. Those who are targeted by racism can experience tension, deprivation, as well as a range of mental health consequences. The long-term effects of stress may persist for a long time and cause cumulative damage. Moreover, racism and discrimination are major contributing factors to health and mental health disparities. Daily racial microaggressions can affect mental health particularly when they have become cumulative over time, thus making a person vulnerable to poor health.[34]

Black men routinely experience daily racial microaggressions by being treated as if they are a physical threat or being treated as if they are invisible. Racial microaggressions are related to depression, anxiety, and the decline in physical health. Daily encounters with racism in the form of racial microaggressions emerge from individual and institutional racism and are reinforced through racial stereotypes that prompt and allow people from all racial groups to treat Black men as dangerous, criminal, or uneducated. Chronic stress for Black Americans is routinely caused by systemic racism (institutional and structural racism) through restricted housing, segregation, and limited economic opportunity and access to social participation. Stressful life events most commonly produce depression and anxiety. Unemployment, discrimination, poverty, sudden death, marriage, war zone combat, assault, accidents, and natural and technological disasters are some stressful life events routinely cited. Expanding this model includes events that may be stressful specifically for Black Americans. This includes a minoritized/racialized status, tokenism where a person is the only person from one's racial group in an institution or organization, experiences of discrimination (e.g., being exposed to a racial incident, lack of social or political power), and socialization into a racial dominant group's customs (e.g., marriage customs, etc.). Individuals who embody internalized racial stereotypes or a poor self-concept may not be able to cope or adapt to racialized experiences and may experience a greater level of stress. PTSD is a more severe stress reaction due to the exposure of a life-threatening event compared to life event stress and psychological health. Historically, life event stress and psychological health has focused on major and everyday events such as marriage, moving, or work-related activities, while PTSD has focused on extraordinary and more severe events that are less common. The significant difference between the two is the level of severity of the event and the reaction to it that creates the stress or trauma.[35]

Traumatic Stress

Trauma is a more severe form of stress in terms of both the nature of the stressor(s) and the type of reaction to the stressor(s). Traumatic stress refers to a form of stress resulting from emotional pain as opposed to a life-threatening event or series of events. Trauma can lead to diagnosable *DSM* disorders such as adjustment disorders, acute stress disorder (ASD), or PTSD but does not need to meet *DSM* criteria to be legitimized as trauma. PTSD with its hallmark symptomology of avoidance, intrusion, and hyperarousal is routinely conceptualized as the most extreme form of trauma. The *DSM-5* (2013) criteria for traumatic events related to PTSD comprises of exposure to actual or threatened death, serious injury, or sexual violence that is directly experienced or witnessed. This is problematic and insufficient as this definition does not address an array of experiences that may not threaten death or serious physical injury but can cause traumatic stress reactions as well as many severe stress experiences such as racism, poverty, neglect, emotional abuse, and homelessness. An emotionally painful racial encounter that is sudden and leaves a person feeling powerless can result in reactions that overlap with PTSD symptoms such as hypervigilance, intrusion, or avoidance.[36]

A traumatic event is any event that is perceived or experienced as shocking enough to produce symptoms of intrusion, avoidance, numbing, and hyperarousal. A traumatic event encompasses violence that can either be psychological or emotional and not merely physical and is marked by the intensity of the emotional impact of the event that can be caused by an act of racism or a race-based encounter. A lifespan developmental perspective in the conceptualization of traumatic events is more expansive than a focus on single events and short-term effects. Therefore, race-based events are not merely physical and occur across the lifespan and can reoccur in various situations and contexts that includes intensity and duration. Various reactions, coping responses, and efforts to adapt to race-based encounters are routinely attempted. The perception or subjective appraisal of the event is negative; thus a person's sense of self is either damaged or threatened by the psychological pain of these experiences. An event that occurs suddenly and without warning or provocation is difficult to adapt to compared to an event that is gradual and takes place over time. Further, an event that is experienced as uncontrollable (helplessness) is highly traumatizing as having some form of control over events serves a self-protective function.[37]

Racist experiences (e.g., individual, institutional, and cultural) are routinely negative, uncontrollable (helplessness), and sudden. Racism is an assault on one's sense of self that heightens tension within and between its targets. Black Americans are subjected to various forms and levels of racism, leaving them vulnerable to lifelong exposure, thus experiencing higher rates of poor physical and mental health as well as being exposed to numerous life event stressors with no or minimal societal support or recognition for their social plight. Therefore, racism is a traumatic stressor that routinely is frequent and intense. The intensity of racial trauma is routinely reflected in various areas of life such as work, living, and education that are simultaneously affected. A particularly painful event can contribute to severe and traumatic stress because of various forms of racism across a range of settings. Black Americans have endured and been exposed to chronic and pervasive anti-Black racism for hundreds of years, thus leaving them physically and emotionally vulnerable. Racist incidents routinely are repeated and reoccurring while subtle and covert, which can be reflected through language or symbols. Racist incidents have occurred societally for centuries in the U.S., where racial harassment and discrimination has been sanctioned and made legal. Traumatic stress is invaluable in assessing and recognizing race-based experiences as both stress and trauma.[38]

RACISM AND TRAUMA

In Chapter 1 multiple definitions of racism along with a unified theory of racism (UTR) were provided. Racism creates an emotional and psychological injury, and the stress of that injury produces trauma. Racial encounters can be direct, subtle, ambiguous, occur on an interpersonal level (e.g., racial microaggressions, verbal assaults, use of symbols or coded language), can arise from structural acts, occur on an institutional level, emerge through the deployment of racial stereotypes or as encounters and assault(s), or occur through cultural racism. An example of cultural racism is the failure of the U.S. to recognize and remedy the various harms and damage enacted against Black Americans, whose descendants were held in bondage and denied access and opportunity due to slavery and Jim/Jane Crow.

Carter and Helms (2002) and Carter (2007) have grouped racism into distinct types of racism that encompasses the various levels of *individual, institutional,* and *cultural* racism to connect specific types of racism with emotional and psychological responses, thus reducing ambiguity associated with various kinds of race-based experiences and making it easier to document the mental health impact or injury of racism. In addition, this would assist mental health professionals with the ability to assist those who have been targets of racism and provide them with the opportunity to obtain redress and recovery from the pain of racism. These types of racism are *racial discrimination, racial harassment,* and *discriminatory harassment* and includes *individual, institutional,* and *cultural* levels of racism. Being stopped by the police because of your race (racial profiling) is a form of racial harassment that can produce traumatic reactions of avoidance and intrusion. Being ignored by salespeople in a store or denied housing are examples of racial discrimination that can cause stress, and the stress can become traumatic. The denial of promotion(s) at work or one's abilities and professional skills constantly questioned in subtle ways are examples of discriminatory harassment that can produce stress and trauma. Providing types of racism that includes a range of experiences that occur over long periods of time can be beneficial to understand the mental health effects. Further, it provides language to communicate experiences of those who are victimized and targeted and helps professionals recognize the acts and associated effects on those targeted. Those targeted potentially can obtain knowledge and recognition of the different types of racism that can assist them in developing coping mechanisms and a sense of empowerment as well as helping mental health professionals to advocate on their behalf in seeking redress for any injury suffered due to acts of racism.

Racial Discrimination (Avoidant Racism)

Racial discrimination are types of experiences with avoidant racism that is reflected in behaviors, thoughts, policies, and strategies that include the intentional or nonintentional effect of maintaining distance or minimizing contact between a dominant racial group and subordinate racial group members. This definition of racial discrimination encompasses a group of events, acts, and experiences that aid dominant racial group members in the engagement of racism covertly. Essed (1991) categorized the underlying meaning of everyday racist events into the three categories of *problematizing, containing,* and *marginalization.* Problematizing involves the characterization or expressed belief that Black people have "problems" or defects in their biological makeup and culture. Therefore, social problems are created by these inherent cultural limitations. Black men in the U.S. are routinely confronted with the attribution of superiority on the basis of whiteness with white skin being the marker. Some of Black men's problematizing encounters involve the denigration of their perspectives, experiences, and personality through pathologizing them or projecting/attributing dangerousness and criminality onto them as well as sexually objectifying them. Problematizing also involves denigrating Black culture through assumptions and behavior that convey that Black Americans are uncivilized, backward, or deficient in the use of English language, are lazy, or lack ability.[39]

Containing involves keeping Black Americans in their place. This is achieved by denial of racism through various mechanisms such as only recognizing extreme forms of overt racism, displaying anger towards Black Americans who point out racism, and dealing with differences through a majority rule process as well as cultural nonrecognition, mistrust of Black Americans, etc. Physical and symbolic violence are deployed through intimidation. Moreover, Black Americans are marginalized through withdrawal, centering whites as the normative group, barring access, discouraging achievement, exclusion, withholding information, and the use of deception. Components and experiences of everyday racism can be conceptualized as a form of avoidant racism. Avoidant racism may occur at the individual level such as denial of opportunity or access of a Black person, the structural or institutional level through lack of access to education or mental health care, and the policy and cultural level through standards and practices that exclude Black Americans or ignore or denigrate their contributions and culture.[40]

Racially based discrimination includes exclusion from social and work networks, dismissal or denial of personal achievement(s), and limits or restrictions on opportunities for achievement, such as requiring advanced high school courses for college admission while discouraging Black Americans from enrolling in them. Emotional responses to being discriminated against includes fear, tension, anxiety, depression, sadness, anger, aggression, attempts to overcome barriers, social cohesion, and using adversity as a source of strength. Black Americans have many experiences of discrimination that encompass historical components that provides meaning and salience to symbolic, subtle, verbal, and non-verbal messages that can produce race-based stress.[41]

Racial Harassment (Hostile Racism)

Racial harassment are types of experiences with hostile racism intended to communicate or make salient the target's subordinate or inferior status due to their societal prescribed inferior status and membership in a subordinate racial group that routinely is conveyed through feelings, thoughts, actions, strategies, behaviors, and policies. Racial harassment is similar to the everyday racist event categories of containment and problematization. Explicit and implicit institutional permission to commit acts of racism reflect racial harassment, and examples include absent explicit policies and procedures for the filing and handling of racial harassment claims or failing to address community violence that disproportionately traumatizes Black children.[42]

Racial harassment can take form through institutional racial policies and practices such as quid pro quo pressure to "fall into line" as a condition of continued employment, education, or social participation. A Black person who remains silent and does not act or does not file formal complaints in return for continued access to opportunities is a quid pro quo arrangement and a form of racial harassment. Reporting acts of racism may be influenced by the fear of losing a home, job, or education. Black Americans are expected to grant the "favor" of ignoring racism for the opportunity to work or live. Being followed by security in stores is a form of racial harassment. Racial harassment includes physical, interpersonal, and verbal assaults. This includes the assumption that one is not to be trusted, treating people according to racial stereotypes (e.g., Black Americans are lazy or lack ability), and the assumption that one is a criminal or dangerous. Anger, rage, powerlessness, shame, guilt, helplessness, low self-esteem or persistent self-doubt, suspiciousness, and distrust are common emotional reactions to hostile treatment. Carter and Forsyth (2010) found that racial harassment was associated with more hypervigilance and anxious reactions than racial discrimination (avoidance).[43]

Discriminatory Harassment (Aversive-Hostile Racism)

Discriminatory harassment are types of experiences or encounters with aversive hostile racism and encompasses elements of hostility in thoughts, behavior, actions, feelings, or policies and procedures that are intended to create distance among racial group members after a Black person has gained entry into an environment from which they previously had been excluded. Discriminatory harassment can emerge from structural racism and is a combination and complex mixture of both avoidance (racial discrimination) and hostility (racial harassment). An example would be a Black person who is provided access to an institution (job, etc.) and is avoided in a hostile manner, thus experiencing aversive racism combined with harassment. If it is a job, they might be treated with disdain after being hired and not trained to perform their job duties well in addition to having their qualifications questioned. Further, they are subjected to poor work evaluations and reprimanded for minor infractions. Examples of avoidance would be coworkers and supervisors ignoring or shunning (e.g., isolation at work) the Black employee, and the acts of hostility would be demonstrated through critical feedback and the denigration of their work and presence in the workplace.[44]

Aversive racism may occur at the individual, institutional, and cultural level. Routinely aversive racism is expressed in colorblind beliefs and practices, including expressions of discomfort, disgust, and fear as long as factors other than race are cited in decision-making and behavior by people and organizational leaders. These definitions of three different types of racism can facilitate recognition among those who are targeted and victimized by systematic, covert, subtle, and unconscious forms of racism. Instead of solely providing a general definition of racism or racial discrimination, specific definitions or types of racism are provided in this section as well as Chapter 1 with the intent to begin to capture a taxonomy of everyday anti-Black racism for the purpose of identifying racial trauma. These definitions can provide guidance for mental health professionals in their analysis, assessment, and practice in responding to race-based experiences. Further, those targeted or victimized can be empowered to seek out mental health professionals for psychological help or legal redress.[45]

PSYCHOLOGICAL AND EMOTIONAL INJURY

Harm or injury can occur from race-based events that may be moderate or severe as well as daily slights or racial microaggressions that have a memorable impact or lasting effect or through cumulative or chronic exposure to the various types of racism. Physical attacks may not be the most severe forms of racial trauma. Racism in the form of either racial harassment (hostility), racial discrimination (avoidance), or discriminatory harassment (aversive hostility) can cause a RBTS (racial trauma) injury that manifests as emotional or physical pain or as hypervigilance toward the threat of physical and emotional pain. Racial trauma should be conceptualized as a psychological and emotional injury rather than a mental health disorder(s) as the effects of racism originate from the sociocultural environment and are situational not dispositional (intrapsychic).[46]

A person's psyche and personality can be damaged due to racism in the same way that being subject to community violence, being held captive, or being psychologically tortured can create emotional damage. Mental health professionals routinely focus on how the individual must adjust to their circumstances (resilience) within dominant cultural patterns, thus viewing individual difficulties as dispositional or characterological instead of resulting from situational stress. Problems are typically located in people and their personal failures attributed to dominant American cultural socialization. The situational factors and circumstances that can create stress, emotional distress, pain, and trauma for those targeted and victimized should be conceptualized and assessed as psychological and emotional injury that recognizes the mental health impact of racism. Normal functioning is routinely disrupted, and a person is often left harmed and ill because of racism. Moreover, types of racism can result in psychological and emotional impacts, but the impacts may not necessarily reflect a pathological process. Psychological and emotional pain or injury is a nonpathological process but includes a set of emotional reactions and associated cluster of symptoms and reactions that can impair functioning. Race-based stress or trauma can be assessed to identify reactions and integrate the situational (external) and dispositional (internal) components that are contextual to a person's life history and experiences.[47]

A traumatic reaction is an experience that is perceived to be negative (e.g., cause emotional pain or threat of pain), be sudden, and create a sense of helplessness (uncontrollable). Racist experiences routinely cultivate a trauma reaction. Experiences of racial discrimination, racial harassment, and discriminatory harassment may be indirect, symbolic, or through coded language. The symptomology of RBTS includes reactions of intrusion (reexperiencing), numbing, or avoidance of trauma associated stimuli, and increased hyperarousal (arousal or vigilance). The psychological threat or assault may be characterized by an insult that may trigger racial trauma, but routinely it is manifested in subtle ways and prolonged that represent a "last straw" encounter or experience that expands the level of stress to the threshold of trauma. The reliance on PTSD as a marker of racial trauma is problematic in that the target or victim of racism is pathologized, and their emotional pain is not fully recognized. The strength and intensity of a person's reaction and the symptomology that emerges should determine the severity of a race-based event. Severity may be the consequence of the cumulative effects of numerous racist events that have occurred throughout a person's lifetime. Following a series of accumulated racial incidents, a "last straw" event that may appear to be seemingly innocuous or minor may render a person unable to manage the stress and pain of encounters with racism.[48]

RBTS is an emotional trauma caused by the stress of racism. The RBTS model provides a framework for clients to be able to articulate their experience(s), access mental health services, and seek legal redress. In addition, it provides a framework for clinicians to be able to provide responsive care and advocate on behalf of their clients in seeking legal redress. The limitations of the RBTS framework are that it is a psychological model that is focused on individual and contextual experiences that are within the purview of the narrow definitions of racism (i.e., discriminatory harassment, racial discrimination, and racial harassment) that are fundamental to the RBTS model. Cultural trauma theory is a social process that refers to a collective experience that is historically produced through social phenomenon. The limitation of the cultural trauma framework is that it is a sociological model that focuses on a collective experience. Historical trauma theory is a social epidemiological framework with a primary emphasis on social determinants of health and disease. The limitations of the historical trauma framework are its primary emphasis on social determinants of health and disease. The strengths of RBTS, cultural trauma, and historical trauma theories are also limitations, but all three theories complement each other and, when combined, address the limitations of each theory. Therefore, the IMRT provides a comprehensive alternative to the limitations of each framework.[49]

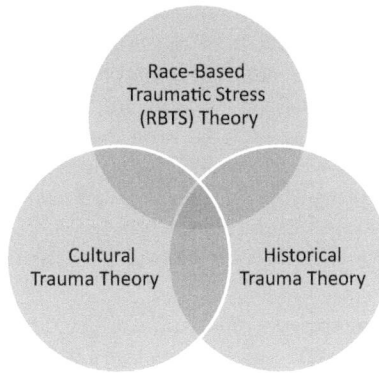

Figure 3.2 Integrated Model of Racial Trauma (IMRT)

CLINICAL IMPLICATIONS

Racial trauma is understudied and ill-defined. The integrated model of racial trauma (IMRT) provides a comprehensive framework to begin to define and study racial trauma and Black men. Furthermore, racial trauma due to police violence may be expressed through anger, sadness, fear, avoidance, dissociation, and hypervigilance among Black males. Vicarious trauma might be experienced by viewing video clips of Black death and dying or other forms of violence directed at Black people on various media and social media platforms. As previously highlighted, Black males (ages 18–24 years old) in Baltimore, Maryland, disclosed witnessing (e.g., witnessing police beat up and injure older Black men) and experiencing (e.g., racial profiling, harassment, physical injury, threats, and verbal aggression) police violence that began in childhood and continued into emerging adulthood, which met the *DSM-5* criteria for trauma exposure and embodied theoretical conceptualizations of racial trauma. The exposures to police violence created distrust and fear of police among Black males and informed appraisals and understandings of their vulnerability (Black male vulnerability to physical, psychological, social, economic, or legal harm) to police violence (i.e., racial profiling, injury, and death) across the life course. In addition, Black males disclosed losing loved ones to police killings, which activated hypervigilance and grief. They were challenged to navigate morbidity, mortality, and traumatic loss as a function of community violence while concomitantly challenged to navigate the chronic risk of exposures to violence and premature death due to police encounters. Young Black men disclosed feeling frustrated, exhausted, embarrassed, anger, shame, and fear. Geller et al.'s (2014) research on aggressive policing (i.e., stop-and-frisk and suspicionless stops and searches) and the mental health of young urban men (80 percent non-white, average age of 22 years, and 78 percent reported no criminal activity) found that more frequent police contact was associated with trauma and anxiety symptoms where the non-consensual encounters were experienced as intrusive with a higher prevalence of PTSD among Black males.[50]

RBTS and cultural trauma can be assessed by using the Race-Based Traumatic Stress Symptom Scale Short Form (RBTSSS-SF), the Carter-Vinson Race-Based Traumatic Stress

Interview Schedule, and the Cultural Trauma Scale (CuTs). But it is recommended that clinicians conceptualize racial trauma from the IMRT framework. The IMRT provides therapists with the option to approach case conceptualization from a multidimensional approach that incorporates psychology, sociology, history, and epidemiology. The RBTS model is sufficient when attempting to assess racial trauma and helping clients articulate their pain. In addition, therapists can advocate for clients to be able to access mental health services and legal redress. A progressive assessment environment is optimal that is supportive where the clinician demonstrates efforts to understand the client's racial and cultural experiences of trauma, including when they are not evident to the client manifesting symptoms or reactions.[51]

According to Carter and Forsyth (2009), those targeted by racism can pursue remedy or redress under the Civil Rights Acts of 1866 (section 1891), the Civil Rights Act of 1964, Civil Rights Act of 1991, Title VII (prohibits discrimination in the workplace) of the 1964 Civil Rights Act, and civil tort law (compensatory damages for intentional infliction of emotional distress). In addition, claims and complaints can be filed and pursued through city and state court systems, and municipal and state departments of human or civil rights. Unfortunately, most plaintiffs (80 percent) in cases of racial harassment do not prevail in the courts and those that do have been exposed to blatant forms (i.e., traditional racism-overt forms of racial discrimination) of racism that included explicit racial animus and hostile treatment for prolonged periods of time. This includes work-related racial harassment cases filed with the Equal Employment Opportunity Commission (EEOC) that progressed to the courts. Chew and Kelley (2006) found that only 1 percent of EEOC racial harassment charges were litigated between 1980 and 1999. Therefore, it is important that therapists are cognizant of these facts when supporting or recommending clients take legal action to address anti-Black racism. Clients need to know that bringing forward a discrimination case does not necessarily result in resolution of their claim(s).

The limited definitions of racism (i.e., discriminatory harassment, racial discrimination, and racial harassment) provide a measurable structure that is fundamental to the RBTS framework but is also problematic as the definitions are narrow in scope. Therefore, it is recommended that clinicians utilize the UTR model along with the IMRT if the therapist is not formally assessing for RBTS or assisting the client in seeking legal redress. The IMRT and UTR afford therapists the ability to integrate a comprehensive biopsychosocial approach. The Index of Race-Related Stress-Brief Version (IRRS-B/Utsey, 1999) surveys anti-Blackness and race-related stress within the domains of cultural racism, institutional racism, and individual racism but is not a measure of racial trauma and does not focus on Black men, while the Cultural Trauma Scale (CuTs/Gregory & Tucker Edmonds, 2023) focuses on Black men's perceptions of cultural trauma. Consequently, it is recommended that an assessment be developed for racial trauma with a focus on anti-Black racism as well as anti-Black misandry that incorporates elements of Black male negation (BMN; see Chapter 6: "The Black Messiah" for details). Racial trauma is a psychological and emotional injury and not a mental health disorder as it originates from the sociocultural environment (environmental stressors). Racial trauma occurs due to events and encounters that are experienced as sudden, out of one's control, and emotionally painful (negative). The symptom cluster includes intrusion (reexperiencing), arousal (hypervigilance), avoidance, and numbing. It is recommended that at least two out of the three symptom clusters be reported by those victimized, and although they are important, they are not required components of racial trauma reactions. In addition, racial trauma may be expressed as a symptom cluster that includes anxiety, anger, rage, depression, low self-esteem, physical reactions, shame, and guilt. Clinicians need to be able to recognize the psychological harm caused by racism and validate their client's racial trauma. Moreover, therapists should inquire about coping efforts, and the results of coping attempts among their clients reporting racial trauma. Racial trauma interventions for Black men may need to include family and community members as well as incorporate spirituality or religion and culture.

NOTES

1 Briere & Scott, 2014.
2 Mlotek & Paivio, 2017; Galatzer-Levy & Bryant, 2013; American Psychiatric Association, 2013; Turnbull, 1998; SAMHSA, 2014; Boone et al., 2003; Carter, 2007; Zoellner et al., 2011; Jones & Cureton, 2014; American Psychiatric Association, 1980; Helzer et al., 1987; McFarlane, 1988; Galatzer-Levy & Bryant, 2013; Chou et al., 2012; Briere & Scott, 2014; Van der Kolk et al., 1996; Paivio & Pascual-Leone, 2010; Abbas et al., 2009; McFarlane, 1988; Janoff-Bulman, 1992; American Psychiatric Association, 2013.
3 Mlotek & Paivio, 2017; Galatzer-Levy & Bryant, 2013; American Psychiatric Association, 2013; Turnbull, 1998; SAMHSA, 2014; Boone et al., 2003; Carter, 2007; Zoellner et al., 2011; Jones & Cureton, 2014; American Psychiatric Association, 1980; Helzer et al., 1987; McFarlane, 1988; Galatzer-Levy & Bryant, 2013; Chao et al., 2012; Briere & Scott, 2014; Van der Kolk et al., 1996; Paivio & Pascual-Leone, 2010; Abbas et al., 2009; McFarlane, 1988; Janoff-Bulman, 1992; American Psychiatric Association, 2013.
4 Mlotek & Paivio, 2017; Galatzer-Levy & Bryant, 2013; American Psychiatric Association, 2013; Turnbull, 1998; SAMHSA, 2014; Boone et al., 2003; Carter, 2007; Zoellner et al., 2011; Jones & Cureton, 2014; American Psychiatric Association, 1980; Helzer et al., 1987; McFarlane, 1988; Galatzer-Levy & Bryant, 2013; Chao et al., 2012; Briere & Scott, 2014; Van der Kolk et al., 1996; Paivio & Pascual-Leone, 2010; Abbas et al., 2009; McFarlane, 1988; Janoff-Bulman, 1992; American Psychiatric Association, 2013.
5 Mlotek & Paivio, 2017; Galatzer-Levy & Bryant, 2013; American Psychiatric Association, 2013; Turnbull, 1998; SAMHSA, 2014; Boone et al., 2003; Carter, 2007; Zoellner et al., 2011; Jones & Cureton, 2014; American Psychiatric Association, 1980; Helzer et al., 1987; McFarlane, 1988; Galatzer-Levy & Bryant, 2013; Chao et al., 2012; Briere & Scott, 2014; Van der Kolk et al., 1996; Paivio & Pascual-Leone, 2010; Abbas et al., 2009; McFarlane, 1988; Janoff-Bulman, 1992; American Psychiatric Association, 2013.
6 Mlotek & Paivio, 2017; Galatzer-Levy & Bryant, 2013; American Psychiatric Association, 2013; Turnbull, 1998; SAMHSA, 2014; Boone et al., 2003; Carter, 2007; Zoellner et al., 2011; Jones & Cureton, 2014; American Psychiatric Association, 1980; Helzer et al., 1987; McFarlane, 1988; Galatzer-Levy & Bryant, 2013; Chao et al., 2012; Briere & Scott, 2014; Van der Kolk et al., 1996; Paivio & Pascual-Leone, 2010; Abbas et al., 2009; McFarlane, 1988; Janoff-Bulman, 1992; American Psychiatric Association, 2013.
7 Mlotek & Paivio, 2017; Galatzer-Levy & Bryant, 2013; American Psychiatric Association, 2013; Turnbull, 1998; SAMHSA, 2014; Boone et al., 2003; Carter, 2007; Zoellner et al., 2011; Jones & Cureton, 2014; American Psychiatric Association, 1980; Helzer et al., 1987; McFarlane, 1988; Galatzer-Levy & Bryant, 2013; Chao et al., 2012; Briere & Scott, 2014; Van der Kolk et al., 1996; Paivio & Pascual-Leone, 2010; Abbas et al., 2009; McFarlane, 1988; Janoff-Bulman, 1992; American Psychiatric Association, 2013.
8 Mlotek & Paivio, 2017; Galatzer-Levy & Bryant, 2013; American Psychiatric Association, 2013; Turnbull, 1998; SAMHSA, 2014; Boone et al., 2003; Carter, 2007; Zoellner et al.,

2011; Jones & Cureton, 2014; American Psychiatric Association, 1980; Helzer et al., 1987; McFarlane, 1988; Galatzer-Levy & Bryant, 2013; Chao et al., 2012; Briere & Scott, 2014; Van der Kolk et al., 1996; Paivio & Pascual-Leone, 2010; Abbas et al., 2009; McFarlane, 1988; Janoff-Bulman, 1992; American Psychiatric Association, 2013.

9 Mlotek & Paivio, 2017; Galatzer-Levy & Bryant, 2013; American Psychiatric Association, 2013; Turnbull, 1998; SAMHSA, 2014; Boone et al., 2003; Carter, 2007; Zoellner et al., 2011; Jones & Cureton, 2014; American Psychiatric Association, 1980; Helzer et al., 1987; McFarlane, 1988; Galatzer-Levy & Bryant, 2013; Chao et al., 2012; Briere & Scott, 2014; Van der Kolk et al., 1996; Paivio & Pascual-Leone, 2010; Abbas et al., 2009; McFarlane, 1988; Janoff-Bulman, 1992; American Psychiatric Association, 2013.

10 Neborsky, 2003; Barbash, 2017.

11 Van der Kolk, 2003, 2005; Cloitre et al., 2009; Mlotek & Paivio, 2017; Resick et al., 2003.

12 Briere & Scott, 2014; Galatzer-Levy & Bryant, 2013.

13 WHO, 2019; Brewin, 2020; Maercker et al., 2013.

14 Foa et al., 2006; Foa & Kozak, 1986; Paivio & Pascual-Leone, 2010.

15 Van der Kolk, 2003; Van der Kolk et al., 1996; Lanius et al., 2004.

16 Eyerman, 2001, 2004; Sotero, 2006; Harrell, 2000; Chae et al., 2021; Carter, 2007; Carlson, 1997; Lebron, 2015; Pierce, 1992, 1995; Bryant-Davis & Ocampo, 2005; Singletary, 2020; Williams-Washington, 2010; Carter & Forsyth, 2010; Bryant-Davis, 1997, 2007; Lazarus & Folkman, 1984; Carter et al., 2017b; Eyerman, 2001, 2004, 2012, 2015; Smelser, 2004; Woods, 2019; Sotero, 2006; McMichael, 1999; Krieger, 2001.

17 Eyerman, 2001, 2004; Sotero, 2006; Harrell, 2000; Chae et al., 2021; Carter, 2007; Carlson, 1997; Lebron, 2015; Pierce, 1992, 1995; Bryant-Davis & Ocampo, 2005; Singletary, 2020; Williams-Washington, 2010; Carter & Forsyth, 2010; Bryant-Davis, 1997, 2007; Lazarus & Folkman, 1984; Carter et al., 2017b; Eyerman, 2001, 2004, 2012, 2015; Smelser, 2004; Woods, 2019; Sotero, 2006; McMichael, 1999; Krieger, 2001.

18 Eyerman, 2001, 2004; Sotero, 2006; Harrell, 2000; Chae et al., 2021; Carter, 2007; Carlson, 1997; Lebron, 2015; Pierce, 1992, 1995; Bryant-Davis & Ocampo, 2005; Singletary, 2020; Williams-Washington, 2010; Carter & Forsyth, 2010; Bryant-Davis, 1997, 2007; Lazarus & Folkman, 1984; Carter et al., 2017b; Eyerman, 2001, 2004, 2012, 2015; Smelser, 2004; Woods, 2019; Sotero, 2006; McMichael, 1999; Krieger, 2001.

19 Eyerman, 2001, 2004; Sotero, 2006; Harrell, 2000; Chae et al., 2021; Carter, 2007; Carlson, 1997; Lebron, 2015; Pierce, 1992, 1995; Bryant-Davis & Ocampo, 2005; Singletary, 2020; Williams-Washington, 2010; Carter & Forsyth, 2010; Bryant-Davis, 1997, 2007; Lazarus & Folkman, 1984; Carter et al., 2017; Eyerman, 2001, 2004, 2012, 2015; Smelser, 2004; Woods, 2019; Sotero, 2006; McMichael, 1999; Krieger, 2001.

20 Eyerman, 2001, 2004; Sotero, 2006; Harrell, 2000; Chae et al., 2021; Carter, 2007; Carlson, 1997; Lebron, 2015; Pierce, 1992, 1995; Bryant-Davis & Ocampo, 2005; Singletary, 2020; Williams-Washington, 2010; Carter & Forsyth, 2010; Bryant-Davis, 1997, 2007; Lazarus & Folkman, 1984; Carter et al., 2017b; Eyerman, 2001, 2004, 2012, 2015; Smelser, 2004; Woods, 2019; Sotero, 2006; McMichael, 1999; Krieger, 2001.

21 Eyerman, 2001, 2004; Sotero, 2006; Harrell, 2000; Chae et al., 2021; Carter, 2007; Carlson, 1997; Lebron, 2015; Pierce, 1992, 1995; Bryant-Davis & Ocampo, 2005; Singletary, 2020; Williams-Washington, 2010; Carter & Forsyth, 2010; Bryant-Davis, 1997, 2007; Lazarus & Folkman, 1984; Carter et al., 2017b; Eyerman, 2001, 2004, 2012, 2015; Smelser, 2004; Woods, 2019; Sotero, 2006; McMichael, 1999; Krieger, 2001.

22 Eyerman, 2001, 2004; Sotero, 2006; Harrell, 2000; Chae et al., 2021; Carter, 2007; Carlson, 1997; Lebron, 2015; Pierce, 1992, 1995; Bryant-Davis & Ocampo, 2005; Singletary, 2020;

Williams-Washington, 2010; Carter & Forsyth, 2010; Bryant-Davis, 1997, 2007; Lazarus & Folkman, 1984; Carter et al., 2017b; Eyerman, 2001, 2004, 2012, 2015; Smelser, 2004; Woods, 2019; Sotero, 2006; McMichael, 1999; Krieger, 2001.

23 Eyerman, 2001, 2004; Sotero, 2006; Harrell, 2000; Chae et al., 2021; Carter, 2007; Carlson, 1997; Lebron, 2015; Pierce, 1992, 1995; Bryant-Davis & Ocampo, 2005; Singletary, 2020; Williams-Washington, 2010; Carter & Forsyth, 2010; Bryant-Davis, 1997, 2007; Lazarus & Folkman, 1984; Carter et al., 2017b; Eyerman, 2001, 2004, 2012, 2015; Smelser, 2004; Woods, 2019; Sotero, 2006; McMichael, 1999; Krieger, 2001.

24 Eyerman, 2001, 2004; Sotero, 2006; Harrell, 2000; Chae et al., 2021; Carter, 2007; Carlson, 1997; Lebron, 2015; Pierce, 1992, 1995; Bryant-Davis & Ocampo, 2005; Singletary, 2020; Williams-Washington, 2010; Carter & Forsyth, 2010; Bryant-Davis, 1997, 2007; Lazarus & Folkman, 1984; Carter et al., 2017b; Eyerman, 2001, 2004, 2012, 2015; Smelser, 2004; Woods, 2019; Sotero, 2006; McMichael, 1999; Krieger, 2001.

25 Eyerman, 2001, 2004; Sotero, 2006; Harrell, 2000; Chae et al., 2021; Carter, 2007; Carlson, 1997; Lebron, 2015; Pierce, 1992, 1995; Bryant-Davis & Ocampo, 2005; Singletary, 2020; Williams-Washington, 2010; Carter & Forsyth, 2010; Bryant-Davis, 1997, 2007; Lazarus & Folkman, 1984; Carter et al., 2017b; Eyerman, 2001, 2004, 2012, 2015; Smelser, 2004; Woods, 2019; Sotero, 2006; McMichael, 1999; Krieger, 2001.

26 Eyerman, 2001, 2004; Sotero, 2006; Harrell, 2000; Chae et al., 2021; Carter, 2007; Carlson, 1997; Lebron, 2015; Pierce, 1992, 1995; Bryant-Davis & Ocampo, 2005; Singletary, 2020; Williams-Washington, 2010; Carter & Forsyth, 2010; Bryant-Davis, 1997, 2007; Lazarus & Folkman, 1984; Carter et al., 2017b; Eyerman, 2001, 2004, 2012, 2015; Smelser, 2004; Woods, 2019; Sotero, 2006; McMichael, 1999; Krieger, 2001.

27 Eyerman, 2001, 2004; Sotero, 2006; Harrell, 2000; Chae et al., 2021; Carter, 2007; Carlson, 1997; Lebron, 2015; Pierce, 1992, 1995; Bryant-Davis & Ocampo, 2005; Singletary, 2020; Williams-Washington, 2010; Carter & Forsyth, 2010; Bryant-Davis, 1997, 2007; Lazarus & Folkman, 1984; Carter et al., 2017b; Eyerman, 2001, 2004, 2012, 2015; Smelser, 2004; Woods, 2019; Sotero, 2006; McMichael, 1999; Krieger, 2001.

28 Eyerman, 2001, 2004; Sotero, 2006; Harrell, 2000; Chae et al., 2021; Carter, 2007; Carlson, 1997; Lebron, 2015; Pierce, 1992, 1995; Bryant-Davis & Ocampo, 2005; Singletary, 2020; Williams-Washington, 2010; Carter & Forsyth, 2010; Bryant-Davis, 1997, 2007; Lazarus & Folkman, 1984; Carter et al., 2017b; Eyerman, 2001, 2004, 2012, 2015; Smelser, 2004; Woods, 2019; Sotero, 2006; McMichael, 1999; Krieger, 2001.

29 Carter, 2007; Taylor, 1999; Kessler et al., 1997; Cohen, 2000; Pearlin, 1989; Kessler, 1997; Slavin et al., 1991; Harrell, 2000.

30 Carter, 2007; Taylor, 1999; Kessler et al., 1997; Cohen, 2000; Pearlin, 1989; Kessler, 1997; Slavin et al., 1991; Harrell, 2000.

31 Carter, 2007; Taylor, 1999; Kessler et al., 1997; Cohen, 2000; Pearlin, 1989; Kessler, 1997; Slavin et al., 1991; Harrell, 2000.

32 Carter, 2007; Taylor, 1999; Kessler et al., 1997; Cohen, 2000; Pearlin, 1989; Kessler, 1997; Slavin et al., 1991; Harrell, 2000.

33 Carter, 2007; Taylor, 1999; Kessler et al., 1997; Cohen, 2000; Pearlin, 1989; Kessler, 1997; Slavin et al., 1991; Harrell, 2000.

34 Carter, 2007; Taylor, 1999; Kessler et al., 1997; Cohen, 2000; Pearlin, 1989; Kessler, 1997; Slavin et al., 1991; Harrell, 2000.

35 Carter, 2007; Taylor, 1999; Kessler et al., 1997; Cohen, 2000; Pearlin, 1989; Kessler, 1997; Slavin et al., 1991; Harrell, 2000.

36 Carter, 2007; Norris, 1992; Carlson, 1997; Lazarus & Folkman, 1984; Carter et al., 2017b.

37 Carter, 2007; Norris, 1992; Carlson, 1997; Lazarus & Folkman, 1984; Carter et al., 2017b.
38 Carter, 2007; Norris, 1992; Carlson, 1997; Lazarus & Folkman, 1984; Carter et al., 2017b.
39 Carter, 2007; Carter et al., 2005; Feagin & McKinney, 2003.
40 Carter, 2007; Carter et al., 2005; Feagin & McKinney, 2003.
41 Carter, 2007; Carter et al., 2005; Feagin & McKinney, 2003.
42 Carter, 2007; Essed, 1991; Carter & Helms, 2002.
43 Carter, 2007; Essed, 1991; Carter & Helms, 2002.
44 Carter, 2007; Carter et al., 2005.
45 Carter, 2007; Carter et al., 2005.
46 Carter, 2007; Herman, 1992; Carlson, 1997; Sotero, 2006; Eyerman, 2001, 2004; Kellerman, 2001; Williams et al., 2003.
47 Carter, 2007; Herman, 1992; Carlson, 1997; Sotero, 2006; Eyerman, 2001, 2004; Kellerman, 2001; Williams et al., 2003.
48 Carter, 2007; Herman, 1992; Carlson, 1997; Sotero, 2006; Eyerman, 2001, 2004; Kellerman, 2001; Williams et al., 2003.
49 Carter, 2007; Herman, 1992; Carlson, 1997; Sotero, 2006; Eyerman, 2001, 2004; Kellerman, 2001; Williams et al., 2003.
50 Smith Lee & Robinson, 2019; Lipscomb et al., 2019; Motley et al., 2020; Carter, 2007; Carter & Pieterse, 2020; Pieterse & Carter, 2007; Helms et al., 2012; Carter et al., 2013; Carter & Sant-Barket, 2015; Utsey, 1999; Gregory & Tucker Edmonds, 2023.
51 Smith Lee & Robinson, 2019; Lipscomb et al., 2019; Motley et al., 2020; Carter, 2007; Carter & Pieterse, 2020; Pieterse & Carter, 2007; Helms et al., 2012; Carter et al, 2013; Carter & Sant-Barket, 2015; Utsey, 1999; Gregory & Tucker Edmonds, 2023.

CHAPTER 4

THE CARCERAL STATE AND BLACK MEN

The carceral state includes formal institutions of the criminal justice system and encompasses ideologies, logics, and social processes (e.g., political and economic) that substantiates dominance and death. Carceral state violence often results in trauma among Black men. The carceral state has contributed to the trauma of Black men through neo-slavery which includes the history of policing in the U.S., construction of Black criminality, police brutality, war on crime, frontlash, criminalization of racial poverty, state terrorism, the prison-industrial complex, death penalty, news and media, and racial surveillance. Therefore, it is imperative that these carceral state mechanisms are explicitly interrogated to articulate their connection to the trauma of Black men.

NEO-SLAVERY[1]

The 13th Amendment states, "Neither slavery nor involuntary servitude, except as a punishment for crime whereof the party shall have been duly convicted, shall exist within the United States, or any place subject to their jurisdiction."

Neo-slavery is a continuation of the enslavement of Black Americans and racial caste under the illusion that slavery has been abolished. Slavery recreates itself continuously under U.S. law. Slavery is not abolished but codified by the 13th Amendment of the U.S. Constitution, where involuntary servitude is permissible against those convicted of crimes thus reconfiguring and continuing slave law. In addition, the 13th Amendment transitions Black Americans from private property to public property. Neo-slavery and racial caste replace the former configuration of slavery as a means of maintaining the structure of slavery where the behavior of Black Americans is heavily regulated. The paradigmatic power relations of white supremacy and anti-Black racism that undergirded chattel slavery continued evolving into other institutionalized structurings that inform contemporary criminalization and carceral apparatuses. What we see is an extension of the same core mechanisms of slavery being instituted again and again that includes domination, exploitation, subjugation, subordination, surveillance, and ultimately death.

The Black codes of 1865–1866 were the first line of defense against Black citizenship while lynching was the second. Black codes included vagrancy laws and convict leasing along with peonage were instituted after slavery was abolished to continue the enslavement of Black Americans. This public-private system of the convict prison lease system negated the freedoms that came with Reconstruction after the Civil War and enforced a new reign of terror over all Black Americans in the South. This vicious and virulent form of slavery resulted in Black Americans being starved and worked to death. States leased out imprisoned Black Americans to individuals and corporations as a labor force. The state-corporate enterprise of the convict prison lease system contributed to the deaths of more Black Americans as public property than when they were private property of individual planters. These practices persisted until World War II. Slavery was outlawed by the U.S. by restricting it to incarcerated criminals that were managed by the state or corporate America followed by legislation (Black codes and Jim/Jane Crow laws). Neo-slavery continued shapeshifting

DOI: 10.4324/9781003430551-5

into various forms and manifestations. This included Jim/Jane Crow, lynching, the Great Migration, the crack epidemic, the war on drugs, and hypercriminalization/incarceration. Therefore, enslavement functions as a 400+ year multigenerational American institution. The revamping, complicating, and enhancing institutions of dominance, hierarchy, and violence broadly reflect the long historical formation of neo-slavery in the U.S. Neo-slavery continues to be a cause of collective trauma for Black communities.[2]

Today, Black Americans are more likely to be stopped by police, detained pretrial, charged with more serious crimes, and sentenced more harshly than white people. Black Americans experience harsher outcomes from police encounters, bail setting, sentence length, and capital punishment in comparison to white people. The deeply punitive and racially unequal nature of the U.S. criminal legal system through the history of the courts, prisons, and police institutions maintains racial hierarchy and caste. The U.S. continues to operate as a slavocracy and is the world leader in incarceration as the prison population is the largest it has ever been since the first penitentiaries were created in the world. The U.S. imprisonment rate in 1925 was close to today's Western European average of approximately 100 per 100,000. Whites represent 70 percent of those arrested for the majority of crimes, but Black Americans are most likely to be overrepresented in arrests (28 percent in relation to their U.S. population percentage). Whites compose the greatest percentage of criminals and convicts, and most crime is committed by whites, but the perception is that most crime is perpetrated by Black men. In the 1930s, Black Americans were three times more likely to be incarcerated than whites, and this ratio increased to more than seven times that of whites in the 1990s. The U.S. law enforcement system includes systematic positive assessments of whiteness (white supremacy) with the simultaneous devaluation of Blackness. The FBI's Uniform Crime Report (UCR) is routinely cited for U.S. crime statistics but is limited to arrests and does not include convictions. In addition, the UCR emphasizes street crime to the exclusion of organized and white-collar crime.[3]

The criminality of Black Americans is routinely dramatized, while white crime statistics are virtually invisible. The idea of Black criminality provides ideological currency where discussions of crime are implicit discussions of Black maleness and race. Blackness and crime are inextricably linked. Racial criminalization in the U.S. involves the stigmatization of crime as *Black* while simultaneously presenting crime among whites as individual failure. Crime among Black Americans is thought of as group pathology, which reinforces and reproduces racial inequality. In addition, the stigma of criminalization is used as a justification for the disposability of Black males. Black criminality is the most significant signifier of Black inferiority in white America that has been ever-present since the dawn of Jim/Jane Crow. For the first time, prison statistics became the basis of national discourse about Black Americans as a distinct and dangerous criminal population with the publication of the 1890 census. The census data indicated that Black Americans made up 12 percent of the population but 30 percent of the nation's prison population. Black criminality became one of the most widely accepted beliefs that justified racial prejudice, racial discriminatory treatment, and the acceptance of white racial violence as necessary for public safety.[4]

As previously mentioned, 1.5 million Black men are missing due to early deaths and hyperincarceration. Black men account for approximately 7 percent of the U.S. population, while Black Americans make up 13 percent of the U.S. population but account for approximately 33 percent of those incarcerated in state and federal prisons. Comparatively, whites make up 60 percent of the population but only 30 percent of prisoners. Black men are impacted more adversely by the criminal justice system at every stage of the process than any other demographic in the U.S. Interestingly, imprisonment rates were stable until the early 1970s. In 1967, approximately 220,000 U.S. residents were incarcerated, and most of them were white. In 2009, 841,000 Black men were incarcerated in state or federal prisons or local jails, while 64,800 Black women were incarcerated in state or federal prisons or local jails. By the end of 2009, the number of Black men in prison or jail, on probation, or on parole roughly equaled the number of enslaved Black Americans in 1850. There has been more Black men incarcerated in the U.S than the total prison populations in Argentina, Canada, England, Finland, Germany, India, Israel, Japan, and Lebanon combined, including more Black men incarcerated in the U.S. than the total number of women incarcerated on the entire planet. The largest and fastest reduction (17 percent) in the overall prison population in American history took place during the first year of the COVID-19 pandemic. This was primarily due to the disproportionate reduction in the white prison population, while the Black and Latino prison population sharply increased. The increase was especially significant among Black people even in the midst of a supposed *racial reckoning*.[5]

Black men also account for 47 percent of those proven wrongfully accused or convicted. Approximately 1,696 Black men have been exonerated (1989–2022) since 1989 due to wrongful convictions of crimes they did not commit. The National Registry of Exonerations lists exonerees who since 1989 (excludes time spent incarcerated prior to conviction) spent time in prison for crimes they did not commit prior to exoneration; approximately 51 percent of the exonerees have been Black men. These men served an approximate combined total of 23,792 years incarcerated. Black Americans who are imprisoned and convicted for murder are 50 percent more likely to be innocent than other convicted murderers. Black Americans who are imprisoned for murder are more likely to be innocent if they were convicted of killing white victims. Only approximately 15 percent of murders by Black Americans are committed against white victims, but 31 percent of innocent Black murder exonerees were convicted of killing white people. A Black person convicted for sexual assault is three-and-a-half times more likely to be innocent than a white sexual assault convict. Assaults perpetrated by Black men against white women are a small minority (approximately 11 percent) of all sexual assaults in the U.S. but account for half of sexual assaults with eyewitness misidentification that led to exoneration. Approximately 70 percent of white sexual assault victims were attacked by white men. Innocent Black sexual assault defendants receive harsher sentences (an average of almost 4.5 years longer in prison before exoneration) than whites upon conviction and face greater resistance to exoneration even in cases that lead to their release. Gross et al. (2017) posit that most wrongful convictions are never discovered, and there is no direct measure of the number of convicted innocent murder defendants and estimates that the numbers significantly eclipse known figures.[6]

The targeting of Black males begins as early as adolescence, where Black boys are consistently harassed by police officers, are routinely stopped, interrogated, and arrested by the police at higher rates than white youth, including on the street, in school, and in stores. Black boys are consistently referred to the juvenile justice system more than any other group of children, and spending time in prison has become an inevitable part of the life cycle for Black boys from working-class communities.[7]

Forty-nine percent of Black men can expect to be arrested at least once by the age of 23 and 1 in 3 Black men born today can expect to be incarcerated during his lifetime compared to 1 in 6 Latino men, 1 in 17 white men, 1 in 18 Black women, 1 in 45 Latina women, and 1 in 111 white women. One in four Black children born in 1990 had an incarcerated parent at some point during their childhood. Black Americans are incarcerated at a rate of 5 times greater than that of white people. The U.S. has the highest incarceration rate in the world. [8]

Contemporary U.S. policing has origins in slave patrols that were established to capture runaway enslaved Black Americans and quell uprisings in colonial Virginia during the 18th century. After slavery was abolished, white dominance was reasserted particularly in the South through police and the advent of the prison-industrial complex. Law enforcement enabled, sanctioned, and participated in the lynchings of Black Americans by white mobs under the pretext of a supposed crime. Further, vagrancy laws, convict leasing, and share-cropping systems were enacted by Southern whites through police force and imprisonment in order to reestablish enslavement (neo-slavery). The "War on Crime" declared by President Lyndon Johnson in 1964 was followed by President Richard Nixon's "Law and Order" and "War on Drugs," which appealed to the fears of supposed Black male criminality. This author refers to this era as phase II of hypercriminalization/incarceration, whereas phase I refers to the Black codes and convict leasing along with Black criminalization by social scientists in the North. This created a sevenfold increase in the size of the incarcerated population with Black Americans incarcerated at five times the rate of white people. Once incarcerated, Black Americans are disproportionally targeted and subjected to solitary confinement (administrative segregation units), which is a more punitive type of confinement that is associated with elevated levels of anxiety, mood disorders, PTSD, and serious psychological distress. One in ten Black men are placed in solitary confinement before the age of 32. This form of deprivation routinely takes place by confinement to a small cell for 23 hours a day with no human contact and sometimes lasts for years and is defined as torture by the United Nations (UN). What is being referred to as the prison-to-solitary pipeline continues racial disparities and extreme state violence that is short of capital punishment. Those who are incarcerated are disproportionately at risk of death after release. Hypercriminalization/incarceration created economic gains for whites through the expansion of prisons in deindustrialized rural white areas by providing employment. In addition, police have been entangled in other forms of structural racism such as the enforcement of racial-residential segregation and racial restrictions in "sundown towns" that excluded Black Americans outside of working hours, which now has continued into the targeting of Black Americans who enter white neighborhoods. A history of structural racism and inequality of opportunity means that Black Americans are more likely to be living in conditions of concentrated poverty, which exposes them to risk factors for both offending and arrests (i.e., criminalization of racialized poverty). A criminal conviction has an adverse impact on both employability and access to housing and public services. Moreover, disproportionately incarcerating Black Americans from poor communities removes economic resources and exacerbates cycles of poverty and justice system involvement as well as normalizing/ritualizing criminal justice contact.[9]

THE HISTORY OF POLICING IN THE U.S. (SLAVE PATROLS)

Contemporary U.S. policing has origins in slave patrols that were established to capture runaway enslaved Black Americans and quell uprisings in colonial Virginia during the 18th century. After slavery was abolished, white dominance was reasserted particularly in the South through police and the advent of the prison-industrial complex. Law enforcement enabled, sanctioned, and participated in the lynchings of Black Americans by white mobs under the pretext of a supposed crime.[10]

Slave patrols formally began in the 1700s as modern-day law enforcement. They began in S. Carolina and spread across the slave states and colonies. Slave patrols were the enforcement arm of slave codes as they emerged during slavery and were bestowed with search powers that the colonists later found objectionable when it was directed towards them from British authorities. Slave codes were laws that regulated slave life, which included where and when Black Americans could gather, what activities they were prohibited from engaging in, and what types of punishment were meted out for violating the codes. All aspects of Black life were surveilled and regulated by patrollers who were routinely white enslavers. Any white person between the ages of 16 and 60 were legally allowed to serve as a slave patroller. Slave patrols would search slave cabins, keep enslaved Black Americans off the roadway, and prevent gatherings of enslaved Black Americans. Slave patrols were designed to preserve the institution of slavery by thwarting any activities that were a threat to the institution of slavery, particularly escapes or uprisings. Patrollers were also authorized to exact punishment and were roving enslavers. Slave patrols remained in force following the Civil War and changed form. Various groups joined what had previously been slave patrols that were now patrols designed to police the movements of newly freed Black Americans during the beginning of Reconstruction. The new, more violent patrols consisted of the state militia, the federal military, and the Ku Klux Klan (KKK). Not only were slave patrols the first uniquely American form of policing but were also the first publicly funded police agencies. American policing was designed to police Black people with a specific focus on Black men.[11]

European institutions served as the slave patrol's institutional forebears. This includes *posse comitatus* in modern England, where bands of men were called out to chase down and arrest fleeing felons in striking similarities to slave patrols, limiting the movements and behavior of enslaved Black Americans. A constable's bellowing *hue and cry* in the wake of elusive criminals would call upon all available men to assist in the capture of the thief or burglar provided a blueprint for chasing down enslaved Black Americans in the New World. Spanish and English settlers combined their knowledge of posses and militia groups and created a new law enforcement institution to supplement the authority of white enslavers, which became slave patrols. Race was the defining feature of this new colonial creation. Slave patrols also supervised the activities of free Black Americans and suspicious whites but mainly focused on enslaved Black Americans. The defining feature of race made Black Americans easy and immediate targets of racial brutality. These racially focused law enforcement groups were considered a new American innovation in law enforcement.[12]

Police work in the South emerged from an early fascination with what enslaved Black Americans were doing by white patrollers. White patrolmen watched (surveilled), caught, and beat enslaved Black Americans. White women who owned enslaved Black Americans were required to provide a substitute for patrol service. Enslaved Africans began running away almost as soon as they landed in S. Carolina. Therefore, colonists used Native Americans to recapture the African runaways. Native Americans would go into swamps and other desolate regions where whites were hesitant to travel. In 1696, S. Carolina's assembly passed a new slave code that took a more comprehensive approach to slave regulation and was a more coercive system of private enforcement. This included the pass system, where enslaved Black Americans were mandated to carry a ticket when away from their white enslaver's plantation as well as the provisions for returning a slave to their owner or to the local jail. Slave patrols were officially created in S. Carolina in 1704 due to fear of a Spanish invasion coupled with rumors of a slave insurrection. The colony created two military forces, which included a militia to repel foreign enemies and a patrol to deter slave revolts. This separate military group would ride from plantation to plantation and round up enslaved Black

Americans who had no ticket from their white enslaver. Slave patrols would include men of high social status, including the wealthy as well as poor slaveless whites and primarily consisted of businessmen and farmers.[13]

Slave patrols and slave catchers shared common interests in capturing runaway slaves, but there were marked differences. Slave patrols functioned as officials of the county or state, whereas slave catchers advertised their ability to capture runaway slaves and were hired by white enslavers for short-term jobs. Whole communities appointed and sometimes compensated patrollers, while individuals hired slave hunters for a specific job (recapturing the enslaved). The tasks of patrollers included searching slave cabins for weapons and dispersing slave meetings, while slave catchers were primarily concerned with capturing fugitive slaves.[14]

Slave patrols along with slave catchers and ordinary citizens who apprehended fugitive slaves to obtain colony or state-mandated rewards all shared common characteristics. Slave patrols eventually gave way to paid police forces in cities such as Richmond, Raleigh, and Charleston, whose primary task was controlling enslaved Black Americans until the Civil War. Slave patrols searched slave quarters, rummaging through an enslaved Black person's dwellings and looking for weapons of revolt such as guns, scythes, and knives as well as writing paper, books, and other indicators of education. In addition, slave quarter inhabitants were scrutinized in search of extra occupants who did not belong on the plantation as well as those who were missing. Slave patrols had the additional responsibility of dispersing any gatherings of enslaved individuals, including religious meetings independently organized by enslaved Black Americans. These patrols were in areas around plantations and within towns, monitoring roads either by riding or walking to maintain control. Enslaved Black Americans who were away from their plantations without permission were questioned and detained by the patrols, and those who were resistant were punished.[15]

Enslaved Black Americans were legally required to carry a pass or a ticket from their white enslaver which permitted them to leave the plantation. The pass stated the enslaved Black person's name, where they had permission to go, on what date, how long the pass was valid (e.g., "to North Hampton Plantation until Sunday night"), and the owner's signature. Slave patrols would begin their inquiry and examine the pass upon an encounter with enslaved Black Americans. Enslaved Black Americans without a valid pass would be beaten by slave patrols, and Black men would receive more severe beatings. Slave patrols in rural areas regularly traveled on horseback, while slave patrols in urban areas regularly worked on foot. Slave patrols relied on instruments of intimidation such as guns, whips, and binding ropes. Enslaved Black Americans who were caught away from their plantations without passes would be beat with whips. Slave patrols employed systematic surveillance methods directed at Black Americans, such as stakeouts that would eventually be adopted by policemen as a part of routine law enforcement. After the Civil War, the new legal iteration of slave patrols were Southern police officers who continued the legacy of urban slave patrolling that was presented as race-neutral but was in reality selectively applied to Black Americans with a specific focus on Black men. This was initially achieved through nightly curfews and vagrancy laws that regulated the movement of Black Americans just as slave patrols had done during the colonial and antebellum eras. Moreover, vigilante groups such as the KKK took on the more random and ruthless aspects of slave patrolling. Very little difference existed between the brutality of slave patrols, white Southern policemen, and the Klan. The work of controlling Black Americans shifted from slave patrols to the Klan and police, and the white community's need for racial dominance continued.[16]

POLICE BRUTALITY

U.S. police kill significantly more civilians than police in other wealthy countries. The legacies of slavery, lynching, and police brutality has continually organized Black life in America, where 21st century policing operates as an instrument of racial terror and social control. The application of excessive force by police is systematically applied to Black males more frequently and severely than white people. The civil liberties of Black males are routinely violated, and they are placed at disproportionate risk for suffering violent injuries or death during police encounters.[17]

The deaths of Trayvon Martin, Michael Brown, Eric Garner, John Crawford, Tamir Rice, Walter Scott, Freddie Gray, Alton Sterling, Philando Castile, Terrence Crutcher, Ahmaud Arbery, George Floyd, and Tyre Nichols have highlighted the disposability of Black men in the U.S. Police killings of civilians are not tracked by any governmental institutions. It was not until 2015 that the two leading newspapers the *Washington* Post and the *Guardian* began to record this data. Police executions of Black men saw a massive spike beginning in the late 1960s.[18]

Black men experience the highest levels of inequality in mortality risk. Over the life course, Black men are 2.5 times more likely to be killed by police than white men, and Black women are 1.4 times more likely to be killed by police than white women. One in 1,000 Black men and boys will be killed by police over the life course. A *New York Times* investigation of car stops over a five-year period that left more than 400 unarmed people dead revealed that police officers often characterized those that they killed as utilizing their vehicle as a weapon. Some officers actually put themselves in danger, while others appeared to not be in danger at all. Black male motorists were overrepresented among those killed.[19]

Research examining police use of nonfatal force found that Black Americans were more likely to experience nonfatal force at the hands of police officers than either Latino/as or whites. Moreover, very little public information is available regarding the prevalence of nonlethal police violence that results in injury or disability. Police and legal systems target, intervene, and utilize the application of force based on race, sex, and age. Research discovered that police in the U.S. killed an estimated 30,800 people between 1980 and 2018. This indicates 17,000 more deaths than reported by the National Vital Statistics System (NVSS), which is a misclassification rate of 55 percent. The deaths of Black Americans were the most likely to be undercounted with 5,670 deaths missing out of an estimated 9,540. Medical examiners in 47 documented cases falsely claimed that sickle cell trait (SCT) was the cause of death of Black men killed by police. The intended purpose of police and prisons is social control of Black men through violence.[20]

WAR ON CRIME

In 1964, President Lyndon Johnson declared a "War on Crime," which was later followed by President Richard Nixon's "Law and Order" and "War on Drugs" that appealed to the fears of supposed Black male criminality. This represented the modern era of hypercriminalization/incarceration (phase II) that was more sophisticated in scope compared to the Black codes and convict leasing along with Black criminalization by social scientists in the North (phase I). Thus facilitating a sevenfold increase in the size of the incarcerated population with Black Americans incarcerated at five times the rate of white people.[21]

During the five summers of Lyndon B. Johnson's presidency, the nation witnessed 250 incidents of urban civil disorder. Policymakers, journalists, and the public termed this violence *riots*, which moved through American cities and resulted in the deaths of more than 200 Black Americans, 13,000 injured civilians and officers, and billions of dollars' worth of property destruction. It began with the killing of an unarmed 15-year-old Black boy by New York City police that sparked the Harlem riot/uprising in July 1964. The uprisings would constitute a prolonged and sporadic conflict that involved more than 100,000 Black participants and law enforcement officials. These uprisings were sparked by the presence of exploitative and exclusionary institutions in Black neighborhoods unlike earlier race riots that were sparked by white hostility towards integration. By the end of the 1960s, the uprisings constituted the greatest period of domestic bloodshed in the U.S. since the Civil War.[22]

The beginning of hypercriminalization/incarceration is often attributed to Barry Goldwater's 1964 presidential election campaign theme of crime and disorder, but the uprisings radically altered the direction of President Johnson's Great Society programs, where he merged anti-poverty programs with anti-crime programs that ultimately laid the groundwork for contemporary hyperincarceration. The linkages between the fighting of crime and the fighting of urban inequality as a result of the urban discord were established in the three pieces of legislation that were the Johnson administration's response to the civil rights movement in early 1965. In March of 1965, the administration presented to Congress the Housing and Urban Development Act that provided the subsidizing of private homes for low-income renters; the Voting Rights Act, which provided Black Americans in the South the opportunity to participate in the electoral process as full citizens; and the Law Enforcement Assistance Act, which established federal influence over local police operations, thus breaking from 200 years of national policy. As Johnson reflected on these three programs, he stated that his hope was that 1965 would not be remembered as the apex of American liberal reform but "as the year when this country began a thorough, intelligent, and effective war against crime." Johnson's "War on Crime" blended opportunity, development, and training programs with surveillance, patrol, and detention programs. These Great Society policies were entanglement programs that allowed law enforcement officials to use methods of surveillance that overlapped with social programs (e.g., anti-delinquency measures framed as equal opportunity initiatives that would supposedly effectively imbue crime-control strategies into the everyday lives of Americans in segregated and impoverished communities). The boundaries of the carceral state expanded beyond penal institutions as a result of domestic social programs that actively participated in national law enforcement. The carceral state had metastasized into a vast network of social programs originally created to combat racial exclusion and inequality by the time Johnson's Omnibus Crime Control and Safe Streets Act passed in 1968. These social programs shifted in purpose toward controlling the violent symptoms (rioting/uprisings) of socioeconomic problems.[23]

Poverty as the root cause of crime was understood by Johnson and many other liberals, but Daniel Moynihan's hugely influential 1965 report *The Negro Family* influenced their view that community behavior and not structural exclusion was the cause of that poverty. The Law Enforcement Act of 1965 won unanimous support in Congress and was different than the previous two centuries of crime-control legislation, where this act created direct funding channels between federal government and the criminal justice system and emphasized training and experimental programs for urban police forces serving low-income communities. Urban police officers were viewed as the "frontline soldier" of the national law enforcement program, and Johnson believed that "we are today fighting a war within our own boundaries." Thus, the Office of Law Enforcement Assistance (OLEA) invested the vast majority of the federal crime-control funds in local police departments, private firms, and social science researchers working to improve urban surveillance and patrol strategies under the direction of Attorney General Nicholas Katzenbach. The single largest group of residents arrested during the national uprisings were Black men between the ages of 15 and 24. Black men came to be viewed as prone to rioting/uprising and, by extension, prone to criminality. Johnson evoked race-neutral terms and the Black criminal/rapist in referencing Black men in Washington, DC, by stating "we're not going to tolerate hoodlums who kill and rape and mug in this city." The OLEA collaborated with local law enforcement to develop new technologies to group preemptive law enforcement methods in statistics, which included building criminal profiles of residents as well as computerized crime prediction programs that anticipated crime with targeted street patrols in urban areas (counterinsurgency). Further, the police were supported by the Johnson administration in building their weapon arsenals in preparation for the ever-looming threat of unrest. Urban police departments were supplied by Katzenbach and his staff with military-grade equipment, which included bulletproof vests, machine guns, M-1 military carbines, walkie-talkies, helicopters, and army tanks and armored vehicles as riot-prevention measures. Social welfare and social control imperatives imposed a soft form of surveillance in vulnerable and isolated communities as many politicians and local authorities worried that Black youth would revolt at any moment. The federal government increased its investment in fighting crime while it pulled back from social welfare programs, which were eventually shuttered during the second half of the 1960s. The War on Poverty that encompassed health, housing, education, and training programs gave way to improving police-community relations during the War on Crime. Moreover, police patrols were assigned to public schools as well as law enforcement officials providing additional supervision in after-school programs as well as during summer months. This liberal reform toward surveillance further inflamed violent civil disorder by the increase in police presence on the streets, in the sky, and within schools and housing projects. During the first two years of the War on Crime, Black residents and activists became more confrontational as a result of the militarization of the police force as well as officers assuming the role of social service providers. Black urban life had long been shaped by police brutality and law enforcement practices. The formation of the Black Panther Party (BPP/1966) as well as other organizations called for community control and armed self-defense in response to law enforcement programs that arose from the Great Society.[24]

During the War on Crime era, urban civil disorder only escalated which culminated in unprecedented destruction and Black civilian casualties in Newark and Detroit during the summer of 1967 and the riots/uprisings in 125 cities following the assassination of Martin Luther King Jr. in April 1968. The expansion of the carceral state was accelerated by state and local authorities who were financially incentivized to increase surveillance and patrols in already-targeted Black urban neighborhoods through the Omnibus Crime Control and Safe Streets Act (1968), which was the capstone of the Great Society. The Omnibus Crime Control and Safe Streets Act shifted the focus from punishing offenders and preventing crime to management and control within isolated and marginalized communities. Moreover, the OLEA was expanded into the Law Enforcement Assistance Administration (LEAA) in which Congress introduced the block-grant system that granted crime-control funds to states with the effect of restoring state autonomy that had been weakened by the dismantling of Jim/Jane Crow. A climate of surveillance and intimidation that often culminated in street warfare between police and residents was generated as a result of tactical forces occupying urban communities. The War on Poverty programs were ultimately dissolved and replaced with the state apparatus of punishment that included law enforcement, criminal justice, and prison systems, which remains a cornerstone of American economic and social policy. The Johnson administration initiated the liberal welfare state's undoing by linking anti-poverty and anti-crime interventions that ultimately expanded and strengthened the carceral state. The scale of resources allocated to federal crime-control measures exploded from $22 million in 1965 to approximately $7 billion before the presidency of Ronald Reagan and by the dawn of hyperincarceration in the 1980s. Ordinary life for a generation of Black males came to involve contact with police, a stay in a juvenile detention center, and a long-term stay in prison. Supervision in segregated urban public schools, housing projects, and within families on welfare became the norm. Black communities and Black male youth were brought into everyday contact with police through these targeted patrol and surveillance programs. Federal grant funds were connected to arrest records which promoted the apprehension of alarming numbers of low-income urban Black Americans and entrapped them into criminal justice supervision where they faced detainment and draconian sentencing guidelines that increased their chances of long prison sentences and becoming hardened criminals.[25]

FRONTLASH

The civil rights movement brought about the passage of the Civil Rights Act of 1964 that included fair housing legislation, federal enforcement of school integration, and the Voting Rights Act of 1965 that outlawed discriminatory voting mechanisms. Moreover, it was during this time that the death penalty was reinstated, felon disenfranchisement statutes from the Reconstruction era were revived, and the chain gang returned. Criminal codes were revised by state and federal governments that effectively abolished parole, imposed mandatory minimum sentences, and allowed juveniles to be incarcerated in adult prisons.[26]

The opponents of civil rights galvanized a powerful elite countermovement in response to the stinging defeats of civil rights. This defeated group who fought vociferously against civil rights shifted their focus and campaign to crime and riots/uprisings. This process is what Weaver (2007) identifies as *frontlash* where formerly defeated groups become dominant and strategic issue entrepreneurs in light of the development of a new issue campaign in order to defeat long-standing political discourse. *Frontlash* is supported by the research of Gilens and Page (2014), who found that economic elites and organized groups who represent business interests wield significant power over U.S. government policy while average citizens and large interest-based groups have very little or no independent government policy influence. This author would argue that the American public sanctions economic elites and business interest groups to act in the interests of the white group (white supremacy ideology) through anti-Blackness. Therefore, the relationship between economic elites and business interest groups is symbiotic and provides symbolic and material rewards for the American public. Crime was fused with the anxiety of ghetto revolts and racial disorder. This was initially defined as a problem of racial disenfranchisement but was redefined as a crime problem and was instrumental in shifting the debate from social reform to punishment particularly between the years of 1965 to 1972. Civil rights and crime were conflated by strategic policymakers who defined racial disorders as criminal, which necessitated crime control and the depoliticization of civil rights grievances. A durable connection between Black activism and crime was created by conservatives who pitted toughness on crime against vigorous advocacy for civil rights. The social uplift approach by liberals collapsed under the weight of this powerful doctrine. Liberals began to move closer to the conservative position in order to not appear as soft on crime and excusing riot-related violence, thus emulating and endorsing conservative doctrine. Conservatives connected civil rights to lawlessness and argued that civil disobedience ignored laws and would ultimately lead to more lawless behavior. Their strategy encompassed depoliticization and criminalization of racial struggle and the racialization of crime. The view they championed was that civil rights demonstrations amounted to violence and created a climate of lawlessness. Therefore, racial struggle whether peaceful or violent was inherently criminal. Conservative strategists set out to discredit the idea that violent racial struggle was an outcome of social conditions and were preoccupied with demonstrating that racial discord was not motivated by police brutality or racial discrimination but simply criminality. One example were looters who were depicted as criminals who pursued their loot simply for self-gain even though looting was a form of protest that usually targeted discriminatory businesses. In 1967, President Johnson established the National Commission on Civil Disorders (Kerner Commission) in response to the riots/uprisings that took place during the long hot summer of 1967. The Kerner Commission found that most racial disorders were instigated by confrontations between the local community and police due to police brutality and excessive force. The common denominator government researchers found among those most likely to riot was that they had either experienced or witnessed an act of police brutality (i.e., direct and vicarious racial trauma). Further, the commission found that the lack of economic opportunity, failed social service programs, racism, and the white-oriented media contributed to the riots/uprisings as well. The Kerner Commission's final report was issued March 1, 1968, in which the report concluded that the U.S. was moving towards two societies, one Black and one white that were separate and unequal. The report identified urban issues being caused by "white racism" and that "white institutions" created the ghetto and maintain it while white society condones it. The report recommended billions of dollars in federal spending to restructure cities. Conservatives were not pleased with the report as it did not validate their explanations that the riots/uprisings were caused by a handful of radicals and that a law and order approach would further incite tension. The social scientists concluded that most Black people were not pleased with their conditions and existence, and those most active in the riots/uprisings were not misfits but were people who voted, read newspapers, and were aware of world events. The report was the first federal report to ever blame white society for the conditions of poor Black neighborhoods. The social scientists who were part of the commission refused to call the disturbances *riots* as the word denoted an irrational outburst rather than a deliberate rational response to the horrid conditions in poor Black neighborhoods and the failure of local government to respond to their needs. The social scientists preferred the word *rebellion* as they believed the responses were rational and justified due to the horrible conditions that Black people were subjected to and lived in daily. The social scientists highlighted how the police either incited violence or overreacted when it occurred. The report indicated that approximately 75 percent of police departments in the country demonstrated "evidence of strong racist attitudes." They identified that in some cities police engaged in daily harassment of ghetto residents with stop-and-frisk tactics and verbal abuse. These "disruptive police activities" played a significant role in initiating violence or escalating it. Moreover, professionalism dissipated, and officers became "avengers of their personal or department pride" once a disturbance erupted. The social scientists indicated that the disturbances were justified and that the police were routinely the responsible instigators of the unrests. The conventional idea being promoted among some of the commissioners was that poverty created the conditions that led to violence, but the social scientists found no direct relationship between poverty and rioting. Poor Black Americans were no more likely to participate in disturbances than middle-class Black Americans. As previously mentioned, the common denominator government researchers found among those most likely to riot was that they had either experienced or witnessed an act of police brutality, which indicates they had either been directly traumatized by police violence and brutality or experienced vicarious trauma from witnessing it. The report originally titled *The Harvest of American Racism* was destroyed, and all but one of the social scientists were dismissed. The final document submitted by the commission blamed the disturbances on white racism and the resulting economic disadvantage. President Johnson refused to accept the watered-down final Kerner Commission report. But many legislators and public commentators continued to construe racial disorders as being committed by professional agitators, Communist Party affiliates, and self-serving looters, hoodlums, and criminals. Crime became the justification for not expanding civil rights and social justice with the nearly 100 pieces of legislation implemented from 1965 to 1969 that made participating in a riot/uprising a federal offense with harsh penalties.[27]

President Richard Nixon was able to inherit a vibrant law enforcement infrastructure created by the Johnson administration and is often credited as spearheading the War on Crime. Richard Nixon's campaign theme was the law and order rhetoric, which was influenced by Ronald Reagan's deployment of the law and order theme in the California gubernatorial election of 1966. Twenty pieces of anti-crime legislation, including pretrial detention, were submitted by the Nixon administration as well as a memo that declared the right of the DOJ to utilize electronic surveillance on any subversive group without permission from the courts. Fear was a prominent feature of President Richard Nixon's speeches, and he blamed crime on the permissiveness of society, parents, and the courts. Johnson increased the federal government's role in crime in scale from zero to a hundred while Nixon moved crime from one side of the spectrum to the other in approach. The Office of Drug Abuse Law Enforcement (ODALE) was formed by Nixon, which created the crime strike forces that greatly increased policing and surveillance in Black communities. In addition, John Ehrlichman, who was counsel and assistant to President Nixon for Domestic Affairs stated that Black people were viewed as an enemy by Nixon and that you could not make it illegal to be Black but that an association between Black Americans and heroine was intentionally fabricated, which allowed them to criminalize Black Americans (Blackness) and disrupt Black communities. Further, Ehrlichman stated that this provided them with the license to arrest Black leaders, raid their homes, break up their meetings, and routinely vilify them on the evening news. Law enforcement continued to expand while poverty programs were reduced or eliminated, and there were almost no new civil rights legislation. The social construction of crime and race (civil rights) was an elite initiative with the public perception of high levels of crime concern that registered changes after elite discourse.[28]

CRIME VARIABLES

The term *criminal predator* is routinely used as a euphemism for *young Black male*. The images of crime are heavily trafficked than the actual dynamics of crime. This includes the image of the young Black male as a violent and menacing street thug. The mythology of Black men has evolved from a petty thief or rapist to an ominous criminal predator. Whites are more likely to characterize Black Americans as violent, more likely to abuse drugs, and more likely to engage in crime than whites and any other racial or ethnic group. Research has demonstrated that more than 50 percent of whites believe Black Americans are prone to violence along with the majority of whites characterizing Black Americans as aggressive. Further, a National Race Survey (1991) found that the majority of whites and Black Americans believed that Black Americans were more aggressive and violent. The public generally associates violent street crime with Black Americans. The public perceives violent crime involvement among Black Americans in greater percentages than what is actually indicated in official statistics.[29]

Serial predatory violence among Black men is actually a rare phenomenon in the U.S. White Americans overestimate the actual share of burglaries, illegal drug sales, and juvenile crime committed by Black Americans by 20–30 percent. The percentage of young Black men in white and Black American neighborhoods is one of the main predictors of the perceived severity of neighborhood crime. Blumstein's (1982) research of the prison population found that 80 percent of prison disparities could be explained by racial differences in arrests. Further, Blumstein (1993) found that the incarceration of drug offenders was significantly less correlated with crime involvement (i.e., estimates of drug use and drug selling). Between 1980 and 1996, it is estimated that only 12 percent (almost all is represented by arrests for drug crimes) of the increase in incarceration is attributed to an increase in crime. Eighty-eight percent of the increasing incarceration rates are a result of changes in crime control policies, which includes a 51 percent increase in the probability of incarceration following arrest and a 37 percent increase in the average length of sentences. Black Americans arrested for violent crime in the U.S. constitute only 1 percent of the Black population and approximately 2 percent of Black males. But the approximate 2 percent of Black males who are arrested for violent crime are used as justification for dominance and discrimination against the Black population and the death of Black males at large where Black maleness equates to criminality.[30]

The incarceration of Black men impacts Black women and families where women are left to raise children alone, thus increasing households headed by women and single parents or individual family members. Wilson (1987) found that the scarcity of employed Black males relative to Black females was directly related to the prevalence of families headed by women in Black communities. Black families headed by women increased over 50 percent between 1970 and 1984. This is identified as family disruption and is substantially related to rates of Black murder and robbery particularly by juveniles. Family disruption is associated with joblessness and poverty. White families headed by females is also related to white juvenile and adult violence. Predictors of white robbery are largely identical in sign and magnitude to those for Black Americans. In addition, research has demonstrated that white men who live in an environment characterized by poverty, unemployment, and single-parent households are more likely to commit homicide and other violent crimes than Black men who face a similar set of structural barriers. Therefore, the effect of Black family disruption on Black crime is independent of cultural factors within the Black community provided the similar and differential effect of white family disruption on white crime. Thus, there is nothing inherent in Black culture that is conducive to crime. The structural linkages between employment, economic deprivation, and family disruption in Black communities significantly contribute to crime. Higher levels of violent crime occur in poor urban neighborhoods regardless of race. Krivo and Peterson (1996) concluded that extremely disadvantaged neighborhoods had considerable rates of violence regardless of race and that structural disadvantage equally influences violent crime in both Black and white neighborhoods. Approximately 70 percent of poor whites lived in non-poverty areas in 1980 compared to only 16 percent of poor Black Americans. Approximately 7 percent of poor whites lived in extreme poverty or ghetto areas compared to 38 percent of Black Americans. The majority of poor Black Americans live in communities characterized by high rates of family disruption, while poor whites live in areas of relative family stability even those from "broken homes." Sampson (2013) found that penal confinement was an additional associated factor in enduring neighborhood poverty. In addition, Eitle (2009) examined the phenomenon of hypersegregation (see Chapter 5: "Starving the Black Beast" for details) and Black homicide rates across 201 metropolitan areas. He found that two indicators of severe segregation (exposure and centralization dimensions) and two measures of hypersegregation (i.e., the number of dimensions of severe segregation that exist in a metro area) were associated with Black homicides. Concentration and centralization were found to be a significant predictor of Black homicide rates. Therefore, racial segregation appeared to mediate the association between racial economic inequality and the Black homicide rate. Racial differences in poverty and family disruption are extremely significant, where the worst urban living conditions of whites are considerably better than the average living conditions of Black communities. Structural racism has created and contributed to Black poverty and family disruption in the inner-city. This includes racial-residential segregation (hypersegregation), Black male joblessness, Black middle-class migration out of the inner-city, and housing discrimination.[31]

POLICE

Black Americans report more negative experiences in police interactions than other groups. Voigt et al. (2017) found that police officers speak less respectfully to Black Americans than white community members in everyday traffic stops regardless of the race of the officer, infraction severity, stop location, and stop outcome. Moreover, Camp et al. (2021) found that during traffic stops, police officers' tone of voice conveyed less warmth, respect, and ease when they spoke to Black men compared to white men. These results were independent of the race or sex of the officers. Research from Cobbina et al. (2019) revealed that when Black men challenged (i.e., verbal resistance through questioning the police and challenging their authority out of suspicion of being targeted) the police, it proved to be harmful and resulted in the threat of or actual use of force where Black males were more likely to be handcuffed/arrested, experience police violence (i.e., assaulted), or jailed. When Black women challenged the police, they were often let go without adverse outcome or at the very worse received a traffic ticket. In addition, they found Black males to be more compliant than Black females who were more likely to question the police.[32]

As the data in Chapter 2 underscores, the majority of Black people killed by police are Black males. On computer-based shooting simulations that involved police officers and undergraduate students, Correll et al. (2002, 2007, 2011) found participants typically shot Black male targets who were armed or unarmed more frequently and quickly than white targets. Moreover, participants shot an armed target who responded correctly more quickly when he was Black. For decisions to shoot criminal suspects on a computerized simulation, Plant et al. (2011) found that white participants demonstrated a pronounced bias toward shooting Black men but a bias away from shooting Black women as well as white men and women. They mistakenly shot unarmed Black male suspects more often than unarmed Black female and unarmed white male and white female suspects. Further, participants were more likely to mistakenly not shoot Black female and white suspects of either sex than Black male suspects who were armed. This provided evidence of a behavioral threat-related response specific to Black men and the associated stereotype of aggression.

Violence and aggression are more strongly applied to Black men than women in the U.S. by white people. This includes the perception emanating from white bias that Black men are a threat (e.g., tendency to project anger in Black men's faces) but not Black women. The interaction of race and sex in the U.S. informs the perception of white people that Black men are more threatening (i.e., violent and aggressive) than white men and both Black and white women. McConnaughy and White (2011) found in their study that 40 percent of white respondents ranked "many or almost all" Black men as "violent," while white men and Black women were approximately half as likely to be described in this manner, and white women were very unlikely to be labeled as violent.[33]

Americans associating young Black men with danger is attributed to racial bias in decisions to shoot. Police use of force including firearms is more frequently applied to young Black men. Official U.S. data on the number of persons killed by police is unreliable due to the long-standing and well-documented resistance of police departments to making these data public and underreporting. Police officers focus disproportionately on Black men in all aspects of drug-law enforcement along with the practice of deliberately charging innocent defendants/victims with fabricated crimes. The police domestically and armed forces internationally protect the way of life of those in power. The law functions to maintain the relative privilege and power of white people, thereby preserving racial hierarchy and reproducing social order. The use of terror is one of the primary means by which racial hierarchy is maintained where state terror is disproportionately directed against Black men with the intent of forcing them into submission while simultaneously reinforcing their inferior position. This legally sanctioned terror is perpetrated by the state's law enforcement and the justice system through public displays of violence and the threat of violence. Terror is primarily exercised through discrimination within the criminal justice system.[34]

The prison-industrial complex is a deliberate and calculated product of the white power structure in the U.S. It reifies the domination and the power disparity between Black Americans and symbolizes a colonial relationship. Incarceration of Black Americans sustains white terror, power, and domination. Black Americans constituted over 50 percent of the prison population in 2005 despite comprising only 13 percent of the U.S. population. In 2014, Black Americans constituted 34 percent (2.3 million) of the total correctional population (6.8 million). States with the highest Black-to-white ratio of incarceration are disproportionately located in the Northeast and Midwest, which includes the leading states of Iowa, Vermont, New Jersey, Connecticut, and Wisconsin.[35]

THE JUDICIAL GHETTO

The incarceration rate of Black males in the U.S. is four times the rate of incarceration of Black males in S. Africa during the Apartheid regime. Pawasarat and Quinn (2013) discovered that Wisconsin had the highest incarceration rate of Black men in the country. In addition, they found that more than half of all Black men in their thirties and forties in Milwaukee County had been incarcerated at some point. It was discovered that over half of Wisconsin's Black neighborhoods are actually prisons. Half of Black Americans report having a close friend or relative currently incarcerated. White Americans tend to attribute criminal behavior to individual/group failure rather than contextual causes (e.g., structural racism), thus viewing the criminal justice system as legitimate. White Americans who associate crime with Black Americans are more likely to support punitive policies such as capital punishment and mandatory minimum sentencing. Black Americans are more likely to be denied bail or imposed a bond that they cannot afford than whites as well as being assessed as higher safety or flight risks due to their lower socioeconomic status, criminal records, and their race. Moreover, the odds that defendants will accept less favorable plea deals increases with pre-trial detention. Almost 60 percent of middle-aged Black men without a high school diploma have served time in prison. Prison counts have fallen nationwide since 2010. Black men are more likely to go to prison than complete college, and Britton (2019) found that state cocaine penalties were associated with decreases in the college enrollment of Black men between the years of 1986 to 1991. Oleson (2016) views hyperincarceration as a modern form of eugenics where Black men are prevented from procreating. Therefore, reproduction rates in the non-incarcerated

Black general population can significantly be negatively impacted along with the control of Black women's reproduction. King (1967) identified the plantation and the ghetto as structural sites of confinement that perpetuated dominance and powerlessness. Wacquant (2000) posits that the ghetto and prison are kindred institutions of forced confinement that are entrusted to enclose a stigmatized group (descendants of U.S. enslavement) in order to neutralize the material and symbolic threat it poses to the surrounding society. The ghetto is a relation of racial control and closure built out of stigma, constraint, territorial confinement, and institutional encasement. This creates a distinct space that contains an ethnically homogeneous population that is forced to develop within it a set of interlinked institutions that duplicates broader society's organizational framework from which that group is banished. The subordinated group is therefore afforded a measure of protection, autonomy, and dignity but at a cost of being locked into a relationship of structural subordination and dependency. Therefore, the ghetto operates as a racial prison that encompasses a racial undercaste whose life chances are extremely curtailed in support of the domination of ideal and material goods or opportunities by the dominant group. The prison is conceptualized as a judicial ghetto. A jail or penitentiary is a reserved space that serves to forcibly confine a legally denigrated population. The judicial ghetto is designed for similar purposes and formed by the same four fundamental elements that make up the ghetto, which are stigma, coercion, physical enclosure, and parallelism and insulation. The ghetto and judicial ghetto protect city residents from the contamination of Black men. There has been several "Peculiar Institutions" that have operationally defined, confined, and controlled Black Americans throughout U.S. history. They include chattel slavery, Jim/Jane Crow, and the ghetto along with the prison-industrial complex which has a joint relationship of structural symbiosis and functional surrogacy. Both the ghetto and prison are institutions of forced confinement where the ghetto is a "social prison" while the prison functions as a "judicial ghetto." America's "Peculiar Institutions" of slavery, Jim/Jane Crow, and the ghetto are all instruments for the conjoint extraction of labor and social ostracization of an outcast group (Black Americans) deemed unassimilable. Black Americans are considered the most unassimilable group in the U.S. by white America due to not having a politically organized nation and an accepted culture outside of the U.S. like the Japanese or Chinese. Even though they have had a significantly longer presence in the U.S. than other ethnic groups who have been thoroughly assimilated. Black Americans are viewed as lacking a cultural past and incapable of a cultural future. The Great Migration led to Black Americans immigrating en mass to booming industrial centers of the Midwest and Northeast where they encountered restrictive covenants that forced them to congregate in a "Black Belt." These areas quickly became overcrowded, never-served, and blighted by crime, disease, and dilapidation. Moreover, they were restricted to the most hazardous, menial, and underpaid occupations in both industry and personal services. Thus, the ghetto became the third vehicle to extract Black labor while keeping Black people at a safe distance for the material and symbolic benefit of white society. The ghetto as a mechanism of racial domination began with the urban riots of 1917–1919 in East St. Louis, Chicago, Longview, Houston, etc. The ghetto was becoming functionally unsuited in accomplishing labor extraction and social ostracization by the end of the 1960s. Labor extraction was no longer needed as there was a shift from an urban industrial economy to a suburban service economy that was accompanied by the dualization of the occupational structure as well as an upsurge in working-class immigrants from Mexico, the Caribbean, and Asia. Black people in the "Black Belts" of the northern metropolis were no longer needed. The institution of the prison was erected which was capable of confining and controlling the entire Black community or at the very least its most disruptive, disreputable, and dangerous members-Black men. The prison is a political institution and a central component of the state. Eventually the Black ghetto was further destabilized by the carceral state and merged to constitute a single carceral continuum of entrapment of young Black men who circulate in a self-perpetuating cycle of social and legal marginality with devastating life-altering consequences.[36]

The carceral system of today is different than the carceral system during slavery, Jim/Jane Crow (convict leasing), and the ghetto of the mid-century in that there is no positive economic mission of recruitment and disciplining of the workforce. Today's carceral system only serves to warehouse working-class Black men who cannot find employment due to a combination of employer discrimination, competition from immigrants, and the refusal to submit to indignity of substandard work of the service economy in peripheral sectors often referred to as "slave jobs." Penalization of poverty through policy gave way to the rise of the penal state that responded to the increase in social insecurity and the collapse of the ghetto as a mechanism of control of poor Black men.[37]

DEATHWORTHY

More than eight in ten American lynchings occurred in the South between 1889 and 1918 and more than eight in ten of the 1,400+ legal executions carried out since 1976 have been in the South. Therefore, the modern American death penalty mirrors the lynching (racial violence) of the past. The majority of whites support the death penalty, while the majority of Black Americans oppose it. Unnever and Cullen (2012) found that racial prejudice against Black Americans was one of the strongest predictors of support for the death penalty. Baldus et al. (1983) demonstrated that race played a key role in the determination of which capital defendants receive the death penalty compared to life imprisonment or a lesser penalty. It is significantly more likely that the perpetrator will be sentenced to death if the victim of a murder is white than when the victim is Black. In addition, Eberhardt et al. (2006) found that the more stereotypically Black a Black male defendant is perceived, the more likely the defendant would be sentenced to death in cases involving a white victim. Black physical traits (i.e., those who are perceived to be more stereotypically Black) are a significant determinant of deathworthiness in death-eligible cases involving white victims by jurors. The criminal jury box has reflected and reproduced racial hierarchy in the U.S. since the end of Reconstruction. The U.S. not only has the world's highest incarceration rate but remains the only Western democracy still utilizing the death penalty. Black defendants are more likely to be sentenced to death than white defendants. The national death row population is approximately 42 percent Black even though the Black population is only 13 percent. More than 170 people who had been wrongly convicted and sentenced to death in the U.S. have been exonerated since 1973. Gross et al. (2014) concluded that if all death-sentenced defendants remained under sentence of death indefinitely that at least 4 percent would be exonerated and that this is a conservative estimate of the proportion of false convictions among death sentences in the United States. The death penalty is a form of state-sponsored terrorism that is primarily directed towards Black males.[38]

NEWS AND MEDIA

The media is a conduit of ideology and culture that shapes consciousness and prescribes behavior to targeted populations. The media encompasses more than mechanisms of transmission and includes ideologies, symbols, imagery, worldviews, language, and value systems that shape identity and social reality as well as provide the scripts through which thoughts are both conveyed and formed. Moreover, media products are the ideology or worldview of those who create and transmit them. This reifies the belief that Black Americans are inferior, and whiteness is superior, which provides the justification for Black death and dying. Further, the media provides parameters for culturally sanctioned thought/knowledge and behavior (i.e., racial scripting) by controlling and dominating the desired forms of expression and popularity. The media does not simply represent the interconnected social realities of crime and justice but actually helps to construct it. Race and crime are deeply connected in American society in that talking about crime is talking about race. The media constructs, traffics, and capitalizes on Black male pathology. An ideological link has been established between crime and young Black males that contributes to negative affect directed towards Black men. Barlow (1998) found that *Time* and *Newsweek* began to produce cover stories in the mid-to-late 1960s that portrayed crime as primarily a problem of urban Black Americans. The August 1964, *Newsweek* cover story on Black violence in Harlem began a barrage of cover stories on crime and Black riots/uprisings from 1964 through 1968, which assisted in forging the symbolic connection between "young Black males" and crime for years to come. *Newsweek* published a cover story titled "Crime in the Streets" in August 1965, which explicitly equated crime with "Negro crime" that conveyed an important ideological message and was the first of the *Time* and *Newsweek* cover stories to do so. In addition, the article helped to put Black political violence (uprisings/riots) in the same category as the problem of general crime and was the first to include statements regarding a *war on crime*. A *Newsweek* cover story in June 1966, titled "Police on the Spot," included an opening statement about rising crime rates, and the article promoted the idea that the role of the police was to control ghetto Blacks. Moreover, the article presented police as a national protective force even though police departments are organized as local entities. *Time* magazine's July 13th, 1970, issue stated that victims of Black crime are overwhelmingly Black and specified that it is primarily *young Black males* who commit the most common interracial crime of armed robbery. This was the first time the phrase *young Black male* was used in relation to crime within *Time* and *Newsweek* cover stories. In addition, the article included a photograph of young Black men in a local crowded jail. Later stories began to indicate Black offenders more indirectly (e.g., references to the high proportion of Black victims of crime and high levels of crime in inner-city neighborhoods). The articles demonstrate a shift from traditional to symbolic racism through the social construction of the Black male criminal who is dangerous and to be feared. The media was able to shape public discourse through ideology and the social construction of making Black male synonymous with crime. Since the 1960s, the criminalization of Black men has been pivotal in the fragmentation and stalling of racial justice and equity for Black men. Public consent for the extreme levels of coercive control and violence applied to a substantial number of the Black male population is connected to the ideological linkages created between "young Black males" and crime. In addition, Black Americans and whites have received, interpreted, and acted upon these ideologies of race and crime in social, political, and economic contexts.[39]

The public's racial misconceptions about crime are reinforced by many media outlets who present Black Americans differently than whites both quantitively and qualitatively. Black Americans are overwhelmingly presented as crime suspects and whites as crime victims by television news programs and newspapers. This exaggeration of Black offending and white victimization not only obscures Black male vulnerability but reifies Black criminality and the dangerous Black beast. Black Americans are routinely presented in an ambiguous and threatening manner such as being unnamed and in police custody, which contributes to the mythology of the Black Boogeyman. The media routinely exaggerates Black male offenders and white female victims even though most homicide is intra-racial crime involving men. Lundman (2003) found that journalists gravitated towards unusual cases where the victims were white women and what is deemed typical cases where the perpetrators were Black men. But reporters choose not to cover the murders of Black Americans by whites or of white men by white women. Therefore, newsworthiness is based on scripted stereotypes grounded in white supremacy and the construction of white fear of Black men. Dixon and Linz (2000a, 2000b) found that television news stories in Los Angeles about crime portrayed Black suspects 37 percent of the time even though they made up only 21 percent of those arrested in the city. Moreover, whites represented 43 percent of homicide victims in the local news but only accounted for 13 percent of homicide victims in crime reports. Whites were only 10 percent of victims in crime reports who had been victimized by Black Americans, but these crimes comprised 42 percent of televised cases. These are nationwide disparities that reinforce Black criminality and simultaneously deny Black male vulnerability. Black Americans are underrepresented as victims of violent crime on TV network and local news while being relegated to a depiction as perpetrators of crime where whites are overrepresented as victims. Whites are overrepresented as homicide victims in comparison to crime reports. Black Americans are more likely to appear as perpetrators in drug and violent crime stories than whites on network news. Chiricos and Eschholz (2002) found that television news presented Black crime suspects in more threatening contexts than whites such as being shown in mug shots and in contexts where the victim was a stranger (Black Boogeyman). Further, Black Americans are more likely to be handcuffed on local news programs than whites. Black defendants are more likely to have prejudicial pretrial information aired about them on local news programs than white defendants, which contributes to jury bias. In addition, police officers on reality-based TV shows including *America's Most Wanted* and *Cops* were more likely to treat Black Americans aggressively. Mass media is a major contributor to American misconceptions of crime and journalists and producers create content that contributes to the social construction of race and crime (Black male criminality).[40]

Social media is another tool of violence and domination, particularly against Black men. It was revealed that Facebook (FB; now referred to as Meta) stokes tension and incites ethnic violence that included genocide in Myanmar and Ethiopia. FB artificial intelligence (AI) has categorized Black men as primates. Moreover, Black men are routinely demonized and denigrated on FB by whites, Black Americans, and other groups who receive positive reinforcement for their behavior(s). It is plausible that this contributes to discrimination, violence, and dehumanization perpetuated against Black men that endorses genocidal logics due to this permissible behavior that is sanctioned on FB and other social media platforms. Traditional media has historically created anxiety regarding victimization risk among non-Black groups by Black males, thus being complicit in contributing to the genocide of Black males.[41]

Neal (2020) defines copaganda as the reproduction and circulation in mainstream media favorable law enforcement propaganda, which has been a tool to delegitimize claims of anti-Black violence. Copaganda encompasses active attempts to prevent police accountability due to malfeasance through the construction of the generally fair and hard-working police officer and the Black criminals who are deserved of brutality. According to Karakatsanis (2022), copaganda includes three primary functions. This includes the use of law enforcement public relations (PR) to manipulate articulations of safety, where crimes of poverty committed by the most societally vulnerable are highlighted, while crimes committed by the wealthy and powerful [e.g., wage theft by employers which eclipses all other property crime combined (burglaries, retail theft, and robberies), tax evasion, Clean Water Act violations] are rendered nearly invisible, which can be argued are more significant threats to safety. The second function involves manufacturing crises or "crime surges" that includes the bombardment of news stories such as the rise in retail theft when current data indicates that there is no significant increase. The third function of copaganda is the manipulation of solutions for public safety with the goal of convincing the public to spend more money on police and prisons (i.e., funding the carceral state) even though research does not support the belief that an increase in cops and prisons decreases crime.[42]

RACIAL SURVEILLANCE (RACIAL PROFILING)

Surveillance technologies of Black people in the U.S. have a long history dating back to enslavement, where Blackness as property was monitored through surveillance mechanisms such as the one-drop rule, quantitative plantation records where enslaved Black Americans were listed alongside livestock and crops, slave passes, slave patrols, and runaway notices. The FBI and CIA utilized surveillance that functioned as state terrorism over notable Black leaders, entertainers, and organizations, including Martin Luther King Jr., Malcolm X, the Black Panther Party (BPP), the Student Nonviolent Coordinating Committee (SNCC), the Southern Christian Leadership Conference (SCLC), the Congress of Racial Equality (CORE), the Deacons for Defense, the Republic of New Africa (RNA), the Freedom Riders, Huey P. Newton, Eldridge Cleaver, Bobby Seale, Stokely Carmichael, Fred Hampton, Kathleen Cleaver, Angela Yvonne Davis, Assata Shakur, James Baldwin, Lorraine Hansberry, Fannie Lou Hamer, H. Rap Brown, Elijah Muhammad and the Nation of Islam, W.E.B. Du Bois, Mumia Abu-Jamal, Richard Wright, Ralph Ellison, Josephine Baker, Billie Holiday, Paul Robeson, Muhammad Ali, Jimi Hendrix, E. Franklin Frazier, and Marcus Garvey and the United Negro Improvement Association, etc. This surveillance included the use of informants and the spread of disinformation by the FBI and CIA. The latest iteration of this surveillance apparatus can be found in what Siegel (2023) describes as the counter-disinformation complex, which includes an alliance between U.S. national security (FBI, CIA, and DHS) and the companies of Facebook, Twitter, Google, and Amazon that is cloaked as a war against disinformation. This alliance also includes journalists, academia, foundations, and philanthropists. The partnership between government and internet companies began to form during the Bush administration but significantly coalesced during the Obama administration and has been expanded under the Biden administration. The primary purpose is for the American ruling class to maintain power by controlling what others can think and say through counterinsurgency tactics such as discrediting individuals and institutions as an apparatus of a state-corporate censorship regime (totalitarian system) with the effect of influencing the American political process. Radical politics is conflated with acts of war in order to support a regime of total information control through surveillance traps (e.g., creating fake online profiles to influence online conversations and disseminate pro-American propaganda) and mass psychological operations. The psychological component includes learning group desires and needs as well as the maintenance of a permanent state of fear and emergency in order to influence and control. The next phase of this information war includes AI and algorithmic pre-censorship that is encoded into the infrastructure of the internet that has the potential to alter the perceptions of billions of people. Surveillance in and of Black life is a fact of anti-Blackness in the U.S., where Blackness is fixed and framed as being out of place/not belonging and thus an object of surveillance. The white gaze functions as a totalizing surveillance where Black men are incessantly looked at and watched, including being objectified or thingified and routinely visually dissected followed by disciplinary and punitive actions that are demonstrations of dominance.[43]

The term *racial profiling* was first used by a *New York Times* article (1990) to describe the New Jersey state police practice of stopping Black men (driving while Black) on the New Jersey Turnpike. Black men are the overwhelming majority of police officer targets of racial profiling. More than four out of ten Black people nationwide have reported that they were stopped by police because of their race, and almost three-quarters of young Black men report having been stopped by police because of their race. New York City police officers performed nearly 700,000 pedestrian stops (stop-and-frisk) in 2011 where a half of all stops involved frisks. Black and Latinos were more likely to be frisked than whites and less likely to be found with a weapon. Black people represented over half of these stops, while Latinos represented one third, and whites represented approximately 9 percent of these stops. Young Black and Latino men were targeted for a hugely disproportionate number of stops even though only accounting for approximately 5 percent of the city's population. Black and Latino men between the ages of 14 to 24 accounted for almost 42 percent of all stops. The number of stops of young Black men entirely exceeded the city population of young Black men (168,126 stops compared to 158,406 population). Ninety percent of young Black and Latino men were innocent. Force was used over 179,700 times against pedestrians, and Black and Latino people represented almost 23 percent of this population. Contraband was only discovered in approximately 2 percent of these stops.[44]

Surveillance technologies instituted through slavery (e.g., slave ledger) tracked Blackness as property and rendered the Black subject unrecognizable and outside the category of human. It operated as an overseeing surveillance apparatus that normalized/ritualized surveillance in Black life. An armed insurrection took place in April 1712, in New York City, where over two dozen enslaved Black Americans congregated in the densely populated East Ward of the city and set fire to a building and killed at least nine whites and wounded others. Over 70 were arrested, and many were coerced into confessions of guilt, where 25 were sentenced to death with 23 of these death sentences carried out. They were burned at the stake, hanged, beheaded, and their publicly displayed corpses were left to decompose. Previously enacted discretionary laws were consolidated into codes that governed Black city life. The "Law for Regulating Negro & Indian Slaves in the Nighttime" was passed by the Common Council of New York City in March 1713. No enslaved Negro or Native American age 14-plus years could appear in the streets of New York City during the nighttime one hour before sunset without a lantern and lighted candle. These *Lantern Laws* stipulated that at least one lantern be carried per three Negroes after sunset and strictly regulated curfews, which regulated mobility and autonomy through the use of the technology of the candle lantern. The law was amended in April 1731, where an enslaved Negro or Native American age 14-plus years who was in the company of a white person or white servant that the enslaved belonged could be out during the nighttime but had to be carrying a lit lantern. The lit candle was a supervisory device that marked Black and indigenous people as security risks that needed supervision after dark. Punishment for any slave convicted of being unlit after dark was a sentence of torture to a public whipping of up to 40 lashes, which was later reduced to 15 lashes. The lantern was a technology that criminalized Blackness and made it possible from dusk to dawn for the Black body to be permanently illuminated through racialized surveillance. The NYPD has continued the practice of Lantern Laws through what is called Omnipresence, where police officers and floodlights are stationed in high-crime housing projects. People are subject to violent illumination through artificial light and the use of high-intensity artificial lights, flood lights, or the flashing police car roof lights throughout the night in certain housing projects. Lantern Laws followed by the Black codes were the precursors to stop-and-frisk policies that overwhelmingly target Black men.[45]

The tracking of Blackness as property informs contemporary surveillance of the Black body from branding during enslavement, which was an early form of biometrics (biometric information technology) that utilizes the body, or parts and pieces of the human body to function as identification through body measurement. Those who are deemed criminals are under the gaze of the media and the public. Correctional authorities closely supervise individuals involved in the correctional system. Some inmates are constantly monitored through video and other forms of surveillance in state-of-art supermax prisons while inmates in minimum security facilities are incessantly supervised, repeatedly counted, and their movements are carefully tracked and documented. Electronic surveillance techniques and regularly scheduled meetings with parole and probation officers are mechanisms in which parolees and probationers are routinely tracked. Black men are routinely stopped by law enforcement, and their information (photo, name, address, physical characteristics, vehicle information, criminal history, etc.) along with any associates information is collected that creates an archive of Black male bodies in order to capture larger and larger amounts of data with the expectation that it will help solve a crime later on. Recent public attention has focused on the predominant surveillance of Black men by white women civilians routinely referred to as a *Karen*, who weaponizes patriarchy and white womanhood through the presentation of frailty and victimhood (i.e., emphasized femininity) while perpetrating violence through the utilization of law enforcement and any other mechanism of domination and control.[46]

Facial recognition algorithms generally work best on middle-aged white men's faces but poorly for Black and brown people, women, children, or the elderly. Buolamwini and Gebru (2018) found that some facial analysis algorithms misclassified Black women nearly 35 percent of the time but almost always got it right for white men. Mac et al. (2021) discovered that a controversial facial recognition tool, Clearview AI, that was designed for policing has been deployed across the U.S. with little or no public oversight. More than 7,000 individuals from nearly 2,000 public agencies nationwide have used Clearview AI to search through millions of Americans' faces, looking for people, including Black Lives Matter protesters. Historically, facial recognition has been inaccurate when it comes to scrutinizing the faces of non-white people. This has led to claims of racial bias and false identifications, where innocent people have been accused of crimes. There are at least six known cases of people being jailed after being falsely identified by facial recognition tools, and all of the victims have been Black with five being Black men. Helicopters, airplanes, and drones logging in at least 270 hours of surveillance were deployed in over 15 cities by the Department of Homeland Security (DHS), where demonstrations took place in response to the murder of George Floyd in June 2020. Further, unmanned drones were flown over Washington, DC, by the U.S. Marshals Service on June 5th and 7th, 2020, in response to Black Lives Matter protests, and the Air National Guard deployed aerial surveillance over multiple cities. Customs and Border Protection (CBP) deployed a Predator drone over Minneapolis in response to demonstrators who protested the murder of George Floyd in May 2020. This military technology is used for the surveilling and killing of terrorists abroad. Twitter-affiliated AI startup Dataminr helped law enforcement digitally monitor protests following the killing of George Floyd by tipping off police to social media posts that informed them of the current whereabouts and actions of demonstrators. Moreover, it was discovered that the Los

Angeles Police Department (LAPD) has been collecting social media data on every civilian they stop.[47]

CONCLUSION

Carceral state violence that results in trauma among Black men is understudied. It is urgent that carceral state mechanisms are explicitly examined and articulated along with their connection to the trauma of Black men. The reconfiguration of slavery continues as neo-slavery under the carceral apparatus. The carceral apparatus is primarily directed at Black males through mechanisms of hypercriminalization/incarceration. The carceral apparatus and Black male criminality is legitimized through the judicial and legal system along with state actors that include politicians and law enforcement. The motivations of the carceral apparatus are not only to maintain a Black undercaste of those who descend from U.S. enslavement but also to retain white dominance through population control that is achieved through either downward social mobility, incarceration, or death. Phase I of the carceral apparatus included the construction of Black male criminality after Emancipation in the South followed by the Black codes and convict leasing along with the social science construction of Black male criminality in the North. Phase II of the carceral apparatus included the *War on Crime, Law and Order,* and *War on Drugs* in response to the Black Civil Rights and Black Power movements and are all euphemisms for an all-out assault on Black men/communities that culminated in present-day police killings and hypercriminalization/ incarceration of Black males. Predatory violence among Black males is actually a rare phenomenon with approximately 2 percent of Black males arrested for violent crime in the U.S. The factors that influence crime in the Black community are economic deprivation/concentrated poverty, unemployment, incarceration, family disruption, and hypersegregation (i.e., racial-residential segregation).

The U.S. news and media is a powerful mechanism of the carceral apparatus that promotes Black male criminality ideology. The news and media is a co-conspirator in the construction of the image of the Black male criminal who is deviant and pathological in nature while simultaneously capitalizing off its own creation. The news and media induced anxiety produced from the Black male criminal creation makes the news and media complicit in the genocide of Black males. The racial surveillance of Black men is a long-standing historical practice that is societally accepted and a part of normalized/ritualized everyday social behavior. The totalizing surveillance of the white gaze on the Black male body is omnipresent and involves capturing an archive of Black male bodies that are stored in law enforcement databases for supposed crime prevention technologies. Those that have been jailed after falsely being identified by facial recognition surveillance have all been Black with the majority of them being Black men. Surveillance, police killings, and the incarceration of Black males sustains white terror, power, and domination that is a deliberate and calculated product of the white power structure. Black males wrongfully accused of criminal offenses are likely to be psychologically impacted by loss of identity, stigma, psychological and physical health, relationships with others, impact on finances and employment, traumatic experiences in custody, and adjustment difficulties. This includes those who have been exonerated or had their convictions overturned. Research from Kukucka et al. (2022) revealed that 80 percent of exonerees experience at least one significant traumatic event while incarcerated, and approximately half reported clinically significant PTSD and depressive symptomology.[48]

NOTES

1 The Great Migration is a part of neo-slavery due to it being a largely involuntary forced migration (i.e., serial forced displacement) that was in response to white terrorism and lack of social mobility. The crack epidemic is a part of neo-slavery not only due to the lack of a public health response from the U.S. government but also the structural racism (e.g., redlining-hypersegregation and unemployment) that contributed to it.

2 Blackmon, 2008; Falter, 2016; Ore, 2019; Rodríguez, 2011; Dollard, 1937; Muhammad, 2010; Sellin, 1928; Ogungbure, 2019a; Liptak, 2008; Hartfield et al., 2018; Welch, 2007; Gilens, 1996; Wolfers et al., 2015; Swaine et al., 2015; Duster, 1997; Milloy, 2018; West, 2010; West et al., 2010; Gross et al., 2017; Maston et al., 2011; Russell-Brown, 2017; Travis & Western, 2017; Pettit, 2012; Tsai & Scommegna, 2012; Bailey et al., 2021; Kutateladze et al., 2014; Knox et al., 2020; Francis, 2017; Cullen, 2018; Gilmore, 2007; Gaston et al., 2020; Binswanger et al., 2007; Hinton et al., 2018; Carson, 2018; The Sentencing Project, 2017; Nellis, 2016; Martin, 2017; Moore, 2015, 2018b; Davis, 2017; Brame et al., 2014; Baumgartel et al., 2015; Beck, 2015; Schlanger, 2013; Alexander, 2010; Mauer, 2017; The National Registry of Exonerations, n.d.; Epp et al., 2014; Crutchfield et al., 2012; Rovner, 2016; Walmsley, 2009; Klein, 2021; Klein et al., 2023.

3 Blackmon, 2008; Falter, 2016; Ore, 2019; Rodríguez, 2011; Dollard, 1937; Muhammad, 2010; Sellin, 1928; Ogungbure, 2019a; Liptak, 2008; Hartfield et al., 2018; Welch, 2007; Gilens, 1996; Wolfers et al., 2015; Swaine et al., 2015; Duster, 1997; Milloy, 2018; West, 2010; West et al., 2010; Gross et al., 2017; Maston et al., 2011; Russell-Brown, 2017; Travis & Western, 2017; Pettit, 2012; Tsai & Scommegna, 2012; Bailey et al., 2021; Kutateladze et al., 2014; Knox et al., 2020; Francis, 2017; Cullen, 2018; Gilmore, 2007; Gaston et al., 2020; Binswanger et al., 2007; Hinton et al., 2018; Carson, 2018; The Sentencing Project, 2017; Nellis, 2016; Martin, 2017; Moore, 2015, 2018b; Davis, 2017; Brame et al., 2014; Baumgartel et al., 2015; Beck, 2015; Schlanger, 2013; Alexander, 2010; Mauer, 2017; The National Registry of Exonerations, n.d.; Epp et al., 2014; Crutchfield et al., 2012; Rovner, 2016; Walmsley, 2009; Klein, 2021; Klein et al., 2023.

4 Blackmon, 2008; Falter, 2016; Ore, 2019; Rodríguez, 2011; Dollard, 1937; Muhammad, 2010; Sellin, 1928; Ogungbure, 2019a; Liptak, 2008; Hartfield et al., 2018; Welch, 2007; Gilens, 1996; Wolfers et al., 2015; Swaine et al., 2015; Duster, 1997; Milloy, 2018; West, 2010; West et al., 2010; Gross et al., 2017; Maston et al., 2011; Russell-Brown, 2017; Travis & Western, 2017; Pettit, 2012; Tsai & Scommegna, 2012; Bailey et al., 2021; Kutateladze et al., 2014; Knox et al., 2020; Francis, 2017; Cullen, 2018; Gilmore, 2007; Gaston et al., 2020; Binswanger et al., 2007; Hinton et al., 2018; Carson, 2018; The Sentencing Project, 2017; Nellis, 2016; Martin, 2017; Moore, 2015, 2018b; Davis, 2017; Brame et al., 2014; Baumgartel et al., 2015; Beck, 2015; Schlanger, 2013; Alexander, 2010; Mauer, 2017; The National Registry of Exonerations, n.d.; Epp et al., 2014; Crutchfield et al., 2012; Rovner, 2016; Walmsley, 2009; Klein, 2021; Klein et al., 2023.

5 Blackmon, 2008; Falter, 2016; Ore, 2019; Rodríguez, 2011; Dollard, 1937; Muhammad, 2010; Sellin, 1928; Ogungbure, 2019a; Liptak, 2008; Hartfield et al., 2018; Welch, 2007; Gilens, 1996; Wolfers et al., 2015; Swaine et al., 2015; Duster, 1997; Milloy, 2018; West, 2010; West et al., 2010; Gross et al., 2017; Maston et al., 2011; Russell-Brown, 2017; Travis & Western, 2017; Pettit, 2012; Tsai & Scommegna, 2012; Bailey et al., 2021; Kutateladze et al., 2014; Knox et al., 2020; Francis, 2017; Cullen, 2018; Gilmore, 2007; Gaston et al., 2020; Binswanger et al., 2007; Hinton et al., 2018; Carson, 2018; The Sentencing Project, 2017; Nellis, 2016; Martin, 2017; Moore, 2015, 2018b; Davis,

2017; Brame et al., 2014; Baumgartel et al., 2015; Beck, 2015; Schlanger, 2013; Alexander, 2010; Mauer, 2017; The National Registry of Exonerations, n.d.; Epp et al., 2014; Crutchfield et al., 2012; Rovner, 2016; Walmsley, 2009; Klein, 2021; Klein et al., 2023.

6 Blackmon, 2008; Falter, 2016; Ore, 2019; Rodríguez, 2011; Dollard, 1937; Muhammad, 2010; Sellin, 1928; Ogungbure, 2019a; Liptak, 2008; Hartfield et al., 2018; Welch, 2007; Gilens, 1996; Wolfers et al., 2015; Swaine et al., 2015; Duster, 1997; Milloy, 2018; West, 2010; West et al., 2010; Gross et al., 2017; Maston et al., 2011; Russell-Brown, 2017; Travis & Western, 2017; Pettit, 2012; Tsai & Scommegna, 2012; Bailey et al., 2021; Kutateladze et al., 2014; Knox et al., 2020; Francis, 2017; Cullen, 2018; Gilmore, 2007; Gaston et al., 2020; Binswanger et al., 2007; Hinton et al., 2018; Carson, 2018; The Sentencing Project, 2017; Nellis, 2016; Martin, 2017; Moore, 2015, 2018b; Davis, 2017; Brame et al., 2014; Baumgartel et al., 2015; Beck, 2015; Schlanger, 2013; Alexander, 2010; Mauer, 2017; The National Registry of Exonerations, n.d.; Epp et al., 2014; Crutchfield et al., 2012; Rovner, 2016; Walmsley, 2009; Klein, 2021; Klein et al., 2023

7 Blackmon, 2008; Falter, 2016; Ore, 2019; Rodríguez, 2011; Dollard, 1937; Muhammad, 2010; Sellin, 1928; Ogungbure, 2019a; Liptak, 2008; Hartfield et al., 2018; Welch, 2007; Gilens, 1996; Wolfers et al., 2015; Swaine et al., 2015; Duster, 1997; Milloy, 2018; West, 2010; West et al., 2010; Gross et al., 2017; Maston et al., 2011; Russell-Brown, 2017; Travis & Western, 2017; Pettit, 2012; Tsai & Scommegna, 2012; Bailey et al., 2021; Kutateladze et al., 2014; Knox et al., 2020; Francis, 2017; Cullen, 2018; Gilmore, 2007; Gaston et al., 2020; Binswanger et al., 2007; Hinton et al., 2018; Carson, 2018; The Sentencing Project, 2017; Nellis, 2016; Martin, 2017; Moore, 2015, 2018b; Davis, 2017; Brame et al., 2014; Baumgartel et al., 2015; Beck, 2015; Schlanger, 2013; Alexander, 2010; Mauer, 2017; The National Registry of Exonerations, n.d.; Epp et al., 2014; Crutchfield et al., 2012; Rovner, 2016; Walmsley, 2009; Klein, 2021; Klein et al., 2023.

8 Blackmon, 2008; Falter, 2016; Ore, 2019; Rodríguez, 2011; Dollard, 1937; Muhammad, 2010; Sellin, 1928; Ogungbure, 2019a; Liptak, 2008; Hartfield et al., 2018; Welch, 2007; Gilens, 1996; Wolfers et al., 2015; Swaine et al., 2015; Duster, 1997; Milloy, 2018; West, 2010; West et al., 2010; Gross et al., 2017; Maston et al., 2011; Russell-Brown, 2017; Travis & Western, 2017; Pettit, 2012; Tsai & Scommegna, 2012; Bailey et al., 2021; Kutateladze et al., 2014; Knox et al., 2020; Francis, 2017; Cullen, 2018; Gilmore, 2007; Gaston et al., 2020; Binswanger et al., 2007; Hinton et al., 2018; Carson, 2018; The Sentencing Project, 2017; Nellis, 2016; Martin, 2017; Moore, 2015, 2018b; Davis, 2017; Brame et al., 2014; Baumgartel et al., 2015; Beck, 2015; Schlanger, 2013; Alexander, 2010; Mauer, 2017; The National Registry of Exonerations, n.d.; Epp et al., 2014; Crutchfield et al., 2012; Rovner, 2016; Walmsley, 2009; Klein, 2021; Klein et al., 2023.

9 Blackmon, 2008; Falter, 2016; Ore, 2019; Rodríguez, 2011; Dollard, 1937; Muhammad, 2010; Sellin, 1928; Ogungbure, 2019a; Liptak, 2008; Hartfield et al., 2018; Welch, 2007; Gilens, 1996; Wolfers et al., 2015; Swaine et al., 2015; Duster, 1997; Milloy, 2018; West, 2010; West et al., 2010; Gross et al., 2017; Maston et al., 2011; Russell-Brown, 2017; Travis & Western, 2017; Pettit, 2012; Tsai & Scommegna, 2012; Bailey et al., 2021; Kutateladze et al., 2014; Knox et al., 2020; Francis, 2017; Cullen, 2018; Gilmore, 2007; Gaston et al., 2020; Binswanger et al., 2007; Hinton et al., 2018; Carson, 2018; The Sentencing Project, 2017; Nellis, 2016; Martin, 2017; Moore, 2015, 2018b; Davis, 2017; Brame et al., 2014; Baumgartel et al., 2015; Beck, 2015; Schlanger, 2013; Alexander, 2010; Mauer, 2017; The National Registry of Exonerations, n.d.; Epp et al., 2014; Crutchfield et al., 2012; Rovner, 2016; Walmsley, 2009; Klein, 2021; Klein et al., 2023.

10 Reichel, 1988; Hadden, 2001; Foner, 1975; Russell-Brown, 2017; Camp, 1998.
11 Reichel, 1988; Hadden, 2001; Foner, 1975; Russell-Brown, 2017; Camp, 1998.
12 Reichel, 1988; Hadden, 2001; Foner, 1975; Russell-Brown, 2017; Camp, 1998.
13 Reichel, 1988; Hadden, 2001; Foner, 1975; Russell-Brown, 2017; Camp, 1998.
14 Reichel, 1988; Hadden, 2001; Foner, 1975; Russell-Brown, 2017; Camp, 1998.
15 Reichel, 1988; Hadden, 2001; Foner, 1975; Russell-Brown, 2017; Camp, 1998.
16 Reichel, 1988; Hadden, 2001; Foner, 1975; Russell-Brown, 2017; Camp, 1998.
17 Durr, 2015; Swaine et al., 2015; Tsai & Scommegna, 2012; Bailey et al., 2021; Krieger
    et al., 2015; Fatal Force: Police Shootings Database, n.d.; Fatal Encounters, n.d.;
    Edwards et al., 2019; Hartfield et al., 2018; Swaine & McCarthy, 2017; Gabrielson
    et al., 2014; Soss & Weaver, 2017; Ward, 2018; Hyland et al., 2015; Mauer, 2017; GBD,
    2021; Kimberley, 2021; Barker et al., 2021.
18 Durr, 2015; Swaine et al., 2015; Tsai & Scommegna, 2012; Bailey et al., 2021; Krieger
    et al., 2015; Fatal Force: Police Shootings Database, n.d.; Fatal Encounters, n.d.;
    Edwards et al., 2019; Hartfield et al., 2018; Swaine & McCarthy, 2017; Gabrielson
    et al., 2014; Soss & Weaver, 2017; Ward, 2018; Hyland et al., 2015; Mauer, 2017; GBD,
    2021; Kimberley, 2021; Barker et al., 2021
19 Durr, 2015; Swaine et al., 2015; Tsai & Scommegna, 2012; Bailey et al., 2021; Krieger
    et al., 2015; Fatal Force: Police Shootings Database, n.d.; Fatal Encounters, n.d.;
    Edwards et al., 2019; Hartfield et al., 2018; Swaine & McCarthy, 2017; Gabrielson
    et al., 2014; Soss & Weaver, 2017; Ward, 2018; Hyland et al., 2015; Mauer, 2017; GBD,
    2021; Kimberley, 2021; Barker et al., 2021.
20 Durr, 2015; Swaine et al., 2015; Tsai & Scommegna, 2012; Bailey et al., 2021; Krieger
    et al., 2015; Fatal Force: Police Shootings Database, n.d.; Fatal Encounters, n.d.;
    Edwards et al., 2019; Hartfield et al., 2018; Swaine & McCarthy, 2017; Gabrielson
    et al., 2014; Soss & Weaver, 2017; Ward, 2018; Hyland et al., 2015; Mauer, 2017; GBD,
    2021; Kimberley, 2021; Barker et al., 2021.
21 Hinton, 2015.
22 Hinton, 2015.
23 Hinton, 2015.
24 Hinton, 2015.
25 Hinton, 2015.
26 Weaver, 2007; Gillon, 2018; Shellow, 2018; Baum, 2016; Cooper, 2015.
27 Weaver, 2007; Gillon, 2018; Shellow, 2018; Baum, 2016; Cooper, 2015.
28 Weaver, 2007; Gillon, 2018; Shellow, 2018; Baum, 2016; Cooper, 2015.
29 Welch, 2007; Scheingold, 2011; Russell, 2002; Sigelman & Tuch, 1997; Sniderman &
    Piazza, 1993; Hawkins, 1987; Hurwitz & Peffley, 1998; Chiricos et al., 2004; Welch
    et al., 2002; Katz, 1988; Beck, 2021; Sampson, 1987; Sullivan, 1989; Wilson et al., 1988;
    Sampson & Wilson, 1995; Morgan, 2017; Neiwert, 2017; Krivo et al., 2009; Clear,
    2008; Quillian & Pager, 2001.
30 Welch, 2007; Scheingold, 2011; Russell, 2002; Sigelman & Tuch, 1997; Sniderman & Piazza,
    1993; Hawkins, 1987; Hurwitz & Peffley, 1998; Chiricos et al., 2004; Welch et al., 2002; Katz,
    1988; Beck, 2021; Sampson, 1987; Sullivan, 1989; Wilson et al., 1988; Sampson & Wilson,
    1995; Morgan, 2017; Neiwert, 2017; Krivo et al., 2009; Clear, 2008; Quillian & Pager, 2001.
31 Welch, 2007; Scheingold, 2011; Russell, 2002; Sigelman & Tuch, 1997; Sniderman & Piazza,
    1993; Hawkins, 1987; Hurwitz & Peffley, 1998; Chiricos et al., 2004; Welch et al., 2002; Katz,
    1988; Beck, 2021; Sampson, 1987; Sullivan, 1989; Wilson et al., 1988; Sampson & Wilson,
    1995; Morgan, 2017; Neiwert, 2017; Krivo et al., 2009; Clear, 2008; Quillian & Pager, 2001.

32 Gross et al., 2017; Robinson & Scaglion, 1987; Harrison & Beck, 2006; Mauer & King, 2007; Sidanius & Pratto, 1999; Sidanius et al., 1998; Bobo & Thompson, 2010; Corley, 2013; Kenney, 2016; Unnever & Cullen, 2009; Epp et al., 2014; Bright, 1995; Stevenson, 2017; Correll et al., 2011; Krieger et al., 2015; Ghandnoosh, 2014; Walmsley, 2013; Western, 2006; Jones, 2013; Navarrete et al., 2009, 2010; Quillian & Pager, 2001; Sidanius & Veniegas, 2000; Maner et al., 2005; Fins, 2016; Mauer, 2017; Wilson, 1987; Death Penalty Information Center, n.d.

33 Gross et al., 2017; Robinson & Scaglion, 1987; Harrison & Beck, 2006; Mauer & King, 2007; Sidanius & Pratto, 1999; Sidanius et al., 1998; Bobo & Thompson, 2010; Corley, 2013; Kenney, 2016; Unnever & Cullen, 2009; Epp et al., 2014; Bright, 1995; Stevenson, 2017; Correll et al., 2011; Krieger et al., 2015; Ghandnoosh, 2014; Walmsley, 2013; Western, 2006; Jones, 2013; Navarrete et al., 2009, 2010; Quillian & Pager, 2001; Sidanius & Veniegas, 2000; Maner et al., 2005; Fins, 2016; Mauer, 2017; Wilson, 1987; Death Penalty Information Center, n.d.

34 Gross et al., 2017; Robinson & Scaglion, 1987; Harrison & Beck, 2006; Mauer & King, 2007; Sidanius & Pratto, 1999; Sidanius et al., 1998; Bobo & Thompson, 2010; Corley, 2013; Kenney, 2016; Unnever & Cullen, 2009; Epp et al., 2014; Bright, 1995; Stevenson, 2017; Correll et al., 2011; Krieger et al., 2015; Ghandnoosh, 2014; Walmsley, 2013; Western, 2006; Jones, 2013; Navarrete et al., 2009, 2010; Quillian & Pager, 2001; Sidanius & Veniegas, 2000; Maner et al., 2005; Fins, 2016; Mauer, 2017; Wilson, 1987; Death Penalty Information Center, n.d.

35 Gross et al., 2017; Robinson & Scaglion, 1987; Harrison & Beck, 2006; Mauer & King, 2007; Sidanius & Pratto, 1999; Sidanius et al., 1998; Bobo & Thompson, 2010; Corley, 2013; Kenney, 2016; Unnever & Cullen, 2009; Epp et al., 2014; Bright, 1995; Stevenson, 2017; Correll et al., 2011; Krieger et al., 2015; Ghandnoosh, 2014; Walmsley, 2013; Western, 2006; Jones, 2013; Navarrete et al., 2009, 2010; Quillian & Pager, 2001; Sidanius & Veniegas, 2000; Maner et al., 2005; Fins, 2016; Mauer, 2017; Wilson, 1987; Death Penalty Information Center, n.d.

36 Voigt et al., 1994; Weber, 1978; Myrdal, 1944; Wacquant, 2009; Bobo & Thompson, 2010; Corley, 2013; Kenney, 2016; Unnever & Cullen, 2009; Epp et al., 2014; Bright, 1995; Stevenson, 2017; Correll et al., 2011; Krieger et al., 2015; Ghandnoosh, 2014; Walmsley, 2013; Western, 2006; Jones, 2013; Navarrete et al., 2009, 2010; Quillian & Pager, 2001; Sidanius & Veniegas, 2000; Maner et al., 2005; Fins, 2016; Sidanius et al., 1998; Mauer, 2017; Darity, 2005; Pettit & Western, 2004; Death Penalty Information Center, n.d.

37 Voigt et al., 1994; Weber, 1978; Myrdal, 1944; Wacquant, 2009; Bobo & Thompson, 2010; Corley, 2013; Kenney, 2016; Unnever & Cullen, 2009; Epp et al., 2014; Bright, 1995; Stevenson, 2017; Correll et al., 2011; Krieger et al., 2015; Ghandnoosh, 2014; Walmsley, 2013; Western, 2006; Jones, 2013; Navarrete et al., 2009, 2010; Quillian & Pager, 2001; Sidanius & Veniegas, 2000; Maner et al., 2005; Fins, 2016; Sidanius et al., 1998; Mauer, 2017; Darity, 2005; Pettit & Western, 2004; Death Penalty Information Center, n.d.

38 Bobo & Thompson, 2010; Corley, 2013; Kenney, 2016; Unnever & Cullen, 2009; Epp et al., 2014; Bright, 1995; Stevenson, 2017; Correll et al., 2011; Krieger et al., 2015; Ghandnoosh, 2014; Walmsley, 2013; Western, 2006; Jones, 2013; Navarrete et al., 2009, 2010; Quillian & Pager, 2001; Sidanius & Veniegas, 2000; Maner et al., 2005; Fins, 2016; Sidanius et al., 1998; Mauer, 2017; Frampton, 2018; Death Penalty Information Center, n.d.

39 Williams et al., 2010; McQuail, 2000; Harrell, 1999; Ani, 1994; Drummond, 1990; Hall, 1981; Dixon & Linz, 2002; Romer et al., 1998; Dixon et al., 2003; Entman & Rojecki, 2000; Oliver, 1994; Ghandnoosh, 2014; Entman, 1992, 2006; Smiley & Fakunle, 2016; Dukes & Gaither, 2017; Hutchinson, 1994; Mozur, 2018; Cornish et al., 2021; Sawyer, 2018; Jones, 2021; Mull, 2021; Koerth, 2020; Alexander, 2010.

40 Williams et al., 2010; McQuail, 2000; Harrell, 1999; Ani, 1994; Drummond, 1990; Hall, 1981; Dixon & Linz, 2002; Romer et al., 1998; Dixon et al., 2003; Entman & Rojecki, 2000; Oliver, 1994; Ghandnoosh, 2014; Entman, 1992, 2006; Smiley & Fakunle, 2016; Dukes & Gaither, 2017; Hutchinson, 1994; Mozur, 2018; Cornish et al., 2021; Sawyer, 2018; Jones, 2021; Mull, 2021; Koerth, 2020; Alexander, 2010.

41 Williams et al., 2010; McQuail, 2000; Harrell, 1999; Ani, 1994; Drummond, 1990; Hall, 1981; Dixon & Linz, 2002; Romer et al., 1998; Dixon et al., 2003; Entman & Rojecki, 2000; Oliver, 1994; Ghandnoosh, 2014; Entman, 1992, 2006; Smiley & Fakunle, 2016; Dukes & Gaither, 2017; Hutchinson, 1994; Mozur, 2018; Cornish et al., 2021; Sawyer, 2018; Jones, 2021; Mull, 2021; Koerth, 2020; Alexander, 2010.

42 Williams et al., 2010; McQuail, 2000; Harrell, 1999; Ani, 1994; Drummond, 1990; Hall, 1981; Dixon & Linz, 2002; Romer et al., 1998; Dixon et al., 2003; Entman & Rojecki, 2000; Oliver, 1994; Ghandnoosh, 2014; Entman, 1992, 2006; Smiley & Fakunle, 2016; Dukes & Gaither, 2017; Hutchinson, 1994; Mozur, 2018; Cornish et al., 2021; Sawyer, 2018; Jones, 2021; Mull, 2021; Koerth, 2020; Alexander, 2010.

43 Browne, 2015; Sullivan, 1990; Newton, 1980; Hersh, 1978; Davis, 2017; Newport, 1999; NYCLU, 2012; Scannell, 2018; Garcia-Rojas, 2016; Pettit, 2012; Rhodes, 2004; Crockford, 2020; Grother et al., 2019; Hvistendahl, 2021; Brayne, 2020; Kanno-Youngs, 2020; Biddle, 2020, 2021; Koebler et al., 2020; Levin, 2021; Hill, 2020.

44 Browne, 2015; Sullivan, 1990; Newton, 1980; Hersh, 1978; Davis, 2017; Newport, 1999; NYCLU, 2012; Scannell, 2018; Garcia-Rojas, 2016; Pettit, 2012; Rhodes, 2004; Crockford, 2020; Grother et al., 2019; Hvistendahl, 2021; Brayne, 2020; Kanno-Youngs, 2020; Biddle, 2020, 2021; Koebler et al., 2020; Levin, 2021; Hill, 2020.

45 Browne, 2015; Sullivan, 1990; Newton, 1980; Hersh, 1978; Davis, 2017; Newport, 1999; NYCLU, 2012; Scannell, 2018; Garcia-Rojas, 2016; Pettit, 2012; Rhodes, 2004; Crockford, 2020; Grother et al., 2019; Hvistendahl, 2021; Brayne, 2020; Kanno-Youngs, 2020; Biddle, 2020, 2021; Koebler et al., 2020; Levin, 2021; Hill, 2020.

46 Browne, 2015; Sullivan, 1990; Newton, 1980; Hersh, 1978; Davis, 2017; Newport, 1999; NYCLU, 2012; Scannell, 2018; Garcia-Rojas, 2016; Pettit, 2012; Rhodes, 2004; Crockford, 2020; Grother et al., 2019; Hvistendahl, 2021; Brayne, 2020; Kanno-Youngs, 2020; Biddle, 2020, 2021; Koebler et al., 2020; Levin, 2021; Hill, 2020.

47 Browne, 2015; Sullivan, 1990; Newton, 1980; Hersh, 1978; Davis, 2017; Newport, 1999; NYCLU, 2012; Scannell, 2018; Garcia-Rojas, 2016; Pettit, 2012; Rhodes, 2004; Crockford, 2020; Grother et al., 2019; Hvistendahl, 2021; Brayne, 2020; Kanno-Youngs, 2020; Biddle, 2020, 2021; Koebler et al., 2020; Levin, 2021; Hill, 2020.

48 Brooks & Greenberg, 2021.

CHAPTER 5

STARVING THE BLACK BEAST

PART I

The trauma that Black men experience due to economic deprivation is profound and unacknowledged. The economic deprivation of Black men is analyzed through institutional decimation, political economy of niggerdom, employment, occupations, income/wage, wealth, Black relationships and families, plantation politics and the decadent veil, racial-residential segregation (hypersegregation), and gentrification. The economic deprivation of Black men must thoroughly be examined to have a clear understanding of its relationship with trauma.

THE INSTITUTIONAL DECIMATION OF BLACK MEN

The research of Kraus et al. (2017) found that whites and Black Americans from the top and bottom of the national income distribution overestimated the progress of Black-white economic equality. The overestimates outstripped reality by approximately 25 percent and were connected to a greater belief in a just world and social network racial diversity specifically among Black Americans. In addition, an *Economist/YouGov* (2018) poll indicated that 40 percent of whites believed that Black Americans could be just as well off as whites if they tried harder (protestant work ethic). These profound misperceptions and misplaced optimism regarding societal racial economic inequality can have deleterious public policy consequences.[1]

Stewart and Scott (1978) refer to the institutional decimation of Black American men as a coordinated operation of various institutions in American society which systematically removes Black men from the civilian population. Black men are programmatically eliminated from the Black community and society at large. Black men can become associated with crime (e.g., the underground economy) as an attempt to counter economic impositions from institutions, especially the labor market. Moreover, anti-Black misandry in the labor market can be characterized as a form of ethnic warfare.[2]

Unemployment and underemployment are primary conditions that generate economic distress among Black men. The public assistance industrial complex, the educational system, and the health care system produce comparable economic distress that encourages participation in crime. These frustrations and distress also contribute to the overrepresentation of Black Americans in the enlisted ranks of the military. The long-term effect of the decimation process is the reduction in the probability of Black male survival in comparison to non-Black males and other groups. Since World War II, the ratio of Black unemployment compared to white unemployment has been approximately 2:1 consistently. The official figures understate the magnitude of the problem as a result of undercounting and a large number of Black Americans who have abandoned the search for employment (i.e., discouraged workers). Moreover, young Black men experience significantly higher unemployment rates than the Black population as a whole. The unemployment rate among Black men in some urban areas falls within the 15 to 35 percent range.[3]

Economic distress that is experienced by Black men who participate in the American labor market is comparable to Black men who are unemployed. Black men who are

DOI: 10.4324/9781003430551-6

employed are routinely crowded into low-status occupations along with associated wage rates that are inadequate in providing a standard of living significantly above the poverty level. Black men are disproportionately employed as service workers. Full-time employment for a significant number of Black men who are heads of households is not significant to generate an income that provides a minimum acceptable standard of living. Therefore, other household family members are more likely to participate in the labor market in order to augment family income than are members of families headed by white males. Often, the wife is the family member who augments the labor force participation of Black families. In addition, it is not uncommon for teenaged offspring to participate in the labor market as well in order to augment the earnings of Black families. The inability of a large number of Black males to earn an adequate income through labor force participation forces Black families to disproportionately rely on public assistance in order to augment earnings in the labor market. Thus, the economic distress of Black men is amplified through the need for other family members to enter the labor market and the dependence on public assistance to augment their earnings. Further, economic distress is experienced by teenage Black males who are unable to obtain employment to mitigate the economic hardships faced by both male-headed and female-headed Black families.[4]

The majority of Black Americans in the U.S. are accepted into the lowest-paying jobs, tolerated in public housing, and permitted to join the unemployment lines but are barred from effective power within the corporate and political ruling (slavocracy) class. Black workers consistently experience workplace exploitation and racist assaults against their humanity. Black Americans are concentrated in the lowest paid, blue collar, unskilled, and service sectors of the labor force and are generally the last hired and first fired during periodic recessions. The American economy is segmented into primary and secondary sectors. Monopolistic and oligopolistic firms comprise the primary sector, which pays relatively high wages, generate high profits, are often unionized with good working conditions, and offer a high degree of job security. Small firms in competition with other small firms comprise the secondary sector of the economy, where wages are low, unions are nonexistent or weak, employee turnover is high, frequent lay-off occur, and there is very little opportunity for advancement. The labor market structure is distinctive for each sector associated with it. Black Americans and teenagers are disproportionately found in secondary labor markets. The deleterious economic condition of the Black male worker includes low-wages, fewer weeks of work per year, higher unemployment rates, and greater dependence on public assistance in comparison to other groups. This is largely caused by the systematic bifurcation of the American economy and a set of mechanisms that keep Black Americans trapped in the secondary sector of the economy. A large percentage of Black Americans are excluded from participating in the primary labor market as most of the training for primary sector jobs takes place on the job and not in schools or government training programs. Therefore, the acquisition of necessary skills requires the "social acceptance" of coworkers. Hiring decisions by the primary sector routinely entails the social acceptability of an individual that includes characteristics such as race, sex, and personal appearance, which operate against Black men due to the persistence of anti-Black misandry. Thus, the decision to drop out of high school becomes an economically sound decision for many Black males. The existing arrangement of the structure of the secondary sector of the economy and the inaccessibility of the primary labor market to Black males with no more than a high school diploma perpetuates itself and reinforces patterns of economic distress due to this institutional arrangement. Black males who are able to enter into the primary labor market experience earning disparities where they are among the lowest paid, thus experiencing a new set of economic distress.[5]

Further, racism experienced on the job is an important contributing factor in deciding to abandon stable employment. Policies that would appear to provide a partial solution to the situation of Black males situated within the structure of the secondary labor market routinely have the opposite effect. An example would be the effect of increasing the statutory minimum wage, which increases the income of some workers in the secondary labor market but inadvertently leads to the elimination of large numbers of secondary sector jobs over time, thus increasing public assistance dependence. Institutions that provide public welfare are interconnected with the labor market mechanism.[6]

According to Cloward and Piven (1971), public assistance serves the two functions of quelling civil disorders and reinforcing the protestant work ethic. The public assistance system is expanded during periods of civil unrest to relieve some of the economic distress that underlie the discontent. The system is contracted once the threat of social upheaval is contained, and many recipients are forced to re-enter the labor market and reexperience the accompanying economic distress. This process ensures that economic distress experienced by Black Americans does not approach levels that produce violence and an uprising directed at the society at large.[7]

Economic distress leads to the incarceration of Black men in penal institutions, which forcibly removes them from the Black community. Rusche and Kirchheimer (1939) posit that the prison system is an institution designed to manage surplus labor. Therefore, the prison constitutes a geographical solution to socioeconomic problems that is politically organized by the state. The growth in hypercriminalization/incarceration is attributed to demands that stem from prison guard unions, construction interests, and private security and prison firms that are financially invested in the prison-industrial complex/enterprise. In addition, working-class Black men turn to crime as a means of economic survival in a post-industrial economy. Black men are disproportionately arrested for offenses which have a functional relationship to economic distress relative to the proportion of arrests of Black Americans for all offenses. An example would be Black men participating in underground economies such as the sale of crack cocaine during the height of the crack epidemic in response to being locked out of the labor market and unemployed due to deindustrialization, hypersegregation, relocation of manufacturing plants and various employers, and a new economy that required advanced education and computer literacy.[8]

The educational industrial complex determines civilian labor market functionality. Black males who are deemed to have no degree of functionality for nonmenial occupations in the civilian labor market are pushed out of the educational system without any support into removal mechanisms such as the school-to-prison pipeline where they are removed from the Black civilian population. Consequently, the socioeconomic deprivation that contributes to Black men being in the penal correction system also contributes to Black men enlisting in the military. Black men who are not functioning in the labor market may still be functional in military establishments. The military represents an alternative to civilian employment for some Black men. In the past, military drafts represented a forced separation of Black males from the Black civilian population. The channeling of Black males into the military complements the public assistance system in mitigating violence and protests/uprisings as a result of economic distress experienced by civilian Black Americans.[9]

The dynamic between economic distress and inadequate health care contributes to a high mortality rate (i.e., brutal mortality regime) among Black men. Black men are temporarily and permanently removed from the civilian population through the operation of labor market mechanisms, the education system, the health care delivery system, the public assistance industrial complex, and the institution of crime. The Black male in America is situated within a political socioeconomic milieu that produces economic distress and the response to the distress initiates the elimination of Black men from the population. Research from Austin (2021) supports the institutional decimation thesis and found that Black males are excluded from the workforce due to racist hiring practices as well as being killed and incarcerated at significantly higher rates than other groups. This anti-Black misandry costs the U.S. economy $50 billion annually. Closing this Black-white jobs gap could add $30 billion annually to Black communities (i.e., children, family members, & partners) and significantly reduce Black poverty. In order to close the employment gap, 947,000 jobs (based on 2014 year figures of "moderate" unemployment) would be required for Black men to have a comparable employment-to-population ratio (EPOP) to that of white, Latino, and Asian men.[10]

THE POLITICAL ECONOMY OF NIGGERDOM

According to Travis and Western (2017), violence and poverty have been the two great markers of racial injustice for the past 150 years since Emancipation. Coined by Curry (2017), the political economy of niggerdom is defined by Ogungbure (2019) as a system that applies various methods of anti-Black misandry (sexualized racism) and the stereotype of criminalization as the foundation for racial and economic discrimination against Black males. The political economy of niggerdom encompasses the victimization of Black males by two significant tools of patriarchal economics, which are genocidal logics and emasculation (economic isolation) as grounds for social exclusion. It involves a pattern of economic discrimination and victimization directed towards Black males that excludes them from participation in America's capitalist political economy. Economic access is more of a myth than reality for Black men in America's political economy. This is supported by the foundational myth of democratic capitalism, which has never applied to all groups in America. The democratic capitalism phantasm perpetuates the pathological treatment of Black males within the U.S. economy. Black men experience economic isolation and racialized discrimination in the U.S. from a political economy that deliberately confines them to poverty. This includes the historic exploitation of Black male labor while concomitantly rationalizing their death as a consequence of their deviance and undesirability in U.S. society.[11]

The political economy of niggerdom has its foundations in the historical, as well as the pathological, prejudiced, and caricaturized portrayal of Black people as *niggers* in which Black males are targeted for constituting a threat to the social, economic, and political power of the dominant white males. Thus, the white American imagination constructs and labels Black men as an unwanted being, a social deviant, and brute. The domain of niggerdom is reserved for Black males and includes exclusion, outsideness, and social ostracization. The political economy of niggerdom negatively impacts the Black family through the establishment/maintenance of hypercriminalization/incarceration, underemployment, unemployment, and poverty among Black males. The political economy manifests through the pernicious stigma of criminalization (Black criminality) where the media projects negative images of Black males as a tool to sustain the myths that legitimize white supremacy and the construction of the racialized "other" in the white racial imaginary. The stigma of criminalization serves as the justification for the disposability of Black males, thus ensuring their lack of participation in the U.S. economy. This niggerization and criminalization of Black males has become a dominant concretized global image that entails the idle Black male on the street corner. The racial implications of niggerization includes the mapping of hatred, delinquency, and derogatory portrayals onto Black male bodies, which is used to justify their decimation by the state. Genocidal logics are utilized through the weaponization of poverty, where the oppression of Black males is perfected by constricting them to a life of penury, which ensures a lifetime of economic hardships. The restriction of Black male participation in the economy implies that Black men do not deserve to live. The theoretical lens of the political economy of niggerdom exposes the dynamic between racism, economic injustice, and sex-based discrimination (anti-Black misandry).[12]

EMPLOYMENT

Black men represent approximately 45 percent of the Black labor force, while Black women represent 55 percent. The labor force participation rate of Black men is the lowest among all race and ethnic groups. Since 1970, all racial/ethnic minoritized groups have increased their labor force participation with the exception of Black men. Black Americans are laid off in numbers that are disproportionate to their labor force participation. The unemployment rates experienced by Black Americans during the past 50 years would be considered recessionary if experienced by the entire U.S. population. Leading up to World War II, Black Americans suffered the twin afflictions of segregation (education, housing, transportation, and public accommodations) and employment discrimination that included lower earnings, entry barriers to numerous occupations and industries, and greater exposure to the business cycle and homeland and overseas competition. Post-World War II labor market conditions decreased job barriers and narrowed pay differentials as a result of the demand for goods and services, relatively improved labor quality of Black workers, civil rights legislation, and supportive court decisions. Therefore, the relative earnings of Black Americans increased from 1940 to 1970. The Black/white earning gap narrowed until the mid-1970s and has since stagnated. Darity et al. (2001) found the sharpest decline in labor market discrimination against Black Americans occurred between the years of 1960 and 1980. Moreover, labor market discrimination against Black men was greater in all census years after 1880 until 1970. Labor market discrimination against Black women increased after 1880 and peaked in 1920 and declined continuously thereafter with the sharpest reduction in discrimination taking place between 1960 and 1980.[13]

Labor-force participation of Black men has been relatively low since the 1950s and was considered relatively stable for both Black and white men between 1940 and 1970, but they both experienced sharp declines in participation rates after 1970. The decline was significantly larger for Black men particularly those of prime working age. This included Black men 36 to 45 years old with a decline of approximately 6 percentage points compared to a decline of one percentage point for white men in the same age group. The decade of the 1970s saw the labor-force participation of Black men ages 46 to 54 decline almost 10 percentage points compared to a significantly smaller decline of approximately four percentage points for white men in the same age group. The ratio of Black to white unemployment (male and female) hovered around 2 in the early 1970s and briefly jumped to almost 2.5 in the late 1970s and steadily fell to 2.2 in 1982. By the end of the 1980s, the ratio was in excess of 2.5. Unemployment rates of Black Americans fell from almost 19 percent in 1982 to 11 percent in 1989 while for whites it fell from almost 9 percent to almost 5 percent during the economic expansion of the 1980s.[14]

Joblessness among Black men throughout the 1970s and 1980s was partly due to the decrease in demand for less-skilled labor, which disproportionately affected Black men.

Bound and Holzer (1991) found industrial shifts worsened the relative employment position of Black men. Their research on 52 metropolitan areas found that manufacturing shifts accounted for as much as 10 to 30 percent of the employment declines of Black men while 35 to 50 percent of the employment decline was experienced by Black male dropouts between the ages of 16 to 24 between 1970 and 1980.

Waiters, bellmen, kitchen helpers in restaurants, farm workers, and messengers were jobs that had traditionally been reserved for Black Americans but began to go to the influx of undocumented workers entering the U.S. from Latin America and Asian countries. Employment rates among immigrants with substantially lower educational attainment and language skills are significantly higher than native-born young Black men. It has been posited that immigrants are more likely to accept low-wage jobs in the service sector as well as employers preferring immigrants over native-born Black men while actively recruiting immigrants into many key sectors such as construction and some parts of manufacturing. Employers believe immigrants to be more productive workers and view them as more tractable labor. Opportunities became limited for Black men as the reliance on immigrant networks ensure that labor market information is confined to immigrant communities. Further, the research of Borjas et al. (1991) on the effects of immigration on less-educated youths found that up to one-third of the observed change between college- and high-school-level labor potentially can be attributed to the labor-supply effects of immigration and trade during the 1980s.

Beginning in the late 1970s, Black males were brought into competition or noncompetition with the large numbers of white women entering and re-entering the labor force through the economic expansion in private sector technology and service industries. Being Black and male has been found to have a consistent negative effect on earnings, which indicates the persistent presence of anti-Black wage discrimination that severely impacts Black men. Employment discrimination against Black Americans substantially declined during the years immediately after the passage of the Civil Rights Act of 1964. It was not exterminated but maintained and stabilized by the mid-1970s, and it is after this point that progress ceased for Black men in the labor market. The convergence of labor market outcomes for Black Americans and whites ceased, and a reverse movement erased some of the post-World War II gains that ensued during the 1970s. Further, Black men suffered close to a 15 percent loss in earnings due to discrimination in both 1980 and 1990. Wage inequality research routinely ignores the high rates of joblessness among Black men and primarily focuses on employer discrimination and skills distribution among workers. The Black-white income gap inadequately reflects the relative economic standing of Black men who suffer from a high rate of joblessness. Since 1970, severe increases in incarceration, labor force non-participation, and unemployment have devastated the working lives of poor Black men. During the Great Recession, approximately 38 percent of prime aged Black men were not working compared to approximately 19 percent of white men. Western and Pettit (2005) found that factoring in labor inactivity that includes prison and jail incarceration in 1999 led to a 7 to 20 percent increase in the Black-white income gap among working-age men. Further, the Black-white income gap increased by as much as 58 percent among Black men ages 22–30 in 1999, and incarceration accounted for approximately 31 percent of all joblessness in the same year. Thus, the supposed improvement in the economic position of young Black men is a consequence of rising joblessness fueled by the growth in incarceration during the 1990s. When incarcerated Black men are factored in unemployment statistics, the Black-white income gap significantly increased as well as unemployment statistics among Black men. In addition, incarceration is associated with a 40 percent decrease in annual earnings after release from prison. Assessments of wage inequality include very few low-skilled Black men due to a high jobless rate and low potential earnings. Therefore, the Black-white income gap is a distortion due to the sample selection that causes overestimates of earnings, which gives the impression that it is a gap and not a gulf. The appearance of relative wage gains is the result of declining employment opportunities among low-skilled men who are not factored in the analyses of wage inequality and the labor market. Low-skilled young Black men were removed from the general population (i.e., institutional decimation) due to the growth and expansion of the U.S. penal system through the 1980s and 1990s. Over 40 percent of young Black male high school dropouts were in prison or jail compared to 10 percent of young white male dropouts by 1999. The effect was the concealment of poor young Black men in labor force statistics because of the high incarceration rates. Western and Beckett (1999) contend that the usual measures of employment overstated the U.S. labor market gains through the 1990s economic expansion. The Black-white ratio in joblessness among Black men increased by 20 percent due largely to the rise in incarceration rates.[15]

The high rates of hypercriminalization/incarceration of young Black men contribute to a reduction in employment prospects among Black men with no criminal background. Incarceration significantly contributes to selection bias in the estimation of Black relative wages and thus is a significant source of employment inequality. Moreover, incarceration may directly contribute to labor market inequality by reducing the earnings of ex-offenders. Therefore, using the Black-white wage gap as an indicator of the relative economic status of Black Americans in four decades from 1980 is problematic and distorts Black progress for Black families and specifically Black men. As job applicants, Black men receive fewer job offers than any other race/sex group. Neckerman and Kirschenman (1991) found that employers view inner-city Black youth as having poor skills, bad work habits, and no work ethic. Moreover, they found that addresses in large public-housing projects were a potential negative signifier as well as deeming inner-city public schools as a poor place for recruitment. Job recruitment was centered on specific neighborhoods. Fix and Struyk (1993) discovered through audit studies that discrimination that entailed the preference of white over Black applicants for employment occurred in one in every five audits with job applicants with identical qualifications. Bendick et al. (1994) found through job audits in Washington D.C. that whites were more likely to receive interviews than Black applicants; 50 percent of whites interviewed received job offers compared to 11 percent of Black interviewees; whites who were offered employment were offered higher pay compared to Black Americans who were offered employment; and Black Americans were disproportionately "steered" toward lower level positions after a job offer, while whites were disproportionately considered for higher level unadvertised positions. Black Americans are twice as likely to be unemployed compared to whites and earn 25 percent less when they are employed. Wilson (1996) discovered that a substantial number of Chicago-area employers considered inner-city Black males to be uneducated, uncooperative, unstable (unreliable), or dishonest. Black men are perceived as dangerous or threatening, thus experiencing consistent employment rejection. Black men are effectively screened out of employment opportunities in favor of white or Latino men. Moreover, Black men compete with women and immigrants in the low-wage service sector where they are the least desired.[16]

Employer's refusal to hire qualified Black male workers in desirable jobs may stem from their aversion (i.e., anti-Black misandry) to interacting with Black males, misperceptions (i.e., stereotypes) regarding productivity of Black male workers, or a fear of negative reactions from customers or current non-Black employees if Black males are hired. Employer aversion to hiring Black men has been well documented particularly in service jobs in smaller establishments that mostly serve white customers. Quillian et al. (2017) found through meta-analysis of field experiments conducted since 1989 that labor market racial discrimination against Black Americans has not declined over the past 25 years. They found no change in the level of hiring discrimination against Black Americans but found evidence of a decline in discrimination against Latino/a groups. Bertrand and Mullainathan's (2004) research discovered that people with "Black-sounding" names (e.g., Lakisha, Jamal, etc.) received 50 percent fewer callbacks for interviews compared to people with white-sounding names (e.g., Emily, Greg, etc.). In addition, they found a significant gap in sales occupations between Black men and women where Black women received significantly more callbacks than Black men (52 percent compared to 22 percent). This field experiment included responding to 1,300 employment ads with approximately 5,000 résumés in sales, administrative support, clerical, and customer services job categories. The ads that were responded to ranged from cashier work at retail establishments, clerical work in a mail room, and office and sales management positions. The number of callbacks that a "white name" generates is equivalent to an additional eight years of experience on a résumé. Racial gaps in callback were statistically indistinguishable across all the occupation and industry categories covered in the research study. Federal contractors who are thought to be heavily regulated by affirmative action laws do not treat Black résumés favorably, nor do larger employers or employers who explicitly claim that they are "Equal Opportunity Employers" and are in fact associated with a larger racial gap in callback. There was no evidence that Black Americans benefit any more than whites from living in a whiter and more educated zip code. Experience or computers skills are considered measures of job quality that do not predict the extent of the racial gap. In addition, communication or other interpersonal skills requirements have no bearing on the racial gap either. It was found that all occupation and industry categories included a positive white/Black gap in callbacks with the exception of the transportation and communication industries. The effect is Black Americans receiving relatively lower returns on their credentials, poor labor market participation, and impact on income and social mobility.[17]

Patterson and Wildeman's (2015) research on hyperincarceration and the life course indicates that the label of ex-prisoner or felon (not in prison) deprives Black males 11 years (approximately 27 percent) of their working lives (ages 18 to 64). Combined with the average time spent in prison (4 percent), Black men spent an average of approximately 31 percent of their working lives either imprisoned (in a state prison) or struggling to overcome the negative outcomes that are associated with an ex-prisoner or felon label (i.e., stigma/marked status). Pager et al. (2009) conducted a field experiment in the low-wage labor market (e.g., restaurants and independent retailers) of New York City with white, Black, and Latino male applicants with matched demographic characteristics and interpersonal skills. Black male applicants were half as likely as whites to receive a callback or job offer and fared no better than white applicants who had just been released from prison with a criminal record. This supports Pager's (2003) previous research that found that a Black male applicant with no criminal background experienced job prospects that were similar to the job prospects of a white felon.

Further research indicates that white male applicants with a criminal record actually experience greater job prospects than Black male applicants with no criminal background. This research confirms that Black maleness confers the same disadvantage as a felony conviction. Pager et al. (2009) found that white applicants received a callback or job offer 31 percent of the time, Latino applicants 25 percent, and Black applicants 15 percent. This indicated a clear racial hierarchy with white men at the top and Black men at the bottom but an overall preference for white and Latino job applicants. Previous research has indicated a consistent employer preference of Latino/a groups over Black Americans as Latino/a workers are viewed as more flexible, reliable, and hard-working. Further, their research indicated that a Black male applicant has to search twice as long for a job before receiving an employer callback or job offer compared to an equally qualified white male applicant. In addition, their research found that employers treated Black men less positively.

Three categories of discriminatory behavior stood out in their research that they referred to as categorical exclusion, shifting standards, and race-coded job channeling. Categorical exclusion entailed automatic rejection of a Black male candidate in favor of a white applicant which occurred early in the application process. Moreover, rarely did employers reveal signs of racial animus or hostility toward the Black male applicants, but race appeared to be the sole or primary criterion for employer decision-making. Shifting standards entailed a dynamic process of decision-making, where employers' evaluation of Black male applicants similar (in relation to white male applicants) qualifications or deficits are constructed through a racialized lens thus varying in relevance of the Black male applicant. Whiteness conferred the benefit of doubt even with white applicants who were recently released from prison. Race-coded job channeling moves beyond the hiring decision and focuses on job placement, where employers steer Black men toward particular job types that are often characterized by greater physical demands (hard labor) and reduced customer contact that is recognized as menial labor with less skill and customer contact. This supports Wilson's (1996) research that found that Black men were channeled into low-wage occupations that were dirty, physically demanding, and uninteresting. Further, white male applicants were sometimes encouraged by employers to apply for different jobs (i.e., upward channeling/e.g., that were typically higher-level management jobs) than the job that was advertised or the job that the white applicant had initially inquired about. This indicated that employers prefer white men for certain positions and Black men for others (i.e., downward channeling). These processes are not mutually exclusive and can operate simultaneously. Black men were held to a higher standard than white men in which they were more readily disqualified or reluctantly hired, while white men were viewed as having more potential and a better fit for more desirable jobs.[18]

Stockstill and Carson (2021) conducted two experiments on Amazon's Mechanical Turk (crowdsourcing website for business) where white participants evaluated the professional websites of fictitious job applicants with identical résumés but varied by "distinctly Black" (e.g., Tanisha & Jamal) or "indistinctly Black" names as well as race/color which included white, lighter-skinned Black, medium-skinned Black, or darker-skinned Black. The participants evaluated applicant competence, ability to be hired, promotability, and recommended a salary. What they found was an anti-Black racism that included sex-based colorism via salary recommendations where white participants offered a darker-skinned Black man with a distinctly Black name less salary while offering more salary to a darker-skinned Black woman with a distinctly Black name. Dark-skinned Tanisha received the highest salary recommendation while dark-skinned Jamal received the lowest salary recommendation. Stockstill and Carson's (2021) findings indicate how white people *value* a Black person's skills and posit that white people's anti-Black racism varies in relation to both sex and racial markers. Moreover, Howard and Borgella (2020) discovered that Black Americans are less likely to be selected for an interview or offered a job, and they are subjected to more negative evaluations compared to African immigrants. Kline et al. (2021) conducted a massive nationwide correspondence experiment that was designed to measure patterns of discrimination by large U.S. companies. Eighty-three thousand job applications were sent in response to job vacancies that were posted by 108 Fortune 500 employers. Racially distinctive Black and white names were randomly assigned to job applications. Twenty-three individual companies were found to discriminate against Black applicants, while firms in the top 20 percent of racial discrimination were responsible for nearly half of lost contacts to Black applicants (meaning half of the Black applicants were not contacted). Most firms exhibited what Kline et al. (2021) refers to as *mild discrimination* against Black applicants, and a few exhibited very large biases while all 108 firms *weakly* favored white applicants. Their findings established that systemic illegal discrimination is concentrated among specific large employers. Further, they found no significant penalty for membership in a lesbian, gay, bisexual, transgender, or queer (LGBTQ) club. Pedulla (2014) conducted an online experiment where respondents evaluated résumés for a job opening where the race and sexual orientation of the applicants were manipulated and found that gay Black men were favored over straight Black men. Gay Black applicants received higher salary recommendations than straight Black applicants. Pedulla (2014) indicated that these two different evaluations are attributed to the variation in the perceived threatening nature of the gay and straight Black male applicants.

Research from Mong and Roscigno (2010) evaluated verified employment discrimination cases from 1988 to 2003 and found that Black men experience significant discriminatory firing, on-going racial harassment, and discriminatory promotion and hiring practices. Black men were systematically targeted for oversight by supervisors. Racial stereotyping (i.e., caricatures) was often used as the justification for anti-Black misandry and gatekeepers within organizations often relied on the use of "soft skills" criteria to exclude and inhibit mobility. Moreover, they found a pattern of disparate policing and discretionary sanctioning as well as holding Black men to higher performance standards than whites followed by punitive sanctioning for policy violations that were not applied to similarly situated white employees which again served an identical function of exclusion and blocked mobility. Black male professionals continually challenge and encounter stereotypes regarding Black male inferiority. Many of these stereotypes are assessments questioning if Black men possess a thug or "ghetto-centered" mentality, or if they are violent, and whether their occupational position is a result of merited hard work. These dehumanizing assaults convey that Black men do not belong. The demonstration of intelligence or other agentic behaviors by Black male CEOs are perceived as dangerous threats to whites. Moss and Tilly's (2001) research indicates that during job interviews, Black males are viewed as lacking soft skills (lacking social skills) and less intelligent (lacking cognitive skills) than their female counterparts irrespective of their actual level of education. Wingfield (2007) found that Black professionals who are hired experience sex-based forms of racism while at work where Black men are stereotyped as angry or criminal (angry Black man or the Black criminal caricature) and Black women are stereotyped as excessively devoted to the job (the Black mammy caricature). White employers tend to view Black women as less threatening than Black men. Black male professionals consistently attempted to appear less threatening (non-threatening or militant) or angry through the surveillance of their own behavior (i.e., double-consciousness), speech, mannerisms, and general demeanor. Moreover, Black men were significantly more likely to be excluded from work-related events as well as have very few office allies compared to Black women. Black men were presumed to be intimidating and fearsome people whom coworkers preferred minimal contact with, preventing them from cultivating necessary inter-office friendships and socializing that often is essential for occupational advancement. Black women were able to vocalize and speak out regarding their treatment from colleagues' and supervisors as a result of being perceived as less threatening, while Black men were not able to unless risk eliciting the frightening and angry Black man caricature. Therefore, Black men had to repress emotions, statements, and behaviors that could be interpreted as militant, angry, or belligerent. Thus, Black men are left with very few outlets at work where they can advocate against racial hostilities and emotionally express how they have been impacted by anti-Black misandric behavior which potentially can affect their health and lives outside of work. Black men often become emotionally detached to cope at work and minimize their anger toward the anti-Black misandry they experience that is directed towards them. The implicit messaging is that Black male anger/rage toward anti-Black misandry is not legitimate (i.e., unjustified paranoia) while simultaneously reinforcing the perception that Black men are a threat and danger to the social order. Hiring related experiments indicate that anti-Black racism is both nuanced and persistent where ultimately Black men are severely punished through socioeconomic deprivation and institutional decimation. Black men are permanently removed from the labor market as they are no longer valued and needed for their labor by whites, which leads to their removal from the civilian population. Willhelm (1986) refers to this institutional decimation of Black men as conditional genocide as this structural arrangement (political economy of niggerdom) threatens the very survival of Black Americans.[19]

OCCUPATIONS

Research from Du Bois (1899) of almost 2,000 businesses with over $500 in capital discovered that the majority of these businesses evolved from occupations dictated by slavery. House servants evolved into barbers, restaurant keepers, and caterers; field hands evolved into gardeners, grocers, florists, and mill owners. Plantation craftsmen evolved into builders and contractors, brick masons, painters, and Blacksmiths. The 1890 census indicated there were 17,000 barbers, 420 hotel keepers, and 2,000 restaurant keepers. During the early 20th century; the majority of Black men (88 percent) worked in agriculture, forestry, and domestic service occupations. Black Americans were heavily concentrated in agriculture and forestry in the South while being heavily concentrated in domestic and personal service jobs outside the South. Further, the majority of Black Americans were farmers until the Great Depression of the 1930s. Franklin (1939) found that most jobs available to Black men were low-skilled and low-paying such as bricklayers, shoemakers, and butchers within various Black communities in the Southern and Northern territories during the turn of the century. Moreover, they had to compete with other working-class groups for these jobs such as immigrant European labor. Black Americans were concentrated in the lowest-paying and least skilled occupations in 1940 that included domestic service and farm positions. In the 1940s and 1950s, Black men moved out of agricultural work into blue-collar operative jobs later followed by more skilled blue-collar positions.

By the 1960s, Black men were highly concentrated in low-paying jobs such as file clerks, mail handlers, messengers and office boys, postal clerks, and sanitation labor. In 1964, only 9 percent of Black Americans held professional or managerial positions compared to approximately 25 percent of whites. Blau and Duncan's (1967) research discovered downward mobility in occupations between Black fathers and their sons than among whites. Black males appeared to be destined to end up in the lower manual sector of the economy regardless of their father's occupational standing. According to Hamilton et al. (2011), 87 percent of U.S. occupations can be classified as racially segregated for Black men that is not a result of racial differences in occupational preferences. Black males are overrepresented in 38 percent of certain occupations and underrepresented in 49 percent of other occupations. Black male workers are denied employment in more desirable high-wage occupations (particularly in management and professional occupations) and crowded into less-desirable low-wage occupations. They are underrepresented as chief executives and legislators and are employed at only 32 percent of their expected level of employment in these occupations.

Black males are severely underrepresented in construction, extraction, and maintenance occupations. Almost 50 percent of working Black men are represented in the two occupational groups of *Service and Production* and *Transportation and Material Moving*. These two occupational clusters have the lowest earnings. Black men are significantly underrepresented in the *Management* and *Professional* category. The occupational clustering of Black men in the lower wage categories has not changed in two decades; therefore, they are more likely to be absorbed into low-skill, low-wages, and low-status occupations. Black men represent 31 percent of security guards, 22 percent of personal care aids, and 21 percent of couriers and messengers.[20]

INCOME/WAGE

According to Piketty (2014), income inequality from labor in the U.S. is at an unprecedented level, which has not been seen anywhere in the world at any point in history. For every dollar paid to white men, Black men are paid 51 cents, Latinas are paid 55 cents, Native American women are paid 60 cents, Black women are paid 63 cents, white women are paid 79 cents, Asian American women are paid 87 cents, Native American men are paid 91 cents, Latino men are paid 91 cents, and Asian American men are paid $1.15. The evolution from an industrial to an information economy over the last half-century is routinely provided as an explanation for the wage inequality experienced by Black men. Card and DiNardo (2002) found that this skill-biased technological change (SBTC) hypothesis, associated with new computer technologies, fails to explain sex and racial wage gaps. A persistent feature of the U.S. labor market entails a large gap in the relative earnings of Black and white men since the end of slavery. Black men are paid a wage that denotes their skills are less than they actually are, which points to a race- and sex-specific price penalty and is theft of their labor. The median Black-white earnings gap narrowed from 1940 to the mid-1970s but has since significantly grown to where it was in 1950. Thus, the relative position of Black men in the earning's distribution has remained essentially constant. Black men would have achieved parity by the year 2020 had the narrowing rate of 1950 to 1980 continued. There has been little change in the economic gap between Black Americans and whites since the 1970s. In 1978, Black households earned 59 cents for every dollar earned by whites (median household income), and very little has changed since that time. It fell as low as almost 55 cents in 1982 due to substantial changes in national social and economic policies and did not return to at least 59 cents until the early 1990s. The narrowing of the Black-white income gap and the expansion of the Black middle-class was greatest in the 1960s and this economic progress was halted in the mid-1970s.[21]

Since 1960, the Black-white family income ratios have remained in a relatively narrow band between 60 and 64 percent. Therefore, the Black-white per capita income ratios have experienced very little change for more than a century as Black income was 59 percent of white income in 1880. Black men earn considerably less income than whites at comparable levels of education. Darity et al. (1997) found that the dramatic increase in literacy rates among Black males between 1880 and 1910 simultaneously coincided with proportionate losses in occupational status due to discriminatory treatment. Further, Darity et al. (2001) discovered that labor market discrimination and imposed schooling deficits experienced by Black Americans between 1880 and 1910 significantly weighed down the occupational attainment of their descendants a century later in 1980 and 1990. The median household income of Black Americans is $39,500, while the median household income of whites is $65,000. The Black-white income gap is entirely driven by large differences in wages and employment rates between Black and white men that do not exist between Black and white women. Real earnings have fallen by 19 percent for the median white man from $52,200 in 1970 to $42,100 in 2014, while it has fallen 32 percent for the median Black man from $30,800 in 1970 to $21,000 in 2014. Chachere and Chachere (1990) found that from 1929 to 1969, whites gained $1.6 trillion due to labor market discrimination where 40 percent of racial income inequality was attributable to discrimination. Chetty et al. (2018) reviewed de-identified longitudinal data that covered almost the entire U.S. population from 1989 to 2015 for their research on the sources of racial and ethnic disparities in income and found that family characteristic differences such as parental marital status, education, and wealth as well as differences in ability do little to explain the Black-white income gap and the lack of intergenerational mobility of Black men. The Black-white income gap persisted even among boys who grew up in the same neighborhood resulting in downward mobility for Black males. Black boys who grew up in the same geographic areas (include growing up on the same block) as white boys and in families with comparable incomes had lower incomes in adulthood compared to white boys in 99 percent of Census tracts, making them the least likely of any group to experience upward social mobility leading to profound income disparities that persist across generations.[22]

Twenty-three percent of Black men are employed in the public sector, while 77 percent are employed in the private sector. Grodsky and Pager (2001) found that occupations with large racial gaps in wages were client-based professions in the private sector that relied upon social networks for success. Many of these occupations relied on developing a profitable clientele for success and included securities and financial services, insurance sales, managers in properties and real estate, actuaries, lawyers, and physicians. Grodsky and Pager (2001) posit that Black Americans and whites in the same occupations likely have segregated social networks where whites benefit from access to a wealthier pool of potential white clients. Which can contribute to the earning disparities between white and Black men in the same high-earning occupations. In addition, whites are able to advance in their companies by using intra-company social and business relationships with white peers and superiors, while Black Americans have to primarily rely on their educational credentials and job performance to attempt to professionally advance. Assari et al. (2021) found that higher levels of income provide protection for white men against perceived discrimination but not for Black men who, regardless of their income levels, perceived higher levels of discrimination. Educational attainment and household income are socioeconomic status (SES) indicators that protect most populations from poor health but returns from SES are significantly smaller for Black Americans compared to whites, a phenomenon referred to as minorities' diminishing returns (MDRs), or the Black tax, which refers to the hidden costs of being Black in America. Race/ethnicity is a fixed identifier for discrimination regardless of social position. It is not uncommon for high-SES Black Americans to report more experiences of racial discrimination due to increased contact with whites. Increasing income and educational attainment does not protect the physical and mental health of Black men against adverse health outcomes. In addition, SES and racial discrimination directed towards Black men may be more pronounced as they are routinely the primary target of discrimination by white people.[23]

WEALTH

Wealth data has become more accessible in recent decades. Prior to wealth data becoming available, racial inequity was mainly viewed from income inequality. Racial identity for Black households is a stronger predictor of wealth attainment than occupational sector.

Black Americans are not able to earn themselves out of the racial/lineage wealth gap. Income refers to the periodic flow of resources, while wealth (net worth) refers to the stock of financial resources (assets minus debts) and is an indicator of family financial security. But it is important to note that whites are able to use white debt (i.e., promotes agency and opportunities for future investment for positive outcomes) as an asset that represents an agreement between whites and financial industries, where each party gains materially while Black debt (i.e., higher interest with lower returns and negative outcomes) represent a negative balance sheet that must be prioritized and addressed. The extractive mechanism of Black debt converts assets into white wealth (i.e., racial capitalism). White wealth is preserved through the stock market, banks, corporations, foundation tax havens, associations, and elite schools. Whites and Black Americans are stratified into the economy in a vastly different manner. Anti-Black racism (i.e., racial caste) ensures that Black Americans experience debt as crushing, and whites experience it as an opportunity. Wealth typically is a more stable indicator of a family's economic position compared to income. Wealth provides a more complete measure of household capability and functioning than income, which is more limited. Wealth and income are poorly correlated for Black households compared to white households. In addition, income is a weak analysis of racial inequality in comparison to wealth and an inadequate indicator of economic well-being, mobility, and security but is used by researchers, practitioners, advocates, and policymakers to describe local economic conditions and influence policy decisions. Income assists families to cover their current expenses, while wealth provides them with the opportunity to make investments in a home, education, or business. Greater financial security and stability is achieved the more that wealth is passed down from generation to generation, which has the effect of asset accumulation over time. The cumulative effect of wealth across generations (intergenerational transfers) provides families with greater financial resources to make wealth transfers to offspring along with the purchase of assets that increase wealth. Wealth offers better opportunities for future generations by allowing families to make investments in homes, education, child well-being, and business development. In addition, it provides economic security that cultivates the ability to take risks and shield against financial loss over a lifetime. Common assets include savings accounts, stocks and bonds, retirement accounts, and property. This affords families with the ability to pay for unexpected expenses or address budgetary shortfalls without having to rely on friends or familial networks, credit cards, or predatory lenders such as payday loan sites and other financiers that charge exorbitant interest rates, thus thwarting hardship in the long-term. Wealth can assist in averting a financial crisis such as a car breaking down, losing a job, or medical needs, as well as the stress/health-related consequences.[24]

Black families who have higher incomes often have greater transfer demands from their less-well-off kin networks, which contributes to a reduction in resources earmarked for savings compared to their white peers. Wealth in the U.S. is grossly unequally distributed and in contrast to income is starkly more unevenly distributed. Income is not a key determinant of wealth and is primarily earned in the labor market, while wealth is created by the transfer of resources across generations that includes the maintenance of higher wealth positions among parents and grandparents for their children and grandchildren. Ninety percent of Black Americans were enslaved until Emancipation. They were a source of wealth for whites but were deprived of the capacity to acquire wealth themselves. Fifty-six percent of all wealth in the U.S. was owned by the upper 5 percent of all wealth holders by the mid-1980s. Moreover, the top 1 percent of the wealth distribution possessed approximately a 39 percent share, while the bottom 40 percent held only 0.2 percent of the nation's wealth. Home equity generally is the most significant component of wealth for most Americans with positive net worth. The bottom 80 percent of wealth holders obtained 66 percent of their net worth from home equity. This contrasts with the top 1 percent of wealth holders whose net worth generated by home ownership is only 6 percent. The majority of their portfolios consists of a wide array of financial assets. Further, approximately 13 percent of the nation's financial assets are held by the bottom 90 percent of the wealth distribution. The primary sources of personal wealth in the U.S. are a combination of *in vivo* transfers (e.g., gifts living parents give to adult children) of wealth and inheritance. Inheritances tend to be significantly larger, but *in vivo* transfers are pivotal as wealth-maintaining and wealth-increasing mechanisms due to the timing of such transfers during the course of the life cycle. Affluent parents have multiple avenues that can boost their children's prospects such as gifts of superior education, cultural experiences, and social contacts that can translate into higher salaries and increased saving. In addition, exposure and comfort with different investments can be cultivated by their financial knowledge they instill in their children. These intergenerational transfers take place during markers of important events such as college admission, graduation, marriage, and the birth of children, grandchildren's schooling, and include the purchase of a first home. The intergenerational transfers of wealth (*in vivo* and inheritances) are pivotal to the preservation of racialized economic stratification in the U.S. and a link that connects the present with the racialized past of enslavement, extermination, and expropriation. Moreover, the racial/lineage wealth gap is a reminder of the U.S. white supremacist legacy as well as its continual future reproduction. Intergenerational wealth transfers (*in vivo* and bequests) contribute between 50–80 percent of the wealth position of subsequent generations. Inherited wealth (non-merit resources) provides additional resources for education, insurance against emergencies, greater opportunities for self-employment and business ownership, ability to reside in higher-amenity neighborhoods, access to better legal representation, and the political influence to protect one's self-interests. The racial/lineage wealth chasm is primarily comprised of inheritances, bequests, and intra-family transfers than any other demographic and socioeconomic indicators such as education, income, and household structure.[25]

The wealth/lineage gap is a defining feature of America's racial divide that spawned the historic anti-Black discrimination and present-day suffering of Black Americans. Black Americans have considerably less wealth than whites, which is linked to slavery and historic discrimination. Mortgages were created to subsidize the slave trade and during enslavement, Black Americans constituted property for others and were not allowed to acquire property of their own. During Emancipation, the U.S. government failed to compensate Black Americans for their enslavement and provide a property base as they were propertyless. This includes the denial of the promised 40 acres and a mule (Sherman's Special Field Orders No. 15). By the start of the 20th century, Black Americans were able to acquire 15 million acres of land that was located primarily in the South through an extraordinary feat of effort and perseverance. But a progressive decumulation of Black-owned land from 1920 on through outright seizure by white terrorists, fraud, theft, and the manipulative use of partition sales tactics by whites with the intention to appropriate the property took form. Thus, literally destroying the foundation of wealth in the Black community over the course of the 20th century. Black Americans possessed about one million acres of land in the South by the 1980s. Black Americans have a significantly smaller stock of wealth due to this sustained historical pattern of deprivation of the capacity to accumulate property, specifically land. In addition, seizure of Black-owned land and other property by whites became a common action. There are at least 406 cases documented of Black landowners who had 24,000 acres of farms and timberland stolen from them during the first three decades of the 20th century.

These 406 cases could be established due to existing records but is a limitation as the perpetrators of Black property theft often included the collusion of local, state, and even the federal government in their efforts to defraud Black Americans of their property. Evidence of Black land ownership illegally obtained by white terrorists often would be destroyed in wholesale burnings of courthouses, Black churches, and homes. During Jim/Jane Crow, night riding white terrorists would confiscate land from vulnerable Black Americans. There are 239 cases recorded in Mississippi alone between the years of 1890 and 1910. Moreover, lynching across the U.S. entailed stolen property from lynching victims and their families who were landowners. Jim/Jane Crowism at its height was an engine for the destruction of Black wealth that included the literal annihilation of prosperous Black communities, including Danville, Virginia, in 1883; Wilmington, N. Carolina, in 1898; Atlanta, Georgia, in 1906; Tulsa, Oklahoma, in 1921; and throughout Florida in the 1910s and 1920s (e.g., Rosewood, etc.). In addition, fraudulent and semi-fraudulent legal means were used to appropriate Black-owned land during the period of Jim/Jane Crow and beyond. Partition sales were used as a primary method to de-cumulate Black-owned property. Urban renewal or highway expansion would later become a mechanism to abolish Black-owned commercial districts. The U.S. economy has functioned as an instrument of routinized destruction of Black wealth and maintenance of a racial/lineage income gap causing socioeconomic deprivation that severely impacts Black Americans who are descendants of U.S. enslavement.[26]

Middle-class wealth significantly declined under the Obama presidency, and the average wealth of the bottom 99 percent decreased by $4,500 between 2007–2016, which was especially concentrated among the housing wealth of Black Americans. Moreover, the top 1 percent's average wealth increased by $4.9 million during this time. The decline in wealth was a direct result of policies enacted by President Barack Obama. President Obama's housing policies regarding foreclosures led to millions of families losing their homes with Black families suffering particularly harsh losses and was a disastrous failure. Obama had the ability to sharply ameliorate the foreclosure crisis and even prevent it and chose not to use the power, money, legislative tools, and legal leverage he had at his disposal. The homeownership rate during the Obama presidency crashed by 4 percentage points, which ultimately erased the increase of the mortgage bubble, and the homeownership rate fell to its lowest level since 1965 before a slight rebound. This was the greatest destruction of middle-class wealth since the Great Depression that disproportionately impacted Black wealth. There was a strong demand for subprime mortgages because of the mortgage bubble that specifically preyed upon and victimized Black families. Subprime loans were disproportionately handed out to Black lower-income people who were not in a financial position to pay them back by mortgage originators who also steered Black middle-class families into subprime loans who would have qualified for ordinary mortgages. Practices that harken back to Jim/Jane Crow and redlining where contract sellers would brutally prey (contract for deed) on and exploit Black families that managed to scrape together enough money to buy a house by loading them up with unpayable fees, repossessing the house, and repeating this process on the next unsuspecting Black family. Black families in Chicago who were presented with a "contract for deed" arrangement were overcharged between $3.2 billion and $4 billion (2019 dollars) between the years of 1950 to 1970. The real estate agents and investors were almost exclusively white who profited from what amounts to a direct transfer of wealth. Former Wells Fargo employees indicated that the bank deliberately deceived middle-class Black families whom they referred to as "mud people" into subprime "ghetto loans." From 2004–2008, 21 percent of Black borrowers with a credit score of 660 and up received subprime mortgages, while 6 percent of white borrowers with a credit score of 660 and up received a subprime mortgage. The percentage of Black homeowners with negative equity exploded from 0.7 percent to 14 percent and continued to increase through 2013 unlike white families. Home ownership makes up a significantly larger percentage of Black wealth than it does white wealth as well as contributing to a larger percentage of middle-class wealth in all racial groups. Leading up to the recession, middle-class families held 50 percent to 70 percent of their wealth in home equity while the wealthiest 10 percent of families held 15 to 30 percent of their wealth in home equity, and the top 10 percent of white families held approximately 15 percent of their wealth in housing. The wealthiest 10 percent of white families saw their wealth increase by an average of $1.2 million (approximately 22 percent) followed by the next wealthiest 10 percent of white families who increased their net worth by an average of $141,000 (approximately 16 percent) between 2007 and 2016. Obama's response was to bail out financial assets while allowing homeowners to drown, which resulted in further national wealth concentration into the hands of the richest white families. In fact, Obama received an inheritance from his white grandmother when she died in late 2008 valued at almost $500,000. His grandmother left him stock in the Bank of Hawaii. The side effects of the foreclosure crisis on the rest of the economy included people being at greater risk of job loss and falling into poverty, psychological problems such as suicide, and nearby homes losing value because of damaged and blighted foreclosed properties, which causes declines in tax revenues. It is estimated that properties in proximity to a foreclosure lost $2.2 trillion in value, and half of this loss was in Black and brown communities. *The Color of Wealth in Los Angeles* (2016) reviewed data on assets and debts among subpopulations according to race, ethnicity, and country of origin. What they found was that white households in L.A. had a median net worth (wealth) of $355,000; U.S. Blacks (Black Americans/descendants of U.S. enslavement), $4,000; Mexicans, $3,500; Japanese, $592,000; Asian Indian, $460,000; Chinese, $408,200; African Blacks (African immigrants), $72,000; other Latino/a groups, $42,500; Koreans, $23,400; Vietnamese, $61,500; and Filipinos, $243,000. Black Americans and Mexican households had 1 percent of the wealth of whites in L.A. The median liquid assets of white households were $110,000; Black Americans, $200; Mexicans, $0; other Latino/a groups, $7; and African immigrants, $60,000.[27]

White families in the U.S. hold 90 percent of the national wealth, Latino/a families hold 2.3 percent of the national wealth, and Black families hold approximately 2 percent of the national wealth. Black Americans have gone from a nearly wealthless group (0.5 percent of wealth) during the Emancipation Proclamation (1863) to only approximately 2 percent of the total U.S. wealth over a 150 years later, while whites have increased their wealth many times over during this period and almost doubled their wealth ($63 trillion to $115 trillion) in the past decade. Black households have approximately seven cents for every dollar held by white households. This becomes one cent if the household car is removed from the net worth calculation. The white household living near the poverty line has approximately $18,000 in wealth, while Black households near the poverty line have approximately a median wealth of almost zero. Thus, many Black families have a negative net worth. In addition, the poorest white households (lowest 20 percent of the income distribution) have a greater median wealth than all Black households combined. The median Black family has $24,100 in wealth, while median white family (approximately 42 million white households) has $188,200 in wealth. Contrasting Black and white wealth at the mean (average household) indicates that Black households have $142,500 in wealth, while white households have $983,400 in wealth. Ninety-nine percent of white wealth is held by households with a net worth above the national median (approximately $100,000). Only a mere 4 percent of Black households have a net worth in excess of $1 million in contrast to 25 percent of white households. This is in contrast to the nearly 50 percent of

Black households (approximately 10 million Black households) that have a zero or negative net worth. Black households on the other end of the American economic spectrum constitute approximately 2 percent in the top 1 percent of the nation's wealth distribution, while 96 percent of the wealthiest Americans are constituted by white households. The 99th percentile white family is worth over 12 million dollars, while the 99th percentile Black family is worth merely $1,574,000. This translates to 870,000 white families having a net worth above 12 million dollars, while fewer than 380,000 Black families (approximately 2 percent) out of the 20 million Black families in the U.S. are even worth a single million dollars. While only 5 percent of Black families (1 million Black homes) have more than $350,000 in net worth, which puts them into the 95th percentile of Black wealth, while this amount of net worth puts white families in the 72nd percentile of white wealth. In contrast, over 25 million white families have more than $600,000 in net worth, and another 13 million white families out of the 85 million white families in the U.S. are millionaires or more. Black Americans constitute approximately 13 percent of the U.S. population but collectively own approximately 2 percent of the nation's total wealth. Approximately 73 percent of whites own a home compared to 42 percent of Black Americans. White homeowning households have approximately $140,000 more in net worth than comparable Black homeowning households. Black non-homeowning households have $120 in net worth. The average white household with a head who has a college degree has $268,000 in wealth compared to a Black household with a comparable educated head, who has $70,000 in wealth. The Wall Street Journal (2021) reported that the median net worth of Black households with college graduates who are in their thirties has fallen over the past three decades from $50,400 to $8,200, while their white peers median net worth grew 17 percent to $138,000. The white parents of the baby boomer generation who accumulated considerable wealth due to the assistance of the Federal Housing Administration (FHA), home mortgage interest deduction, and other governmental policies passed to their adult children the largest wealth transfer in U.S. history. In addition, boomers received a massive wealth transfer from the government in the amount of $129 trillion due to government policy since the 1980s. This will be passed down to millennials over the next 30 years in what is being referred to as the *Great Wealth Transfer*. Millennials will be five times wealthier by 2030 than they are today. White household wealth is 20 times that of Black Americans. It was reported by the federal government that U.S. household wealth increased to a record $136.9 trillion due to rising equity markets that added to household assets as well as rising real estate values that contributed to an overall U.S. household wealth increase of $5 trillion. White America has $115 trillion of this amount, which has almost doubled since 2010 ($63 trillion), while Black America has only $6.33 trillion.[28]

Immigrant groups such as Jewish, West Indian, Japanese, and Chinese Americans are distinguished by class background and not national culture. The socioeconomic origins of immigrants reflect lateral rather than *upward* mobility. The wealth position of specific immigrant groups is influenced by their socioeconomic status prior to entering the U.S. After the passage of the 1965 Immigration Act, the majority of immigrants who have come to the U.S. are highly educated, possess higher levels of wealth than the average American, and are highly skilled professionals who tend to hold jobs with higher-earning levels. The economic achievement of Japanese Americans is due to selective immigration, return migration, family formation that is combined with intergenerational transmission of socioeconomic status. The Vietnamese are an exception as they came to the U.S. as refugees usually with limited financial resources. An example of this juxtaposition is the relatively better economic status of African immigrants compared to Black Americans. This is further elucidated by the wealth position outcomes of more successful Asian Indian and Chinese households compared to their Vietnamese counterparts. *The Color of Wealth in Miami* (2019) found that the median wealth of white households was estimated at $107,000; Black Americans, $3,700; Puerto Ricans, $3,940; South Americans, $1,200; other Latino/a groups, $10,500; Caribbean Blacks, $12,000; and Cubans, $22,000. The median liquid assets of white households were $10,750; Black Americans, $11; Puerto Ricans, $200; Caribbean Blacks and South Americans, $2,000; Cubans, $3,200; and other Latino/a groups, $5,000. Latino/a census respondents self-classified as either racially white or "other," while a small percentage chose a Black racial identity which proved to be more predictive of socioeconomic position as Black Latino/a groups fared worse economically. *The Color of Wealth in Boston* (2015) found that the median wealth of white households was $247,500; Black Americans, $8; Dominicans, $0; Caribbean Blacks, $12,000; Puerto Ricans, $3,020; and other Latino/a groups, $2,700. The median liquid assets of white households were $25,000; Black Americans $670; Dominicans $150; Caribbean Blacks $3,500; Puerto Ricans $20; Cape Verdeans $150; and other Latino/a groups $700. *The Color of Wealth in the Nation's Capital* (2016) found that the median wealth of white households was $284,000; Black Americans, $3,500; African immigrants, $3,000; Latino/a groups, $13,000; Chinese, $220,000; Koreans, $496,000; Vietnamese, $423,000; and Asian Indians, $573,000. The median liquid assets of white households were $65,000; Black Americans, $5,000; African Immigrants, $2,100; Latino/a groups, $2,700; Chinese, $30,000; Koreans, $32,000; Vietnamese, $75,000; and Asian Indians, $22,000. The liquids assets include their vehicles and is pre-COVID-19 data, which has disproportionately impacted Black Americans and Latino/a groups. These reports are the first of their kind to disaggregate wealth data between Black Americans with a lineage of U.S. enslavement and Black immigrants. In addition, Brown (2016) found that the majority of Black home (brownstone) owners in Harlem and Brooklyn are disproportionally West Indian. The data from these reports highlight how Black Americans and Black immigrants are racialized differently in the U.S. in relation to wealth and overall stratification.[29]

Darity et al. (2021) has called for wealth to be used as a standard for identification of middle-class status as empirical identification of the middle-class has been through markers of income, occupational status, and educational attainment. Wealth establishes a superior standard for the distinction of the middle-class and can be useful for identification of the middle-class within subaltern (i.e., marginalized) communities. The concept of the middle-class and its associated characteristics in U.S. society is a white-centered narrative. To be middle-class in the Black community based on the Black wealth distribution is the equivalent of wealth poverty based on U.S. wealth distribution standards.

Black Americans are marked at birth in the U.S racial caste system as inequalities persists over the life course where educational attainment and labor market returns almost never translate into wealth related social mobility. The 100 richest people in America control more wealth than the entire Black population (46 million Black Americans). In addition, Jeff Bezos net worth is $211 billion, while Black America combined has $270 billion in private business wealth. White America is worth $115 trillion with 20 percent ($23 trillion) of it only in pensions, while Black America is worth $6.33 trillion with nearly 41 percent of it in pensions and 35 percent in real estate primarily held by baby boomer retirees. White America has $11.33 trillion in private business in contrast to the $270 billion in private business wealth that is held by Black America. White America has $29.98 trillion in corporate equities and mutual fund shares, while Black America has $370 billion in corporate equities and mutual fund shares. White America has $4.88 trillion in just consumer durables (e.g., family car, blankets, clothes, TVs, couches, etc.), while Black America has $400 billion in consumer durables, but white America's wealth in consumer durables is close to the overall wealth ($6.33 trillion) of Black America. White America has nearly $50 trillion just in liquid wealth (e.g., corporate equities and mutual fund shares, private businesses, and other assets), while Black America has approximately $800 billion in liquid wealth. White America has $115 trillion in wealth, while Black America has $6.33 trillion in wealth; not only is this insignificant in comparison to white wealth, but 41 percent of this figure are pensions. There are a total of 85 million white households in the U.S. along with 20 million Black households, which is a 1:4 ratio. The 2 percent of wealth that is owned by Black America in the U.S. is owned by the top 20 percent of Black families who control over 80 percent of this 2 percent of wealth. And as previously mentioned, the bottom 50 percent of Black America has negative net worth. The majority of Black businesses have only one employee, and business ownership is so infinitesimal that it barely registers on the landscape of corporate America where only 2 percent of U.S. businesses are Black-owned. The 2.58 million Black-owned U.S. businesses generated $150 billion in total revenues in 2016. Walmart in contrast grossed $480 billion in total revenues during the same year. Further, Walmart employed 2.2 million more employees than the entire Black Enterprise Top 100 Black-owned firms. The total assets of the five largest Black-owned banks were $2.3 billion, while the total assets of JPMorgan Chase were $2.2 trillion; the Black-owned banks total assets were approximately 0.1 percent of the total assets of JPMorgan Chase. In addition, the five top landowners (Ted Turner, etc.) in the U.S. together own more land than all of Black America combined.[30]

Winship et al. (2021) conducted an analysis of the Black-white gap in intergenerational poverty across three generations. Poverty was defined as being in the bottom fifth of the income distribution. They found that Black families were 16 times more likely to experience three generations of poverty than white families. Three-generation poverty is experienced by one in five Black adults compared to one in 100 whites. Forty-one percent of Black Americans are more likely to be in third-generation poverty than white adults are to be poor. The grandparents of Black adults had significantly lower incomes than the grandparents of white adults. This is coupled with lower rates of subsequent Black upward mobility out of poverty and significant Black downward mobility. Thus, significant differential family poverty trajectories are formed between Black and white adults. Just 8 percent of poor whites in the bottom fifth of the income distribution had parents and grandparents who were also poor compared to half (51 percent) of Black Americans. Sixty-five percent of Black Americans had a poor grandparent among all Black Americans and whites in their late thirties. Eighty-three percent of Black Americans are in their third generation of poverty compared to 17 percent of whites among all Black and white adults who are in their third generation of poverty. It is rare for white Americans to inherit poverty across multiple generations, while it is common among Black Americans. Sharkey (2009) found that among Americans born between 1955 to 1970; 62 percent of Black Americans grew up in neighborhoods where at least a fifth of residents were poor compared to 4 percent of whites. Sixty-six percent of Black Americans born between 1985 and 2000 compared to 6 percent of whites grew up in such neighborhoods 30 years later. In addition, Black Americans account for more than 40 percent (225,735) of the homeless population (567,715) and 52 percent of all of the homeless families even though they make up 13 percent of the general U.S. population. Men account for 70 percent of the homeless population as well as unaccompanied male youth (Racial Inequalities in Homelessness, by the Numbers, 2020).

The median wealth of Black Americans is predicted to fall to zero by the year 2053. Common myths that proliferate the discourse on the racial/lineage wealth gap in the U.S. include conventional ideas regarding greater educational attainment, harder work, racial homeownership, buying and banking Black, Black people saving more, greater financial literacy/better financial decisions, entrepreneurship, emulating successful racialized/minoritized groups, improved "soft skills," and "personal responsibility" – all will close the racial/lineage wealth gap, while the growing numbers of Black celebrities demonstrate that the racial/

lineage wealth gap is closing, and Black family disorganization is the cause of the racial/ lineage wealth gap. Although some of these ideas and recommendations can be helpful to most people, they are grossly inadequate to address the racial chasm in wealth. In addition, these myths point to dysfunctional Black behaviors (Black pathology) as the cause of incessant racial inequality that includes the Black-white wealth disparity. Black Americans cannot close the racial/lineage wealth gap by altering their individual behavior (i.e., assuming "personal responsibility" or acquiring "financial literacy" and the associated portfolio management insights) if the structural sources of racial inequality remain unchanged. There are no unilateral actions that Black Americans can take that will have a significant effect on reducing the racial/lineage wealth gap. These myths and harmful narratives along with unequal access to assets contributes to the maintenance of our nation's underlying economic structure.[31]

It was revealed that 93 percent of neighborhoods in major U.S. cities were unaffordable to the majority of local Black residents at the beginning of the COVID pandemic. Only 7 percent of zip codes in the top 100 metro areas had rents that were affordable to Black residents, while 69 percent were affordable to white residents. The majority of the zip codes that were affordable to Black households were areas that suffered from disinvestment and lacked high-quality schools, clean air, parks, safe streets, and good jobs and were classified as *low opportunity* neighborhoods. Wealth is now calcified inside of whiteness where there does not need to be explicit everyday actions taken by whites (e.g., picketing Black Americans moving into white neighborhoods or Black Americans being allowed to attend private schools, etc.) that keep Black Americans out of specific neighborhoods or from having access to any wealth generating mechanisms as Black people are simply locked out of wealth, which prevents them from accessing housing, employment, education, health care, etc. Therefore, whites can appear as non-racists, while their wealth does their bidding. Further, the costs of living in America are set by white wealth. Black Americans were the labor and the currency that white Americans used to create wealth. In 1860 there were 4 million enslaved Black Americans worth approximately $3.5 billion, which made them the single largest financial asset in the entire U.S. economy and was worth more than all of the railroads and manufacturing combined. But later Black wealth was destroyed and positioned where Blackness became a contagion to wealth accumulation. The cause of the racial/lineage wealth gap can be found in structural characteristics of the American economy.[32]

The U.S. will have to undergo a comprehensive social transformation through the adoption of bold national policies that address the long-standing consequences of slavery, Jim/Jane Crow years that followed, and ongoing present-day societal anti-Black racism and discrimination. Black wealth will need to be built through a significant redistributive effort or a major public policy intervention that addresses racial/lineage wealth inequality. Greater wealth distribution in the U.S. would spur economic growth nationally and regionally. This could be in the form of a specific transformational reparations program for the descendants of U.S enslavement that incorporates compensation for the legacies of slavery and Jim/Jane Crow.

* Wealth data includes the family car, and if you remove it from wealth calculations, Black wealth is disproportionately altered.

NOTES

1 Marcin, 2018; Stewart & Scott, 1978; Darity, 1988; Marable, 1983; Pettit, 2012; Beckett, 1997; Western, 2006; Gilmore, 1999.

2 Marcin, 2018; Stewart & Scott, 1978; Darity, 1988; Marable, 1983; Pettit, 2012; Beckett, 1997; Western, 2006; Gilmore, 1999.

3 Marcin, 2018; Stewart & Scott, 1978; Darity, 1988; Marable, 1983; Pettit, 2012; Beckett, 1997; Western, 2006; Gilmore, 1999.

4 Marcin, 2018; Stewart & Scott, 1978; Darity, 1988; Marable, 1983; Pettit, 2012; Beckett, 1997; Western, 2006; Gilmore, 1999.

5 Marcin, 2018; Stewart & Scott, 1978; Darity, 1988; Marable, 1983; Pettit, 2012; Beckett, 1997; Western, 2006; Gilmore, 1999.

6 Marcin, 2018; Stewart & Scott, 1978; Darity, 1988; Marable, 1983; Pettit, 2012; Beckett, 1997; Western, 2006; Gilmore, 1999.

7 Marcin, 2018; Stewart & Scott, 1978; Darity, 1988; Marable, 1983; Pettit, 2012; Beckett, 1997; Western, 2006; Gilmore, 1999.

8 Marcin, 2018; Stewart & Scott, 1978; Darity, 1988; Marable, 1983; Pettit, 2012; Beckett, 1997; Western, 2006; Gilmore, 1999.

9 Marcin, 2018; Stewart & Scott, 1978; Darity, 1988; Marable, 1983; Pettit, 2012; Beckett, 1997; Western, 2006; Gilmore, 1999.

10 Marcin, 2018; Stewart & Scott, 1978; Darity, 1988; Marable, 1983; Pettit, 2012; Beckett, 1997; Western, 2006; Gilmore, 1999.

11 Ogungbure, 2019; Baradaran, 2018; Donaldson, 2015; Du Bois, 1903.

12 Ogungbure, 2019; Baradaran, 2018; Donaldson, 2015; Du Bois, 1903.

13 Toossi & Joyner, 2018; Byars-Winston et al., 2015; Alexis, 1998; Williams & Collins, 2004; Gottschalk, 1997; Darity & Myers, 1995; Darity et al., 1996, 1997; Testa et al., 1993; Wilson & Neckerman, 1986; Bishop, 1980; Mare & Winship, 1991; Wilson, 1987, 1996; Fairlie & Sundstrom, 1999; Chetty et al., 2018; Bayer & Charles, 2018; Western & Pettit, 2005; Western, 2006; Pettit, 2012; Pager, 2007; Holzer & Offner, 2006; Holzer, 1996, 2007; Pinkney, 1984; Staples, 1985; Field & Winfrey, 1997; Smith et al., 2011; Wingfield, 2007; St. Jean & Feagin, 1998; Willhelm, 1986; Livingston & Pearce, 2009; Kirschenman & Neckerman, 1991; Waldinger, 1997; Waldinger & Lichter, 2003; Pager, 2007.

14 Toossi & Joyner, 2018; Byars-Winston et al., 2015; Alexis, 1998; Williams & Collins, 2004; Gottschalk, 1997; Darity & Myers, 1995; Darity et al., 1996, 1997; Testa et al., 1993; Wilson & Neckerman, 1986; Bishop, 1980; Mare & Winship, 1991; Wilson, 1987, 1996; Fairlie & Sundstrom, 1999; Chetty et al., 2018; Bayer & Charles, 2018; Western & Pettit, 2005; Western, 2006; Pettit, 2012; Pager, 2007; Holzer & Offner, 2006; Holzer, 1996, 2007; Pinkney, 1984; Staples, 1985; Field & Winfrey, 1997; Smith et al., 2011; Wingfield, 2007; St. Jean & Feagin, 1998; Willhelm, 1986; Livingston & Pearce, 2009; Kirschenman & Neckerman, 1991; Waldinger, 1997; Waldinger & Lichter, 2003; Pager, 2007.

15 Toossi & Joyner, 2018; Byars-Winston et al., 2015; Alexis, 1998; Williams & Collins, 2004; Gottschalk, 1997; Darity & Myers, 1995; Darity et al., 1996, 1997; Testa et al., 1993; Wilson & Neckerman, 1986; Bishop, 1980; Mare & Winship, 1991; Wilson, 1987, 1996; Fairlie & Sundstrom, 1999; Chetty et al., 2018; Bayer & Charles, 2018; Western & Pettit, 2005; Western, 2006; Pettit, 2012; Pager, 2007; Holzer & Offner, 2006; Holzer, 1996, 2007; Pinkney, 1984; Staples, 1985; Field & Winfrey, 1997; Smith et al., 2011; Wingfield, 2007; St. Jean & Feagin, 1998; Willhelm, 1986; Livingston & Pearce, 2009; Kirschenman & Neckerman, 1991; Waldinger, 1997; Waldinger & Lichter, 2003; Pager, 2007.

16 Toossi & Joyner, 2018; Byars-Winston et al., 2015; Alexis, 1998; Williams & Collins, 2004; Gottschalk, 1997; Darity & Myers, 1995; Darity et al., 1996, 1997; Testa et al., 1993; Wilson & Neckerman, 1986; Bishop, 1980; Mare & Winship, 1991; Wilson, 1987, 1996; Fairlie & Sundstrom, 1999; Chetty et al., 2018; Bayer & Charles, 2018; Western & Pettit, 2005; Western, 2006; Pettit, 2012; Pager, 2007; Holzer & Offner, 2006; Holzer, 1996, 2007; Pinkney,

1984; Staples, 1985; Field & Winfrey, 1997; Smith et al., 2011; Wingfield, 2007; St. Jean & Feagin, 1998; Willhelm, 1986; Livingston & Pearce, 2009; Kirschenman & Neckerman, 1991; Waldinger, 1997; Waldinger & Lichter, 2003; Pager, 2007s.

17 Toossi & Joyner, 2018; Byars-Winston et al., 2015; Alexis, 1998; Williams & Collins, 2004; Gottschalk, 1997; Darity & Myers, 1995; Darity et al., 1996, 1997; Testa et al., 1993; Wilson & Neckerman, 1986; Bishop, 1980; Mare & Winship, 1991; Wilson, 1987, 1996; Fairlie & Sundstrom, 1999; Chetty et al., 2018; Bayer & Charles, 2018; Western & Pettit, 2005; Western, 2006; Pettit, 2012; Pager, 2007; Holzer & Offner, 2006; Holzer, 1996, 2007; Pinkney, 1984; Staples, 1985; Field & Winfrey, 1997; Smith et al., 2011; Wingfield, 2007; St. Jean & Feagin, 1998; Willhelm, 1986; Livingston & Pearce, 2009; Kirschenman & Neckerman, 1991; Waldinger, 1997; Waldinger & Lichter, 2003; Pager, 2007.

18 Pager et al., 2009.

19 Toossi & Joyner, 2018; Byars-Winston et al., 2015; Alexis, 1998; Williams & Collins, 2004; Gottschalk, 1997; Darity & Myers, 1995; Darity et al., 1996, 1997; Testa et al., 1993; Wilson & Neckerman, 1986; Bishop, 1980; Mare & Winship, 1991; Wilson, 1987, 1996; Fairlie & Sundstrom, 1999; Chetty et al., 2018; Bayer & Charles, 2018; Western & Pettit, 2005; Western, 2006; Pettit, 2012; Pager, 2007; Holzer & Offner, 2006; Holzer, 1996, 2007; Pinkney, 1984; Staples, 1985; Field & Winfrey, 1997; Smith et al., 2011; Wingfield, 2007; St. Jean & Feagin, 1998; Willhelm, 1986; Livingston & Pearce, 2009; Kirschenman & Neckerman, 1991; Waldinger, 1997; Waldinger & Lichter, 2003; Pager, 2007.

20 Seder & Burrell, 1971; Baradaran, 2018; Marable, 1979; Kaplan et al., 2008; Ogungbure, 2019; Harris, 2013; Porter, 2021; Byars-Winston et al., 2015; Hochschild, 1995; Pinkney, 1984.

21 Rothstein, 2017; Leonhardt, 2020; National Partnership for Women & Families, 2020; Miller, 2020; Bayer & Charles, 2018; Becker, 1967; Alexis, 1998; Williams & Collins, 2004; Chetty et al., 2018; Phelan et al., 2010; Assari, 2018; Farmer & Ferraro, 2005; Wilson et al., 2017c; Shapiro, 2004; Darity & Mason, 1998; Vedder et al., 1990; Staples, 1987b.

22 Rothstein, 2017; Leonhardt, 2020; National Partnership for Women & Families, 2020; Miller, 2020; Bayer & Charles, 2018; Becker, 1967; Alexis, 1998; Williams & Collins, 2004; Chetty et al., 2018; Phelan et al., 2010; Assari, 2018; Farmer & Ferraro, 2005; Wilson et al., 2017c; Shapiro, 2004; Darity & Mason, 1998; Vedder et al., 1990; Staples, 1987b.

23 Rothstein, 2017; Leonhardt, 2020; National Partnership for Women & Families, 2020; Miller, 2020; Bayer & Charles, 2018; Becker, 1967; Alexis, 1998; Williams & Collins, 2004; Chetty et al., 2018; Phelan et al., 2010; Assari, 2018; Farmer & Ferraro, 2005; Wilson et al., 2017c; Shapiro, 2004; Darity & Mason, 1998; Vedder et al., 1990; Staples, 1987b.

24 Shapiro & Kenty-Drane, 2005; Darity, 1989, 2005, 2008, 2021; Darity & Mullen, 2020a; Darity & Nicholson, 2005; Wolff, 2001; Rose, 2000; Blau & Graham, 1990; Shapiro, 2001a, 2001b; Darity & Frank, 2003; Lewan & Barclay, 2001; Barclay, 2001; Darity et al., 1997, 2018; De La Cruz-Viesca et al., 2016; Oliver & Shapiro, 2006; Hamilton & Chiteji, 2013; Aja et al., 2019; Muñoz et al., 2015; Williams, 2017; Baradaran, 2018; Wolff, 2001; Rose, 2000; Blau & Graham, 1990; Darity & Frank, 2003; Lewan & Barclay, 2001; Barclay, 2001; Grossman, 1997; Dailey, 2000; Umfleet, 2005; Mixon, 2005; Brophy, 2002; Ortiz, 2005; Mitchell, 2001; Addo & Darity, 2021; Seamster, 2019; Cooper & Bruenig, 2017; Shear & Hilzenrath, 2010; Coates, 2014; Powell, 2009; Austin, 2012; Baptiste, 2014; Rosner, 2001; Houle & Light, 2014; Center for Responsible Lending, 2013; Dettling et al., 2017; Percheski & Gibson-Davis, 2020; Moore & Bruenig, 2017; Hamilton et al., 2015; Moore, 2015a, 2015b, 2017; De La Cruz-Viesca et al., 2016; Takaki, 1989; Suzuki, 2002; Aja et al., 2019; Muñoz et al., 2015; Rugaber, 2013; Kijakazi et al., 2016; Shapiro & Kenty-Drane, 2005; Hoffower, 2019; Saphir, 2021; Survey of Consumer Finances, 2019; Harkinson, 2015;

Hahn, 2021; Sahm, 2020; The Federal Reserve-DFA, 2021; Conley, 2010; Ensign & Shifflett, 2021; Whitehouse, 2019; Asante-Muhammad & Devine, 2021; McKim, 2021; Hamilton, 2019; Folmar, 2022; Stewart, 2018; Levin, 2022.

25 Shapiro & Kenty-Drane, 2005; Darity, 1989, 2005, 2008, 2021; Darity & Mullen, 2020a; Darity & Nicholson, 2005; Wolff, 2001; Rose, 2000; Blau & Graham, 1990; Shapiro, 2001a, 2001b; Darity & Frank, 2003; Lewan & Barclay, 2001; Barclay, 2001; Darity et al., 1997, 2018; De La Cruz-Viesca et al., 2016; Oliver & Shapiro, 2006; Hamilton & Chiteji, 2013; Aja et al., 2019; Muñoz et al., 2015; Williams, 2017; Baradaran, 2018; Wolff, 2001; Rose, 2000; Blau & Graham, 1990; Lewan & Barclay, 2001; Barclay, 2001; Grossman, 1997; Dailey, 2000; Umfleet, 2005; Mixon, 2005; Brophy, 2002; Ortiz, 2005; Mitchell, 2001; Addo & Darity, 2021; Seamster, 2019; Cooper & Bruenig, 2017; Shear & Hilzenrath, 2010; Coates, 2014; Powell, 2009; Austin, 2012; Baptiste, 2014; Rosner, 2001; Houle & Light, 2014; Center for Responsible Lending, 2013; Dettling et al., 2017; Percheski & Gibson-Davis, 2020; Moore & Bruenig, 2017; Hamilton et al., 2015; Moore, 2015a, 2015b, 2017; De La Cruz-Viesca et al., 2016; Takaki, 1989; Suzuki, 2002; Aja et al., 2019; Muñoz et al., 2015; Rugaber, 2013; Kijakazi et al., 2016; Shapiro & Kenty-Drane, 2005; Hoffower, 2019; Saphir, 2021; Survey of Consumer Finances, 2019; Harkinson, 2015; Hahn, 2021; Sahm, 2020; The Federal Reserve-DFA, 2021; Conley, 2010; Ensign & Shifflett, 2021; Whitehouse, 2019; Asante-Muhammad & Devine, 2021; McKim, 2021; Hamilton, 2019; Folmar, 2022; Stewart, 2018; Levin, 2022.

26 Shapiro & Kenty-Drane, 2005; Darity, 1989, 2005, 2008, 2021; Darity & Mullen, 2020a; Darity & Nicholson, 2005; Wolff, 2001; Rose, 2000; Blau & Graham, 1990; Shapiro, 2001a, 2001b; Darity & Frank, 2003; Lewan & Barclay, 2001; Barclay, 2001; Darity et al., 1997, 2018; De La Cruz-Viesca et al., 2016; Oliver & Shapiro, 2006; Hamilton & Chiteji, 2013; Aja et al., 2019; Muñoz et al., 2015; Williams, 2017; Baradaran, 2018; Wolff, 2001; Rose, 2000; Blau & Graham, 1990; Lewan & Barclay, 2001; Barclay, 2001; Grossman, 1997; Dailey, 2000; Umfleet, 2005; Mixon, 2005; Brophy, 2002; Ortiz, 2005; Mitchell, 2001; Addo & Darity, 2021; Seamster, 2019; Cooper & Bruenig, 2017; Shear & Hilzenrath, 2010; Coates, 2014; Powell, 2009; Austin, 2012; Baptiste, 2014; Rosner, 2001; Houle & Light, 2014; Center for Responsible Lending, 2013; Dettling et al., 2017; Percheski & Gibson-Davis, 2020; Moore & Bruenig, 2017; Hamilton et al., 2015; Moore, 2015a, 2015b, 2017; De La Cruz-Viesca et al., 2016; Takaki, 1989; Suzuki, 2002; Aja et al., 2019; Muñoz et al., 2015; Rugaber, 2013; Kijakazi et al., 2016; Shapiro & Kenty-Drane, 2005; Hoffower, 2019; Saphir, 2021; Survey of Consumer Finances, 2019; Harkinson, 2015; Hahn, 2021; Sahm, 2020; The Federal Reserve-DFA, 2021; Conley, 2010; Ensign & Shifflett, 2021; Whitehouse, 2019; Asante-Muhammad & Devine, 2021; McKim, 2021; Hamilton, 2019; Folmar, 2022; Stewart, 2018; Levin, 2022.

27 Shapiro & Kenty-Drane, 2005; Darity, 1989, 2005, 2008, 2021; Darity & Mullen, 2020a; Darity & Nicholson, 2005; Wolff, 2001; Rose, 2000; Blau & Graham, 1990; Shapiro, 2001a, 2001b; Darity & Frank, 2003; Lewan & Barclay, 2001; Barclay, 2001; Darity et al., 1997, 2018; De La Cruz-Viesca et al., 2016; Oliver & Shapiro, 2006; Hamilton & Chiteji, 2013; Aja et al., 2019; Muñoz et al., 2015; Williams, 2017; Baradaran, 2018; Wolff, 2001; Rose, 2000; Blau & Graham, 1990; Lewan & Barclay, 2001; Barclay, 2001; Grossman, 1997; Dailey, 2000; Umfleet, 2005; Mixon, 2005; Brophy, 2002; Ortiz, 2005; Mitchell, 2001; Addo & Darity, 2021; Seamster, 2019; Cooper & Bruenig, 2017; Shear & Hilzenrath, 2010; Coates, 2014; Powell, 2009; Austin, 2012; Baptiste, 2014; Rosner, 2001; Houle & Light, 2014; Center for Responsible Lending, 2013; Dettling et al., 2017; Percheski & Gibson-Davis, 2020; Moore & Bruenig, 2017; Hamilton et al., 2015; Moore, 2015a, 2015b, 2017; De La Cruz-Viesca et al., 2016; Takaki, 1989; Suzuki, 2002; Aja et al., 2019; Muñoz et al., 2015; Rugaber, 2013; Kijakazi et al., 2016; Shapiro & Kenty-Drane, 2005; Hoffower, 2019; Saphir, 2021; Survey of Consumer Finances, 2019; Harkinson, 2015;

Hahn, 2021; Sahm, 2020; The Federal Reserve-DFA, 2021; Conley, 2010; Ensign & Shifflett, 2021; Whitehouse, 2019; Asante-Muhammad & Devine, 2021; McKim, 2021; Hamilton, 2019; Folmar, 2022; Stewart, 2018; Levin, 2022.

28 Shapiro & Kenty-Drane, 2005; Darity, 1989, 2005, 2008, 2021; Darity & Mullen, 2020a; Darity & Nicholson, 2005; Wolff, 2001; Rose, 2000; Blau & Graham, 1990; Shapiro, 2001a, 2001b; Darity & Frank, 2003; Lewan & Barclay, 2001; Barclay, 2001; Darity et al., 1997, 2018; De La Cruz-Viesca et al., 2016; Oliver & Shapiro, 2006; Hamilton & Chiteji, 2013; Aja et al., 2019; Muñoz et al., 2015; Williams, 2017; Baradaran, 2018; Wolff, 2001; Rose, 2000; Blau & Graham, 1990; Lewan & Barclay, 2001; Barclay, 2001; Grossman, 1997; Dailey, 2000; Umfleet, 2005; Mixon, 2005; Brophy, 2002; Ortiz, 2005; Mitchell, 2001; Addo & Darity, 2021; Seamster, 2019; Cooper & Bruenig, 2017; Shear & Hilzenrath, 2010; Coates, 2014; Powell, 2009; Austin, 2012; Baptiste, 2014; Rosner, 2001; Houle & Light, 2014; Center for Responsible Lending, 2013; Dettling et al., 2017; Percheski & Gibson-Davis, 2020; Moore & Bruenig, 2017; Hamilton et al., 2015; Moore, 2015a, 2015b, 2017; De La Cruz-Viesca et al., 2016; Takaki, 1989; Suzuki, 2002; Aja et al., 2019; Muñoz et al., 2015; Rugaber, 2013; Kijakazi et al., 2016; Shapiro & Kenty-Drane, 2005; Hoffower, 2019; Saphir, 2021; Survey of Consumer Finances, 2019; Harkinson, 2015; Hahn, 2021; Sahm, 2020; The Federal Reserve-DFA, 2021; Conley, 2010; Ensign & Shifflett, 2021; Whitehouse, 2019; Asante-Muhammad & Devine, 2021; McKim, 2021; Hamilton, 2019; Folmar, 2022; Stewart, 2018; Levin, 2022.

29 Shapiro & Kenty-Drane, 2005; Darity, 1989, 2005, 2008, 2021; Darity & Mullen, 2020a; Darity & Nicholson, 2005; Wolff, 2001; Rose, 2000; Blau & Graham, 1990; Shapiro, 2001a, 2001b; Darity & Frank, 2003; Lewan & Barclay, 2001; Barclay, 2001; Darity et al., 1997, 2018; De La Cruz-Viesca et al., 2016; Oliver & Shapiro, 2006; Hamilton & Chiteji, 2013; Aja et al., 2019; Muñoz et al., 2015; Williams, 2017; Baradaran, 2018; Wolff, 2001; Rose, 2000; Blau & Graham, 1990; Lewan & Barclay, 2001; Barclay, 2001; Grossman, 1997; Dailey, 2000; Umfleet, 2005; Mixon, 2005; Brophy, 2002; Ortiz, 2005; Mitchell, 2001; Addo & Darity, 2021; Seamster, 2019; Cooper & Bruenig, 2017; Shear & Hilzenrath, 2010; Coates, 2014; Powell, 2009; Austin, 2012; Baptiste, 2014; Rosner, 2001; Houle & Light, 2014; Center for Responsible Lending, 2013; Dettling et al., 2017; Percheski & Gibson-Davis, 2020; Moore & Bruenig, 2017; Hamilton et al., 2015; Moore, 2015a, 2015b, 2017; De La Cruz-Viesca et al., 2016; Takaki, 1989; Suzuki, 2002; Aja et al., 2019; Muñoz et al., 2015; Rugaber, 2013; Kijakazi et al., 2016; Shapiro & Kenty-Drane, 2005; Hoffower, 2019; Saphir, 2021; Survey of Consumer Finances, 2019; Harkinson, 2015; Hahn, 2021; Sahm, 2020; The Federal Reserve-DFA, 2021; Conley, 2010; Ensign & Shifflett, 2021; Whitehouse, 2019; Asante-Muhammad & Devine, 2021; McKim, 2021; Hamilton, 2019; Folmar, 2022; Stewart, 2018; Levin, 2022.

30 Shapiro & Kenty-Drane, 2005Darity, 1989, 2005, 2008, 2021; Darity & Mullen, 2020a; Darity & Nicholson, 2005; Wolff, 2001; Rose, 2000; Blau & Graham, 1990; Shapiro, 2001a, 2001b; Darity & Frank, 2003; Lewan & Barclay, 2001; Barclay, 2001; Darity et al., 1997, 2018; De La Cruz-Viesca et al., 2016; Oliver & Shapiro, 2006; Hamilton & Chiteji, 2013; Aja et al., 2019; Muñoz et al., 2015; Williams, 2017; Baradaran, 2018; Wolff, 2001; Rose, 2000; Blau & Graham, 1990; Lewan & Barclay, 2001; Barclay, 2001; Grossman, 1997; Dailey, 2000; Umfleet, 2005; Mixon, 2005; Brophy, 2002; Ortiz, 2005; Mitchell, 2001; Addo & Darity, 2021; Seamster, 2019; Cooper & Bruenig, 2017; Shear & Hilzenrath, 2010; Coates, 2014; Powell, 2009; Austin, 2012; Baptiste, 2014; Rosner, 2001; Houle & Light, 2014; Center for Responsible Lending, 2013; Dettling et al., 2017; Percheski &

Gibson-Davis, 2020; Moore & Bruenig, 2017; Hamilton et al., 2015; Moore, 2015a, 2015b, 2017; De La Cruz-Viesca et al., 2016; Takaki, 1989; Suzuki, 2002; Aja et al., 2019; Muñoz et al., 2015; Rugaber, 2013; Kijakazi et al., 2016; Shapiro & Kenty-Drane, 2005; Hoffower, 2019; Saphir, 2021; Survey of Consumer Finances, 2019; Harkinson, 2015; Hahn, 2021; Sahm, 2020; The Federal Reserve-DFA, 2021; Conley, 2010; Ensign & Shifflett, 2021; Whitehouse, 2019; Asante-Muhammad & Devine, 2021; McKim, 2021; Hamilton, 2019; Folmar, 2022; Stewart, 2018; Levin, 2022; Bruenig, M. (2023, October 23). Wealth Distribution in 2022. *People's Policy Project*. https://www.peoplespolicyproject.org/2023/10/23/wealth-distribution-in-2022.

31 Shapiro & Kenty-Drane, 2005; Darity, 1989, 2005, 2008, 2021; Darity & Mullen, 2020a; Darity & Nicholson, 2005; Wolff, 2001; Rose, 2000; Blau & Graham, 1990; Shapiro, 2001a, 2001b; Darity & Frank, 2003; Lewan & Barclay, 2001; Barclay, 2001; Darity et al., 1997, 2018; De La Cruz-Viesca et al., 2016; Oliver & Shapiro, 2006; Hamilton & Chiteji, 2013; Aja et al., 2019; Muñoz et al., 2015; Williams, 2017; Baradaran, 2018; Wolff, 2001; Rose, 2000; Blau & Graham, 1990; Lewan & Barclay, 2001; Barclay, 2001; Grossman, 1997; Dailey, 2000; Umfleet, 2005; Mixon, 2005; Brophy, 2002; Ortiz, 2005; Mitchell, 2001; Addo & Darity, 2021; Seamster, 2019; Cooper & Bruenig, 2017; Shear & Hilzenrath, 2010; Coates, 2014; Powell, 2009; Austin, 2012; Baptiste, 2014; Rosner, 2001; Houle & Light, 2014; Center for Responsible Lending, 2013; Dettling et al., 2017; Percheski & Gibson-Davis, 2020; Moore & Bruenig, 2017; Hamilton et al., 2015; Moore, 2015a, 2015b, 2017; De La Cruz-Viesca et al., 2016; Takaki, 1989; Suzuki, 2002; Aja et al., 2019; Muñoz et al., 2015; Rugaber, 2013; Kijakazi et al., 2016; Shapiro & Kenty-Drane, 2005; Hoffower, 2019; Saphir, 2021; Survey of Consumer Finances, 2019; Harkinson, 2015; Hahn, 2021; Sahm, 2020; The Federal Reserve-DFA, 2021; Conley, 2010; Ensign & Shifflett, 2021; Whitehouse, 2019; Asante-Muhammad & Devine, 2021; McKim, 2021; Hamilton, 2019; Folmar, 2022; Stewart, 2018; Levin, 2022.

32 Shapiro & Kenty-Drane, 2005; Darity, 1989, 2005, 2008, 2021; Darity & Mullen, 2020a; Darity & Nicholson, 2005; Wolff, 2001; Rose, 2000; Blau & Graham, 1990; Shapiro, 2001a, 2001b; Darity & Frank, 2003; Lewan & Barclay, 2001; Barclay, 2001; Darity et al., 1997, 2018; De La Cruz-Viesca et al., 2016; Oliver & Shapiro, 2006; Hamilton & Chiteji, 2013; Aja et al., 2019; Muñoz et al., 2015; Williams, 2017; Baradaran, 2018; Wolff, 2001; Rose, 2000; Blau & Graham, 1990; Lewan & Barclay, 2001; Barclay, 2001; Grossman, 1997; Dailey, 2000; Umfleet, 2005; Mixon, 2005; Brophy, 2002; Ortiz, 2005; Mitchell, 2001; Addo & Darity, 2021; Seamster, 2019; Cooper & Bruenig, 2017; Shear & Hilzenrath, 2010; Coates, 2014; Powell, 2009; Austin, 2012; Baptiste, 2014; Rosner, 2001; Houle & Light, 2014; Center for Responsible Lending, 2013; Dettling et al., 2017; Percheski & Gibson-Davis, 2020; Moore & Bruenig, 2017; Hamilton et al., 2015; Moore, 2015a, 2015b, 2017; De La Cruz-Viesca et al., 2016; Takaki, 1989; Suzuki, 2002; Aja et al., 2019; Muñoz et al., 2015; Rugaber, 2013; Kijakazi et al., 2016; Shapiro & Kenty-Drane, 2005; Hoffower, 2019; Saphir, 2021; Survey of Consumer Finances, 2019; Harkinson, 2015; Hahn, 2021; Sahm, 2020; The Federal Reserve-DFA, 2021; Conley, 2010; Ensign & Shifflett, 2021; Whitehouse, 2019; Asante-Muhammad & Devine, 2021; McKim, 2021; Hamilton, 2019; Folmar, 2022; Stewart, 2018; Levin, 2022.

CHAPTER 6

STARVING THE BLACK BEAST

PART II

BLACK RELATIONSHIPS AND FAMILIES[1]

The reduction in the supply of economically able men to fill the roles of husband and father are one of the primary causes for the decline in two-parent families in Black communities. Black men are no longer considered useful in the emerging economic order, thus they are socially unwanted, unneeded, and insignificant (political economy of niggerdom). Reductions in the supply of marriageable (unmarried males in the labor force or in school) mates are exacerbated by policies designed to contain or eradicate the unwanted and marginalized Black male population (institutional decimation). Black families headed by women has increased from 25 percent in the 1950s to nearly 50 percent in the 1990s. Black families headed by mothers are significantly impacted by poverty. The high percentage of Black families headed by women result from the fragile economic position of Black men, which is compounded with the inability of Black women to locate marriage partners in significant numbers. In addition, sex ratios (number of males and females in the general population) are a key determinant of the increase in Black female-headed families. There are more Black women than men in every age group over 15, which equates to a surplus of Black women particularly of childbearing ages 15 to 30. This sex gap does not exist in childhood as there are approximately as many Black boys as girls. But the gap begins to appear among teenagers and widens through the twenties and peaks in the thirties while persisting through adulthood.[2]

As previously highlighted, there are 1.5 million Black men missing due to early death and hyperincarceration. This leaves 83 Black men for every 100 Black women not incarcerated. Ferguson, Missouri, and N. Charleston, S. Carolina, had large sex gaps in this ratio. Further, large numbers of Black men are missing from New York, Chicago, Philadelphia, Detroit, Memphis, Baltimore, Houston, Charlotte, N.C., Milwaukee, Dallas, and the states of Georgia, Alabama, and Mississippi. This sex gap is almost nonexistent for whites (99 white men for every 100 white women not incarcerated). Early deaths and hyperincarceration leaves many communities without enough men to be fathers and husbands. As discussed in Chapter 4, changes in incarceration over time were due to changes in policy and not changes in male behavior. Moreover, more than one out of every six Black men who would have been between the prime-age years of 25 and 54 years old has disappeared from daily life. Approximately 600,000 Black men are incarcerated, while approximately 900,000 are dead. Mason's (2006) calculation of the sex ratios for the civilian unmarried population indicated that there are 71 Black males to 100 Black females compared to 119 white males to 100 white females. This figure decreases to 46 Black males to 100 Black females compared to 90 white males to 100 white females if full-time employment is added as a criterion for marriageable males. Marriage is not solely a romantic commitment but an economic institution, thus the ability to be strong economic providers or breadwinners in the household is highly correlated with the attractiveness of males as marriage prospects. In addition, the scarcity of marriageable Black males positions unmarried Black males who are deemed marriageable with the ability to choose highly desired females. As a result of this scarcity,

DOI: 10.4324/9781003430551-7

a large proportion of Black women have participated in the labor force out of necessity. Charles and Luoh (2010) found that women in response to male incarceration increased both their schooling and labor supply. The relative supply of marriageable males in 1980 was 40 percent for Black Americans and 60 percent for whites. It declined to 35 percent for Black Americans and 55 percent for whites by 2010. The ratio of marriageable males to unmarried females for whites is near 3:5 compared to 2:5 for Black Americans. The growing excess of women over men in every age group during the marriageable years significantly contributes to the sharp decline in the probability of marriage for Black women. The cumulative probability of remaining unmarried increases as the sex ratio increases, and this probability increase is higher than the sex ratio increase.[3]

Over 90 percent of Black women historically were married by the age of 44. This figure fell to 75 percent in the 1970s. One-third of Black women had never been married by the age of 44 by 1980. The excess of females over males for whites does not rise until the age of 44, which is beyond major childbearing years. Therefore, the percentage of female-headed white families (never-married, single, teenaged mothers) is significantly smaller than among Black Americans. The surplus of women influences the structures of Black families. High infant and childhood mortality among males, high mortality rate among young Black males, and hyperincarceration contribute to the sex ratio imbalances among Black Americans. Black families are destroyed by hyperincarceration as it removes fathers from homes and leaves Black males disenfranchised (e.g., erosion of human capital, collateral consequences, etc.) and unemployed under America's racial caste system. Further, the family is left to deal with an experience that is similar to the death of a parent or divorce that includes financial instability and emotional and psychological effects on the children and partner along with social stigma. In addition, the absence of jobs for Black men lowers the marriageable pool of Black men and increases the prevalence of Black families headed by females in Black communities. The institutional decimation of Black men manifests through the significant differential mortality rates between Black men and women, the increased institutionalization of Black men, and the withdrawal of Black men from the civilian labor force that includes their increased entry into the armed forces are all contributing factors that have severely impacted marriage and two-parent families. The greatest cause of death for Black men is homicide. The astronomical rates of incarceration of Black men are a human rights and public health issue. Declining employment opportunities have prompted Black men to withdraw from the civilian labor force, and some have entered the armed services at rates that doubled between 1970 and 1990 with significantly more likely to reenlist compared to whites. Further, Black men are crowded into the least desirable jobs within the armed services and experience higher rates of unemployment upon re-entry into civilian life. Thus, military service postpones their entry into the ranks of the unemployed. These mechanisms of institutional decimation create a surplus of unmarried women over marriageable men. The effect has been long-term declines in fertility, increase in divorce, and increases in the percentage of women who have never been married by the age of 24. Black families headed by females was approximately 28 percent in 1970 and increased to 46 percent that were female-headed by 1990. In comparison, white families headed by females was approximately 9 percent in 1970 and increased to 13 percent by 1990. Fifty-five percent of all Black families were female-headed compared to 22 percent of all white families in 2011.[4]

Testa and Krogh (1995) discovered that Black male employment is positively associated with marriage rates. Black men who experienced stable employment were twice as likely to marry. The steepest increase in female-headed Black families occurred between 1970 and 1990. Joe and Yu (1984) found that between 1976 and 1983, the number of female-headed

Black families rose by 700,000 and the number of Black men out of the labor force or unemployed increased by the same number. This trend can be identified in 1960, where approximately 75 percent of Black men were working, and female-headed Black families accounted for 21 percent of all Black families during the same year. But by 1982, only 54 percent of all Black men were in the labor force and female-headed Black families were at 42 percent. Moreover, Black women experienced the largest relative gains in the decade following civil rights legislation. Their occupational opportunities greatly broadened, which translated into economic and social gains in the late 1960s through the 1970s. Black women are the majority of Black Americans who have moved into the middle class since the civil rights movement. The occupational, economic, and social gains brought them closer to parity with white women, which also had the effect of health gains for Black women. The health gains translated into a larger increase in life expectancy (approximately three years) more than any other race-sex group. Black men in contrast did not experience uniformly positive occupational and socioeconomic gains following civil rights legislation to the same degree as their female counterparts. Black men experienced an inconsistent pattern of gains and setbacks that was initiated in the 1940s by an extensive move out of agricultural work into blue-collar operative jobs, which was countered in the 1960s by rising unemployment relative to white men. Therefore, the gains in the 1970s that resulted from the occupational changes in the 1960s had different effects on racial inequality for Black men and women. Black women experienced a decline in income disparity because of their occupational distribution becoming similar to their white counterparts whereas income disparity increased among Black men as the average occupational status of white men increased, moving away from the average status of Black men including a sharp decline in labor market participation among a rising fraction of Black men. Therefore, not only was the impact of civil rights legislation on the occupational and economic pathways minimal for Black men, but the residual improved health that would come about from these types of gains were minimal as well. Kaplan et al. (2008) posits that employer's racial animus toward Black men (anti-Black misandry) and a preference for Black women instead is a plausible explanation for these disparities. This pattern predates civil rights legislation and has been documented by Frazier's (1939) research on Black families from 1860 to 1900. He found that most families he surveyed had a female-head, and Black women had higher employment rates compared to Black men.[5]

The institutional decimation of Black men drives changes in Black family structure through the decrease in the supply of marriageable mates. The decline in sex ratios create disparities between marriage-aged women and men that results in the formation of a substantial number of Black families headed by females. Increased mortality and institutionalization among Black males are the causes of the depletion in the supply of marriageable males, which results in the reduction of two-parent families. Family formation is disrupted, which leads to lower marriage rates and higher rates of childbirth outside of marriage. Black male death significantly lowers the chance for Black women to marry Black men compared to white women who marry white men. Sixty-nine percent of Black children in 2003 were born to an unwed mother. Seventy-two percent of white, 82 percent of Asian American, and 55 percent of Latino/a children are living with two married parents. This is in sharp contrast to only 31 percent of Black children living with two married parents while 54 percent are being raised by a single parent. Research indicates that children have better outcomes and life chances (e.g., better physical and mental health, higher wages and social ties, and college completion) when they grow up in a two-parent, married home. These outcomes may be attributed to greater resources (material and nonmaterial) that may be provided by a two-parent household. Single parent homes have been associated with increased poverty and welfare participation, which can negatively impact the economic and social well-being of children that can eventually lead to adverse adult outcomes. As previously mentioned, approximately 5 percent of Black children grow up in areas with a poverty rate below 10 percent with more than half of Black fathers present, while white children have a starkly alternate existence where 63 percent of them grow up in areas with a poverty rate below 10 percent with more than half of white fathers present. Twenty-one percent of Black households earn less than $12,500 in household income, while approximately 38 percent earn between $12,500 and $37,499 in household income. Moreover, 19 percent earn between $37,500 and $62,499, while 11 percent earn between $62,500 and $87,499 in household income, and approximately 5 percent earn between $87,500 and $112,499 in household income. The *Pew Research Center* (2020) identified $86,600 as median middle-class income. This poses a serious problem as almost 59 percent of Black households earn less than $37,500, and 89 percent of Black families earn less than $87,500 in household income. Thus, most Black families in America are not middle class based on income standards but are the working poor. In addition, income is an inadequate indicator of economic well-being and social positioning, particularly among Black Americans. Further, white women combine their incomes with white men significantly more often than Black women combine their income with Black men. The large percentage of single parent female-headed Black families indicates that Black women have less of an opportunity to combine their incomes with Black men than white women who combine their income with white men.[6]

Marriage for many Black men becomes an economic burden due to the political economy of niggerdom. Many Black men simply cannot financially afford marriage, which results in their inability to meet the patriarchal expectations of being a financial provider and protector of their families. Ogungbure (2019) indicates that the function of the American capitalist economy is to destroy Black families through the exclusion of Black males from the mechanism of wealth creation. The unemployment and underemployment of Black men reflects the persistence of anti-Black misandry in America, where they are permanently removed from the labor market (institutional decimation). Willhelm (1986) posits that enslaved Black Americans did not have a class position, and Black Americans who are not in the labor market have no class standing as well. He states that they are not part of an underclass but a *declassed* people. Since class position establishes life opportunities, he questions if a declassed Black person even has a chance for life (conditional genocide). The Black family structure reflects economic forces that have been reflected in the rise of the female-headed family, which is a consequence of economic oppression. The result is an apatriarchal Black male who is unable to head a household or participate in American capitalist society. The destruction of the socioeconomic status of the Black family is due to the victimization of Black males within America's capitalist and patriarchal political economy through mechanisms of socioeconomic deprivation, institutionalization, and death.[7]

PLANTATION POLITICS AND THE DECADENT VEIL

All skinfolk ain't kinfolk

—Zora Neale Hurston

Plantation politics builds upon the analysis of Malcolm X (1963) where he articulates the relationship between the House slave who worships the white Master (enslaver) and Field slave who is resistant to this dynamic. He indicated that the remnants of the culture of slavery and the plantation economy that is embedded in the racist capitalist structure of America had continued into the 20th century. These relationships/entanglements have endured where Black Americans remain in inferior roles and the Black middle-class with class aspirations worships and emulates white America while harboring animus toward the Black working-class. This mechanism of white sociopolitical organization keeps Black Americans in bondage. Plantation politics is defined by this author as a modern system of subordination and domination that resembles a colonial plantation hierarchy/relationship and a modern-day plantation where Black people are used to control and silence other Black people by white people in power through bestowing rewards and privileges to Black people who support and promote a white supremacist agenda (neoliberal/liberal, moderate, or conservative ideologies/politics). Plantation politics includes the deployment of Black bodies as representation irrespective of the worldviews, positions, histories, and awareness/understandings that they bring into spaces. This includes the positioning of Black immigrants and those who identify as biracial as spokespersons for Black Americans and issues that are unique to the Black community. Groups outside and within the Black community are made "model minorities" in order for the white ruling class to maintain power and control with poor Black working-class men and women who descend from U.S. enslavement serving as the negation of a "model minority." In addition, plantation politics manifests with white America or Black elites (i.e., Black Bourgeoisie/petty bourgeoisie) designating and positioning some Black people to operate as modern-day slave drivers where they get the rest of the unruly Blacks in line for the master of the plantation. Lemelle (1994) describes this dynamic as an institutionally situated professional-managerial class that is charged with the management of the Black undercaste to maintain the status quo. These Black elites (upper levels of the Black middle class) represent a small social stratum that are retained to primarily articulate the various values (e.g., advocating for the myth of meritocracy and Black respectability) and ideas of white America (i.e., Western liberalism), including maintenance of the social order. A professional-managerial agenda is informed by racist customs and traditions that adhere to hard work (i.e., protestant ethic), loyalty, strength, discipline, religiosity, fitness, patriotism, and character. Lemelle (1994) characterizes the professional-managerial class as initiating status degradation ceremonies in response to their assumptions of disreputable Blacks and specifically Black boys. He views the work of the professional-managerial class as one that is similar to that of the missionary in colonized countries (i.e., neo-colonialism) where the goal of both is to transform the heathen culture into a supposed culture of repute (i.e., respectability). According to Frazier (1957), the Black Bourgeoisie/elites suffers from feelings of inferiority and therefore construct a world of "make-believe" to provide psychic insulation from their feelings of inferiority and insecurity. Their self-hatred is demonstrated in their attempts to distance themselves from working-class Black people (attempts to escape their subordinate status) with a pathological struggle for status and a longing for recognition in the white world. Their feelings of emptiness and futility causes them to constantly seek cognitive delusions as a form of escapism, which causes internal confusion and conflict. These groups often promote platitudes of unity and provide examples of success (i.e., tokenism and Black exceptionalism) as well as promoting the Protestant work ethic (i.e., work hard) as the antidote to anti-Black oppression. Another tool to quell dissent is spiritual bypassing that involves focusing on God, forgiveness, and reconciliation that is devoid of any critical analysis.[8]

Allen (1969, 2005, 2010) articulated that a neo-colonial relationship developed in the late 1960s between the white power structure and Black communities in the U.S. The transfiguration of the white power structure to neo-colonialism was motivated by the advent of Black Power militancy and the urban rebellions where the white power structure (locally and nationally) found itself losing control while being progressively challenged and discredited within Black communities. Hegemony of the internal Black colony was maintained by indirect neo-colonial control through Black intermediary groups (e.g., Black Bourgeoisie, Black celebrity, Black academics, and Black politicians) that replaced direct white control in a similar manner to Third World struggles for national independence against colonialism that were replaced with neo-colonialism. The direct white domination emerged from conservative, segregationist (Jim/Jane Crow), Southern ruling class policy while the indirect neo-colonial domination emerged from the liberal white power structure of the North and related policy. The development of an intermediary class (Black middle class) included the promotion of Black professionals, politicians, bureaucrats, and businessmen/women who were co-opted by the white power structure and deployed not only as a buffer but agents in controlling Black communities on behalf of the white power structure. Black celebrities and academics are among these groups. Moreover, a class of Black elected officials dependent on the Democratic Party emerged to serve neo-colonial interests and thus rewarded with a niche in corporate capitalism while concomitantly deflecting and repressing revolutionary Black militancy. The illusion and rhetoric of Black capitalism is deployed as a containment strategy and a tactic to undermine the influence of Black radicals while focusing on capitalistic ventures that do nothing to change the conditions of poor Black people while unemployed young Black males are sacrificed in this process. Bell (1992) examined this apparatus with the selection of Judge Clarence Thomas to the Supreme Court as the replacement to Justice Thurgood Marshall. He compares the selection of Clarence Thomas to the historical practice of slave masters' elevating slaves to plantation overseer and other positions of quasi-power who were willing to mimic the masters' views and execute orders, thus their very presence provided a perverse legitimacy to the oppression they supported and endorsed. Brown (2003) builds upon the analysis of Malcolm X and refers to the parasitical dynamic of the Black academic (i.e., the Black intelligentsia) and political class in relation to the Black underclass as *New Age Racism* where the Black underclass are exploited by Black academics and politicians (referred to as *New Age House Negroes*) for material and symbolic rewards (e.g., *the first Black*) while simultaneously distancing themselves from the struggles of the Black underclass. Du Bois (1960) had previously articulated this dynamic where a splintering occurred that created a stratified racial class structure among Black Americans where the intermediary class (i.e., Black bourgeoisie) joined the white power structure in exploiting and victimizing the Black working class. Frazier's (1962) analysis elucidated that the group of Black intellectuals (academics) actually promoted anti-intellectualism in their quest to achieve white acceptance through conformity to white ideals, values, and patterns of behavior. They embody whiteness and function as a white prototype espousing the common race-related rhetoric of Black progress. Carter G. Woodson examined this apparatus three decades earlier in *The Miseducation of the Negro* (1933). Darity (2011/ *The New (Incorrect) Harvard/Washington Consensus on Racial Inequality*) examined this propensity to endorse Black pathology (framed as cultural factors that traffic cultural determinism) as causation for disadvantage among primarily Black Harvard University academics along with President Barack Obama, who all chose to ignore available rigorous empiricism that demonstrates structural factors as causation.[9]

Coined by Moore (2014), the decadent veil is defined as a veil of economics that masks the economic struggles of Black Americans through the deployment of Black celebrity (i.e., Black celebrity class-professional athletes, music artists, actors, TV personalities/gurus, etc.).

The decadent veil offers an analysis of Black Americans through a group theory lens in order to explain an illusion that was formed over a 30-year timespan of financial deregulation and newfound access to unsecured credit. The veil includes million-dollar sports contracts, Roc Nation partnerships, etc. The decadent veil is social engineering (sociogenic processes) that obscures the reality of Black existence through optics where TV shows such as MTV Cribs through the viewership of Black celebrity homes primes people to believe that Black people as a collective are financially thriving in America despite research that indicates that 14 million Black households are drowning in poverty and debt. The exceptionalism of a few is positioned to represent millions of Black Americans. This mechanism serves the dual function of the desensitization of the masses to Black poverty while being absorbed by Black celebrity. This includes channels such as ESPN or VH1 parading Black celebrities being paid large sums of money to entertain. This also represents plantation politics where the majority of professional sports teams are owned by white men and women who have generational wealth and make an exorbitant amount of money in comparison to the professional athletes (NBA/NFL) whose Black male bodies they control, commodify, have a short shelf life of physical labor, and whose salary/incomes pale in comparison (which does not include approximately 50 percent in federal/state taxes they have to pay as well as agent fees). These celebrities routinely promote Black capitalism (neo-colonialism) as the antidote to Black poverty over collective uplift as well as other myths and zombie ideologies (e.g., Horatio Alger myth/bootstrap theory, Horace Mann myth/education the great equalizer, sensational empowerment/belief in self, positive thinking, etc.) along with disinformation as they are often used as subject matter experts on various issues that impact the Black community even though they do not have the credentials to do so, thus causing mass confusion and distractions. They frequently speak in abstract and self-aggrandizing terms that include statements such as "representing the culture" or "moving the culture forward" and hijack the cognitive space of the Black community through manufactured provocative "conversations" that are not supported by research. Thus, pertinent issues that impact Black working-class people are not addressed through diversions and containment tactics. These Black celebrities deploy this apparatus by using various media platforms whenever they feel a need to regain relevancy by influencing what people pay attention to and believe is important. Black celebrity is often tied to white capital and is promoted by a culture of celebrity worship and includes an allegiance to the American corporate capitalist power structure.[10]

It is important to note that Black celebrity worship (e.g., digital Blackface) does not equate to the absence of anti-Black racism among fans. According to Cleaver (1968), Black leaders are decimated while the images of Uncle Toms and celebrities (entertainers and athletes from the apolitical world of sports and the performing arts) are inflated by the mass media, who is able to channel and control the aspirations and goals of the Black masses. Issues that affect the Black community are removed out of a political, economic, and philosophical context and placed into the context of white "goodwill." This technique is what Cleaver refers to as "negro control." When a racial problem or crisis arises, a Black celebrity is paraded as a great oracle to provide a predictable and conciliatory interpretation of the matter to sell out and contain the Black masses. There is no other ethnoracial group where celebrities are designated as the spokespersons for the group. This apparatus resembles a modern-day plantation system and is often exhibited between sports team owner and professional athlete and the Black community at large. As Black celebrity is deployed to the viewership of millions of people and millions of times, Black existence in the U.S. is muted, and the thrust to address injustice (reparations, redistribution of wealth, transformative public policy, etc.) by the masses is lost. In addition, white and non-Black fans are able to reassure themselves that America is not racist after all. A false claim is generated within the overall American psyche regarding the chasm in Black wealth disparity through the announcements such as Lebron James' $85 million contract or Oprah's sole Black billionaire status. Black celebrity has been positioned as the representation of Black power in the corporate world. Many of the wealthiest Black Americans obtain their wealth from some form of entertainment and are frequently portrayed as major corporate owners without transparency of how much stake or control they have in a given company. But Piketty's (2014) research indicates that 60 to 70 percent of the top 0.1 percent of incomes from 2000 to 2010 belonged to a specific subclass of executives/employees (managers) that he identifies as *supermanagers* at the upper echelons of large firms. Their extremely high salaries perpetuate wage hierarchy and are a central factor in rising wage inequality as they encompass the majority of the top centile. Athletes, actors, and artists of all kinds by comparison make up approximately 5 percent of this group, and it is plausible that the majority of the athletes, actors, and artists within this group are white. Therefore, identifiable Black superstars are props that allow less-publicized white supermanagers to remain almost invisible. There are five Black CEOs (0.1 percent) in the Fortune 500, and there has only been 20 Black CEOs in the entire history of the Fortune 500 list out of 1,800 chiefs who have been primarily white men and white women.[11]

Young Black men in ghettos across America are conditioned to aspire to be a millionaire as a professional athlete or rapper as this larger-than-life illusion is positioned as the only opportunity structure out of poverty. The Black community's vision of an outward larger economic world is distorted by the decadent veil as well as the outside community's view of the actual financial reality of Black America. The media traffics images of young Black men signing million-dollar sports and music contracts while simultaneously displaying videos with Black Americans in expensive cars and houses promoting decadent consumerism and projecting a false image that a larger percentage of Black Americans are wealthy. The interconnected mechanisms of mass media, sports organizations, and a conditioned collective psyche in Black America produces delusions and a false sense of security through the normalization/ritualization of wealth illusion that is projected globally. The result is apathy for Black Americans and the socioeconomic deprivation they have been subjected to for centuries. The decadent veil renders the political economy of niggerdom and the institutional decimation of Black men invisible through wealth fantasy. Black celebrity is a tool of white supremacy in the 21st century which has come to represent Black Americans globally even though they are an infinitesimal group in comparison to the Black population. These larger-than-life individual brands have come to represent Black existence while obscuring the reality of Black life. The projection of Black progress keeps the Black community in a state of containment, where demands for transformative public policy are abated. A central feature of the Black elites/shapeshifters and their variants is an attachment to capitalism and integration/assimilation (hierarchy-enhancing ideology) that ultimately serves an opportunistic anti-Black agenda. They tend to be formally invested in the power structure and institutions of the dominant white group. This apparatus that Black scholars have been interrogating for almost a century is referred to as *out-group favoritism* (i.e., deference) by social dominance theory (SDT) and is a form of *behavioral asymmetry* where racial hierarchy is produced and maintained by subordinates who favor dominants over their own in-group, which is exemplified in Uncle Tom-ing by some Black Americans toward whites. Therefore, the passive and active cooperation of subordinates with their own oppression preserves group-based racial hierarchy which contributes to its resiliency, robustness, and stability.[12]

REDLINING/URBAN RENEWAL/RACIAL-RESIDENTIAL SEGREGATION (HYPERSEGREGATION)

The U.S. government is primarily responsible for the creation of racial-residential segregation as it collaborated with private industry (public-private partnership) to create current conditions. Racial-residential segregation steadily increased from 1880 to the mid-twentieth century, and it has primarily remained at this level since this time. The National Association of Real Estate Boards Code of Ethics (1924) that future President Herbert Hoover helped draft and that emerged from Hoover's Advisory Committee on Zoning stated, "A Realtor should never be instrumental in introducing into a neighborhood a character of property or occupancy, members of any race or nationality, or any individuals whose presence will clearly be detrimental to property values in that neighborhood." Thus, the federal government codified the relationship between racism and real estate with Black people positioned as a detriment to property values. This translates to Black people being made a social contagion to the physical space they occupy which prevents them from accumulating wealth and threatens the wealth of those in close proximity. Racial-residential segregation leads to adverse outcomes for Black Americans. This includes racial disparities in health outcomes as racial-residential segregation perpetuates racial disparities in poverty, education, and economic opportunity that increase disparities in health. The social and spatial marginalization that is produced by segregation concentrates disadvantage by reinforcing substandard housing, underfunded public schools, employment disadvantages, exposure to crime, environmental hazards, and despair.[13]

Racial-residential segregation is defined as the physical separation of the races by enforced residence in restricted areas. Racial segregation is rooted in Jim/Jane Crow law and policy. The ideology of segregation was a conscious and deliberate strategy developed and advocated by white moderates more than 100 years ago and is a dominant system of regulation and control in the U.S. Segregation is a primary structural factor of the perpetuation of Black poverty in the U.S. Residential-racial segregation was imposed by legislation, reinforced by major economic institutions, preserved by federal government housing policies, enforced by the judicial system, and legitimized by white supremacist ideology (advocated by religious and other cultural institutions).[14]

Segregation is a complex interconnected system of control that regulates the lives of Black Americans. The funding of public education is controlled by local government and residence determines which public-school students can attend. Moreover, the quality of the neighborhood school is determined by community resources (e.g., property taxes), thus determining the quality of the neighborhood school. Poor white families tend to be dispersed throughout communities of varying socioeconomic status (SES) with many residing in desirable residential areas while poor Black Americans tend to be concentrated primarily in impoverished communities. Further, middle-class Black Americans compared to white counterparts tend to live in poorer quality neighborhoods with less affluent white neighbors. Approximately 70 percent of poor whites lived in nonpoverty areas in 1980 compared to only 16 percent of poor Black Americans. Approximately 7 percent of poor whites lived in extreme poverty or ghetto areas compared to 38 percent of Black Americans. Racial differences in poverty and family disruption are extremely significant where the worst urban living conditions of whites are considerably better than the average living conditions of Black communities. Segregation also affects employment by limiting access to social networks that could potentially provide job leads or employment opportunities. The quality of life in segregated communities is often poor due to disinvestment of economic resources. Racial differences in the purchasing power of income is altered due to segregation. Withdrawal from segregated urban areas by commercial enterprises is common. Black men experience a continual "spatial mismatch" between where jobs are increasing in number (often in downtown areas of central cities and outlying higher-income suburbs) compared to where most Black Americans live (racially segregated urban neighborhoods or lower-income suburbs).[15]

Hypersegregated Black areas contain fewer services, and those that are available tend to be poorer in quality and at a higher price point. Black Americans on average pay a higher cost than whites for housing, food, groceries, insurance, and other services. In addition, Black Americans pay a *discrimination tax* of approximately $3,000 every time they search for a home to purchase that includes less than optimal economic transactions and extra time and effort dispensed in closing a deal. Black Americans compared to whites experience smaller returns on investment in real estate due to racial-residential segregation where housing equity over time is significantly less in these hypersegregated areas compared to comparable homes in other areas. Cutler and Glaeser (1997) found that integration of Black Americans into nonsegregated communities would increase high school graduation and employment rates, increase earnings, decrease single motherhood, and decrease travel times to work. They estimate that a reduction in segregation by 13 percent would eliminate one-third of the gap of these outcomes between whites and Black Americans. Sixty percent of Black Americans would have to change residences to create an even distribution of races across neighborhoods in the average American city.[16]

Deliberate actions taken by white Americans to isolate Black Americans spatially created the Black urban ghetto in the late 19th and 20th centuries with the effect of social, economic, and political marginalization. The Great Migration was the impetus for the segregation of Black Americans and a calcified residential color line. The residential color line was initially enforced by white-on-Black violence where angry white mobs prevented Black Americans from attempting to enter white neighborhoods by burning crosses, bombings, shootings, and arson. A wave of anti-Black race riots erupted through urban America as a result of the pileup of Black American migrants that spilled over to the white side of the residential color line which culminated in the great Chicago Riot of 1919. The Chicago Riot caused destruction of property which prompted the real estate industry to step in and institutionalize discrimination in housing markets. As previously mentioned, the National Association of Real Estate Brokers adopted an article in its code of ethics in 1924 that stated that a Realtor would not introduce racialized (race or nationality) members into a neighborhood whose presence would be detrimental to property values in that neighborhood (as previously mentioned, future President Herbert Hoover was instrumental in drafting these code of ethics). This clause remained in effect until 1950. A restrictive covenant followed, which was developed in 1927 by the Chicago Real Estate Board and served as a model for neighborhood organizations and real estate boards throughout the U.S. A covenant (deed clauses) represented a private contract between property owners who agreed not to rent or sell homes to Black Americans within a specific geographic area. The contract became binding, and violators could be sued in court for breach of contract after a majority of property owners in a covered area had signed the covenant. Community associations were created before homes were put up for sale by many subdivision developers that made membership a condition of purchase to ensure racially restrictive covenants. Half of Chicago's white residential areas had such racial covenants by 1947. These racial covenants were actively promoted and enforced by all levels of government, including state supreme courts and the U.S. Supreme Court. In addition, churches, universities, and hospitals endorsed racially restrictive covenants while being permitted to retain their tax-exempt status with the Internal Revenue Service (IRS).[17]

Restrictive covenants were a preferred legal tool of institutional segregation until the U.S. Supreme Court case of *Shelly v. Kramer* (1948) declared them unenforceable and contrary to public policy. But state-sponsored segregation was preserved for at least another decade by the FHA and other federal agencies who evaded and subverted the ruling. The FHA in 1937 was tasked with creating a mortgage insurance program that would transform housing and lending markets throughout the U.S. The FHA would insure up to 90 percent of a loan's value against default provided that the mortgage conformed to FHA criteria, which gave banks a risk-free way of making money. This not only created the white middle class but was instrumental in the creation of white middle-class wealth, where small down payments (0 percent down instead of the customary 50 percent over 25 years instead of the customary seven years) and low monthly payments made mass home ownership achievable. It was more affordable to purchase a new suburban home than rent comparable older dwellings in the central city due to the combination of FHA financing and new construction techniques. FHA regulations that preferred new construction, single-family homes, and large lot sizes exacerbated bias that favored the suburbs and resulted in a whites only suburbanization. The FHA and VA used maps developed by the Home Owners Loan Corporation (HOLC) and color-coded neighborhoods according to their creditworthiness and utilized red to indicate risky neighborhoods that were not eligible for federally insured loans. But Fishback et al. (2021) found that the FHA crafted and implemented its own redlining methodology prior to the advent of the HOLC maps and the drafting of the maps did not significantly change this exclusionary pattern. Black neighborhoods or neighborhoods perceived to be in danger of becoming Black were cut off from credit through the institutionalization of the practice of "redlining," which entailed automatically coloring these neighborhoods red. In conjunction, the federal government and the FHA authorized bankers and developers to lead the HOLC. HOLC was responsible for quantifying the risk bankers would take by providing loans to specific people in specific places, which would inform the agreement on rates for FHA loan insurance between the federal government and banks. These decisions were based on HOLC surveyors who went to every residential block in just about every city in the country. They would review a neighborhood and grade it on a scale from A (very safe) to D (very unsafe). The HOLC used three main criteria to determine risk, which was the age of the building stock, the density of housing, and racial composition of residents, which was the most significant of the criteria. While Jews were considered communistic with the probability of going on strike, Italians were branded as dangerous gangsters, and Black Americans were completely written off, and any block where Black Americans inhabited was given a low grade. Further, the FHA lowered risk estimates of mortgage applicants for individual properties with racially restrictive covenants.[18]

The FHA made segregation and suburbanization the *de jure* housing policy of the U.S. under the guise of following the "best practices" of the real estate industry. In addition, the FHA *Underwriting Manual* (1939) stated that properties should be occupied by the same social and racial classes for a neighborhood to retain stability and recommended the application of racially restrictive covenants to safeguard neighborhood stability. Further, the FHA was invested in school segregation and warned that a neighborhood would become less stable and desirable with mortgage lending in such neighborhoods becoming risky if white children were forced to attend schools with large numbers of lower caste Black children. Half of all new mortgages nationwide were being insured by the FHA and VA by 1950. The FHA routinely financed entire subdivisions in the suburbs that were exclusive white enclaves. The

FHA and VA required that builders create entire white suburbs. Tax benefits disproportionately went to white Americans due to the federal government actively subsidizing white
homeownership (1933 to 1977) and systematically discouraging Black people from achieving
homeownership. Moreover, housing opportunities opened up for Black Americans in central
cities as a result of the massive outflow of whites to the suburbs. Ghetto neighborhoods
expanded rapidly in space as urban Black populations continued to grow as a result of mass
migration, and by 1970, entire cities (Atlanta, Baltimore, Detroit, Gary, Newark, and Washington) for the first time became majority Black, while many more cities (Chicago, Philadelphia, St. Louis, New York, and Milwaukee) had large Black populations, which created a
new geography of segregation throughout municipal and neighborhood boundaries.[19]

White elite districts that held their place-bound investments were inevitably threatened
because of the rapid expansion of Black neighborhoods, and they blocked the expansion
of Black settlement toward imperiled zones using urban renewal and public housing programs. Local urban renewal authority was established to regulate land using the power of
eminent domain whenever Black residential expansion threatened a preferred district. This
led to Black neighborhoods being razed for "redevelopment" as a middle-class or commercial residential zone in which at least 550 square miles of U.S. cities were razed. Public
housing was used by federal and local governments to corral Black Americans into urban
ghettos. The geographic concentration of Black poverty was dramatically increased through
the construction of public housing in other Black neighborhoods to house the displaced
Black residents from the "redeveloped" communities. Urban renewal was a form of state
violence where city governments were financially supported by the federal government to
demolish hundreds of Black neighborhoods that were often referred to as "blighted" or
"slum" neighborhoods. Close to 5,000 families (approximately 20,000 residents) in the Western Addition neighborhoods of San Francisco were displaced from rental homes, private
property, and businesses. James Baldwin stated that urban renewal meant "negro removal."
Black communities were destroyed, and their citizenship meant nothing while the government was an accomplice in this destruction. Urban renewal operated from 1949 to 1974
and represented one of the most comprehensive and systematic examples of the modern
destruction of Black property, neighborhoods, culture, community, businesses, and homes.
Entire Black neighborhoods were simply cleared out. By 1962, approximately 800 Black
communities had been displaced. Urban renewal peaked during the mid-1960s and at the
time annually displaced a minimum of 50,000 families with estimates up to 66,000 families.
This took place during the civil rights movement when voting rights were secured and the
desegregation of public and private spaces. A minimum of 300,000 families with estimates
of up to 1.2 million Americans (primarily renters who received no financial relocation assistance) were displaced as a result of federal subsidies that were provided to more than 400
cities, suburbs, and towns for more than 1,200 projects. Black Americans comprised at least
55 percent of those displaced. While urban renewal is often attributed to large cities, the
majority of projects took place in cities with 50,000 residents or less.[20]

Another mechanism to destroy and displace Black communities was through the construction of the federal interstate highway system. State and local governments supported
by the federal government designed interstate highway routes with the intention to destroy
urban Black communities. This method was devised in 1938 by Secretary of Agriculture
and later Vice President Henry Wallace who proposed to President Franklin D. Roosevelt
that highways routed through cities could eliminate "unsightly and unsanitary districts"
while simultaneously considering aid for interstate highways. Mayors and other urban political leaders partook in the process of highway construction that removed Black Americans

from white neighborhoods near downtown districts. The Urban Land Institute was an influential political force on national legislation and administration of the highway system. The Florida State Road Department in 1956 routed I-95 to clear Black Americans from a downtown Miami adjacent area, which upon its completion reduced a Black community of 40,000 Black Americans to 8,000. This state violence involved theft that destabilized Black neighborhoods and communities and destroyed social ecosystems (kinship ties, neighborhood relationships, etc.) through serial forced displacement.[21]

Massey and Denton (1989) coined the term *hypersegregation* to identify the extreme forms of segregation that Black Americans experience along the five dimensions of segregation. The five dimensions of spatial variation in segregation include *evenness, exposure, clustering, centralization,* and *concentration. Evenness* refers to the degree in which the percentage of minoritized/racialized group members within residential areas is equal to the percentage of minoritized/racialized group members citywide; segregation increases as areas retract from the ideal of *evenness. Exposure* refers to the degree of potential contact between minoritized/racialized group members and majority group members. *Clustering* refers to the extent that minoritized/racialized areas border one other; this dimension is maximized when the neighborhoods form one large contiguous ghetto and minimized when they are widely scattered spatially. *Centralization* refers to the degree in which minoritized/racialized group members are settled in and around the center of an urban area (typically defined as the central business district). *Concentration* refers to the relative amount of physical space occupied by minoritized/racialized group members; an increase in segregation indicates the increased concentration of minoritized/racialized group members within a small geographically compact area. According to Johnston et al. (2007), there are two superdimensions of segregation separation (i.e., unevenness, exposure, and clustering) and location (i.e., concentration and centralization). Massey and Denton (1989) found that Black Americans were more segregated than any other group on single dimensions and simultaneously more segregated across all dimensions. In addition, Black Americans were highly segregated on at least four (evenness, exposure, clustering, and concentration) of the five spatial dimensions in a subset of metropolitan areas (hypersegregation). Massey and Denton (1993) discovered there was very little movement toward integration between 1970 and 1980. Rugh and Massey (2014) found that high levels of Black segregation since 2010 are actively supported by restrictive density zoning in suburbs and high levels of anti-Black discrimination across metropolitan areas. Hypersegregation persisted particularly in large areas with older housing stocks characterized by large Black populations who had low levels of income and education compared to whites. Slower declines in segregation took place in metropolitan areas that displayed high levels of anti-Black sentiment, restrictive density zoning regimes, and low socioeconomic status of Black Americans. Milwaukee, Gary, Detroit, Newark, and New York were the five most segregated metropolitan areas in 2010 with no decline in Black segregation. Massey and Tannen (2015) discovered that in 2010, African Americans remained hypersegregated in 21 metropolitan areas (Milwaukee, Detroit, St. Louis, Cleveland, Chicago, New York, Philadelphia, Baltimore, Boston, etc.), and these areas accounted for a third of the metropolitan Black population, while another 21 percent lived under conditions of high segregation (i.e., a high percentage of Black Americans and whites do not share neighborhoods). This indicates that over half of the Black population in the U.S. lives under conditions of residential apartheid (i.e., racial undercaste). Between 1970 and 2010, hypersegregated Black areas declined from 40 to 21, while the number of Black Americans experiencing hypersegregation declined by half. But areas that remained hypersegregated indicated no movement toward integration, and several areas demonstrated increased levels of segregation across the five dimensions. Therefore, the segregation of Black Americans has remained persistent even though there has been substantial decline in some metropolitan areas

Whites are the most spatially isolated group in the U.S. In 2010, the likelihood of a white person sharing a residential space with a minoritized/racialized person was 8 percent, compared to 6 percent for Asian, and 11 percent for Latino/a groups. Many metropolitan areas remain just as segregated as they were in 1968 during the passage of the *Fair Housing Act*. According to Allen (1969, 2005, 2010), the Black community (urban ghettos) is an internal colony within the U.S. that is politically, economically, and militarily subjugated to white America that shares similar characteristics with colonially subjugated colonies in Africa, Asia, and Latin America who were under the direct control of European powers. Structures of domination and subordination are instrumental in the colonial relationship. The internal colonial relationship is still present but was more visible during Jim/Jane Crow.[22]

Audit studies demonstrate that whites continue to be preferred over Black Americans in real estate transactions. Moreover, Black Americans are disproportionately "steered" away from white residential areas and toward segregated or racially mixed neighborhoods. Other audit studies highlight the persistence of mortgage lending discrimination against Black Americans and the continuation of redlining of Black neighborhoods or predatory lending (high interest and high risk loans) of Black borrowers, which is referred to as "reverse redlining." Research has also revealed "linguistic profiling" of callers who speak African American Vernacular English (AAVE) or have a "Black" accent during phone call inquiries regarding the availability of housing in which callers are not informed of housing availability compared to callers who speak Standard American English. Research in Los Angeles indicates that since 1980, homeowners in formerly redlined neighborhoods earned 89 percent less home equity, which equates to $524,000 compared to their counterparts in greenlined neighborhoods. Further, another research study found that neighborhoods that suffered redlining in the 1930s are at an increased risk of flooding due to disinvestment and formerly redlined neighborhoods are hotter than non-redlined neighborhoods sometimes by almost 31 degrees due to more pavement and concrete and fewer trees. Black Americans are twice as likely to die from heat exposure than whites in New York City. A residential complex of 140 affordable housing units opened to controversy in an affluent New Jersey suburb where community residents vociferously protested that it would lower property values, raise crime rates, and increase taxes. Massey et al. (2013) conducted a systematic analysis of the effect this project had on the community and adjacent neighborhoods. No detrimental effects were found, and low-income residents benefitted greatly where residents experienced a reduction in exposure to neighborhood disorder and violence by 81 percent, negative life events reduced by 25 percent, and symptoms of mental distress reduced by 23 percent. In addition, they experienced an increase in employment by 22 percent and an increase in family income by 25 percent. But Chetty et al. (2018) indicated that reducing racial-residential segregation alone may be inadequate in closing the Black-white gap as significant disparities persist within neighborhoods.[23]

GENTRIFICATION

Gentrification is routinely presented as neighborhood revitalization which results in the physical displacement and social disruption of urban working-class Black people. Gentrification is the process by which capital is reinvested in urban neighborhoods and includes the displacement of poorer residents and their cultural products that are replaced by wealthier people and their preferred aesthetics and amenities. These spatial transformations result in low rents significantly increasing. Profit is generated by the eviction of long-term tenants by landlords and speculators. These tenants are forced to live significantly farther from their jobs and communities to the outer geographical limits of metropolitan areas, thus enduring super-commutes, while wealthier people move closer to their central city jobs. These super-commutes can create transportation obstacles and absenteeism and ultimately job loss. Black communities who invested in building up neglected neighborhoods are recasts as outsiders in their own homes and communities in favor of white newcomers. These neighborhoods and communities eventually become cities that only the wealthy can afford with environments engineered according to their preferences. The commercial fabric is recycled and replaced. This includes deeming existing bars, restaurants, coffee shops, supermarkets, hardware stores, and other common urban spots as deficient along with their replacement with new bars, restaurants, coffee shops, supermarkets, and hardware stores. The replacements charge higher prices and pay higher rents thus are deemed superior. Municipal investment is followed by real estate investment.[24]

Gentrification is a third stage in a long-term process of capital flow in and out of space. The preconditions for gentrification were established by the 1934 New Deal legislation that established the FHA with the authority to standardize, regulate, and insure home mortgages. Property owners in Black neighborhoods were shut out of the finance system, and over time, their buildings declined, rents fell, and some landlords abandoned their property. The abandonment of property became a buyer's opportunity in the 1960s, 1970s, and 1980s, where many young urbanites and financiers seized on the opportunity to grab low-cost properties and renovate them. Many of the tenants of these properties were evicted, and the buildings were converted into single-family homes while loft landlords removed remaining industrial tenants in order to convert these buildings into residential spaces. Gentrification provided an alternative option for cities to continue redeveloping their housing stock and increasing land values without initially spending much money. This model proved effective over time, and local governments, banks, and major real estate firms got into the business of financing gentrification through either loans to high-income homeowners in previous redlined areas or by building luxury landscapes in neighborhoods that had long been considered undesirable (e.g., unsafe) for investment. Gentrification became a "spatial fix" for capitalism's urban crisis. Investors were able to find new places to turn money into more money from spaces/ places that previously were considered disasters. The space for real estate's revival was created by deindustrialization, and the spatial patterns for disinvestment and reinvestment were set by redlining and urban renewal. This building-by-building and block-by-block phenomenon of gentrification became a way to transform entire cities from places into products while initially appearing as an opportunistic venture for middle-class movers and profit-seeking landlords.[25]

Police officers are the enforcers of what urban planners and policymakers enact. Planning and police departments are routinely aligned around protecting property and encouraging gentrification even though they are separate entities. Police officers aggressively stop, ticket, arrest, beat, and even kill people accused of low-level infractions like loitering, unpermitted vending, etc. often in gentrifying neighborhoods. Aggressive policing practices are a form of geographical targeting and is neither incidental nor accidental but ensures that the terrain is clear for future investment and makes wealthier white households more comfortable with the idea of living among poor Black men. In addition, aggressive policing tactics are used to boost property values and tax yields. The U.S. Department of Justice found during their investigation of Michael Brown's murder by a police officer that the city of Ferguson's (MO) punitive policing tactics of Black residents was a result of a systemic effort to increase revenue. Moreover, Breonna Taylor's family asserted that the drug raid on her apartment was motivated by the mayor's desire to gentrify an area of Louisville (KY). Gentrification represents neocolonialism with the acquisition of space and place (i.e., white property rights) and the continual underdevelopment of the working-class Black community. While cities are turned into luxury products, Black Americans are not recognized as community assets worth retaining in the gentrification process. The economic well-being or wealth positionality of Black Americans is not changed or transformed but Black Americans are harmed in this process. Gentrification has been a tool of violence that causes dispossession and serial forced displacement of Black Americans, their families, and communities and has even been described as a form of ethnic cleansing and institutional decimation that removes Black Americans from their communities that they have lived in for generations.[26]

CLINICAL IMPLICATIONS

The economic deprivation and the trauma it causes among Black men is understudied. The economic deprivation of Black men must be examined to articulate its relationship with trauma. The issues brought forth in Chapters 5 and 6 are largely systemic (structural and institutional) barriers that are interconnected and require public policy interventions. Therefore, this section will focus on the effects of anti-Black misandry and the relationship between employment, earnings, and mental health. Black men are made to suffer for the failure of the U.S. There is a long history of deliberately preventing the full participation of Black men in the labor market and how that participation is constituted as well as what kind of compensation Black men will receive for their labor. Thus, Black males are among the most vulnerable groups to an unemployment status. The denial of social status results in symbolic violence, which is a form of terrorism that is responsible for the suffering of Black males. Black men experience the highest rates of downward mobility and the highest levels of employment (pre/post-employment) and wage discrimination than any other group in the U.S. (for every dollar paid to white men, Black men are paid 51 cents, which is the lowest amount among all groups). Black men derive their sense of self (identity and self-confidence) through their ability to provide for their families. Moreover, Black Americans report that their greatest source of life satisfaction is their family life, while their jobs are cited as the source of least satisfaction. Racism (anti-Black misandry) experienced on the job is often a significant factor in the decision of many Black males to abandon stable employment. Traditional family life routinely provides a buffer against anti-Black racism more so than any other institution in American life. Black families are able to collectively resist oppression and affirm one another.[27]

In American society, a person's identity is connected to their occupation. An occupation is often an extension of a person's self-concept and can have a spiritual aspect of "giving back" through service, which is a strong value for Black men. Work provides access to resources (e.g., food, shelter, and clothing) that help to ensure continued survival. Black men are subjected to conditional genocide without these life-sustaining resources. Moreover, work provides access to social support and relational connections. Working provides Black men with a sense of connection to the social and cultural fabric of life where they feel more connected to the economic and social welfare of their communities.[28]

In addition, working provides a sense of self-determination, which includes authenticity and the ability to author the direction of one's life. Working conditions that foster autonomy, competence, and relatedness cultivate self-determination. Men in general and Black men specifically are often objectified as success objects who are supposed to provide economic stability for Black women and are denigrated when they don't fit this profile. What does it mean for Black men who historically as a collective have never been allowed to participate willfully in occupations of their choosing but instead have been channeled through an opportunity structure that dictates that their only options are to be a baller, entertainer, unemployed, institutionalized, or dead? How would a formal education enhance their lives if these are the only options? Let alone position them to obtain a consistent living wage.[29]

Earnings and employment are correlated with improved psychological health and well-being as well as provide a means for individual satisfaction and accomplishment. Black Americans are more likely to experience psychological harm from joblessness as a result of being subjected to joblessness more often. Unemployment and low or no income adds additional stressors that impact resilience. Black men experience economic and psychological alienation due to unemployment and underemployment, the public assistance complex, the educational system, and the health care system.[30]

Employment and income predict recovery from PTSD for Black Americans. The psychological impact of the socioeconomic deprivation (institutional decimation and the political economy of niggerdom) that Black men experience from anti-Black misandry can result in anxiety and worry, depression, anger and rage, low self-esteem and self-confidence, low motivation, sleeplessness, relational conflicts and decreased marital stability, substance abuse, alcohol abuse/dependency, criminal activity, suicide, and increased mortality. Moreover, it can result in emotional withdrawal or physical ailments (somatic complaints/chest and stomach pains, headaches, fatigue, etc.). Their energy, time, and space can be consumed with attempts to address (racial battle fatigue) the anti-Black misandry directed towards them, which could have been used to invest in themselves, their communities, or society at large. These uncontrollable experiences can be experienced as an assault on their sense of security and dignity, which leaves Black men with a sense of learned helplessness. Where they believe they have no agency to affect their current situation and their future status, and there is plenty of research to indicate that this assessment is accurate. This helplessness leaves Black men with a sense of not being in control of events (diminished internal locus of control) that affect their lives. Black men may initially react in an attempt to establish control over their lives in response to an uncontrollable event, but learned helplessness emerges as the exposure lengthens and experienced as involuntary. Loss of freedom, social exclusion, and lower satisfaction are the side effects of unemployment. What's obvious is that incarceration prevents one from finding work. Further, the prolonged exposure to the physical or psychological trauma that is endemic to prison environments may further damage a person's ability to work. Socioeconomic deprivation disrupts social and familial relationships.[31]

Continuous rejection from job searches can impact an individual's psychic disposition that ranges from frustration and disappointment to anger/rage, sadness, fear, and shame. The expectation of rejection can produce a fear of rejection which ultimately affects confidence and can lead to defensiveness due to shame or avoidance behaviors to avoid these potentially threatening experiences that can impact work performance and job-seeking behavior. These stigmatizing experiences may result in strained and uncomfortable social interactions, constricted social networks, compromised quality of life, low self-esteem, depressive symptoms, and unemployment and income loss. Black men may come to expect disapproval or rejection while their internal defense mechanisms are activated and vigilant. The stress caused by these interactions can cause Black men to drop out of the labor market altogether, which may serve as a form of self-preservation by providing congruence between one's aspirations and one's achievement or have the effect of internalization of negative self-attributions that result in lowered self-expectations for success. It is recommended that the Black-white jobs gap be closed through robust policy. Darity and Hamilton (2012) recommend a federal job guarantee program for all Americans that would provide the economic security of a job and remove the threat of unemployment. But a specific job guarantee program focused on Black men that intends on closing the Black-white job gap and ensure that Black men have a comparable employment-to-population ratio (EPOP) to that of white, Latino, and Asian men is imperative. Clinicians will need to actively advocate for policies (reparations, etc.) that have the capacity to systemically (structurally and institutionally) transform the lived experiences of Black men regardless of clinical interventions to address the issues raised in Chapters 5 and 6.[32]

NOTES

1 This section focuses on heterosexual marriage markets. The figures of marriageability are likely to be impacted as approximately 4 percent of Black adults identify as LGBT.
2 Cox, 1940; Darity & Myers, 1983, 1984a, 1984b, 1989, 1995; Rodgers & Thornton, 1985; Strobino & Sirageldin, 1981; Darity, 1980; Miller, 1991; Holzer, 2007; Willhelm, 1986; Curry, 2017, 2020; Hamilton et al., 2009; Amato, 2005; McLanahan & Sandefur, 1994; Seltzer, 1994; Geronimus & Korenman, 1992; Hoffman et al., 1993; Sampson, 1987; Chetty et al., 2018; Craigie et al., 2018; McLanahan & Booth, 1989; Fitzgerald & Ribar, 2004; Wilson, 1987; Lichter et al., 1991; South, 1996; Koball, 1998; Watson & McLanahan, 2011; Schneider, 2011; Kaplan et al., 2008; Landry, 1987; Alexis, 1998; Kearney & Levin, 2017; Darity et al., 2018; Pew Research Center, 2015; Wolfers et al., 2015; Stewart & Scott, 1978; Staples, 1985; Cho et al., 2021; Hagan & Dinovitzer, 1999; Pettit, 2012; Hampton, 1980; Blumstein & Beck, 1999; Noël, 2014.
3 Cox, 1940; Darity & Myers, 1983, 1984a, 1984b, 1989, 1995; Rodgers & Thornton, 1985; Strobino & Sirageldin, 1981; Darity, 1980; Miller, 1991; Holzer, 2007; Willhelm, 1986; Curry, 2017, 2020; Hamilton et al., 2009; Amato, 2005; McLanahan & Sandefur, 1994; Seltzer, 1994; Geronimus & Korenman, 1992; Hoffman et al., 1993; Sampson, 1987; Chetty et al., 2018; Craigie et al., 2018; McLanahan & Booth, 1989; Fitzgerald & Ribar, 2004; Wilson, 1987; Lichter et al., 1991; South, 1996; Koball, 1998; Watson & McLanahan, 2011; Schneider, 2011; Kaplan et al., 2008; Landry, 1987; Alexis, 1998; Kearney & Levin, 2017; Darity et al., 2018; Pew Research Center, 2015; Wolfers et al., 2015; Stewart & Scott, 1978; Staples, 1985; Cho et al., 2021; Hagan & Dinovitzer, 1999; Pettit, 2012; Hampton, 1980; Blumstein & Beck, 1999; Noël, 2014.
4 Cox, 1940; Darity & Myers, 1983, 1984a, 1984b, 1989, 1995; Rodgers & Thornton, 1985; Strobino & Sirageldin, 1981; Darity, 1980; Miller, 1991; Holzer, 2007; Willhelm, 1986; Curry, 2017, 2020; Hamilton et al., 2009; Amato, 2005; McLanahan & Sandefur, 1994; Seltzer, 1994; Geronimus & Korenman, 1992; Hoffman et al., 1993; Sampson, 1987; Chetty et al., 2018; Craigie et al., 2018; McLanahan & Booth, 1989; Fitzgerald & Ribar, 2004; Wilson, 1987; Lichter et al., 1991; South, 1996; Koball, 1998; Watson & McLanahan, 2011; Schneider, 2011; Kaplan et al., 2008; Landry, 1987; Alexis, 1998; Kearney & Levin, 2017; Darity et al., 2018; Pew Research Center, 2015; Wolfers et al., 2015; Stewart & Scott, 1978; Staples, 1985; Cho et al., 2021; Hagan & Dinovitzer, 1999; Pettit, 2012; Hampton, 1980; Blumstein & Beck, 1999; Noël, 2014.

5 Cox, 1940; Darity & Myers, 1983, 1984a, 1984b, 1989, 1995; Rodgers & Thornton, 1985; Strobino & Sirageldin, 1981; Darity, 1980; Miller, 1991; Holzer, 2007; Willhelm, 1986; Curry, 2017, 2020; Hamilton et al., 2009; Amato, 2005; McLanahan & Sandefur, 1994; Seltzer, 1994; Geronimus & Korenman, 1992; Hoffman et al., 1993; Sampson, 1987; Chetty et al., 2018; Craigie et al., 2018; McLanahan & Booth, 1989; Fitzgerald & Ribar, 2004; Wilson, 1987; Lichter et al., 1991; South, 1996; Koball, 1998; Watson & McLanahan, 2011; Schneider, 2011; Kaplan et al., 2008; Landry, 1987; Alexis, 1998; Kearney & Levin, 2017; Darity et al., 2018; Pew Research Center, 2015; Wolfers et al., 2015; Stewart & Scott, 1978; Staples, 1985; Cho et al., 2021; Hagan & Dinovitzer, 1999; Pettit, 2012; Hampton, 1980; Blumstein & Beck, 1999; Noël, 2014.

6 Cox, 1940; Darity & Myers, 1983, 1984a, 1984b, 1989, 1995; Rodgers & Thornton, 1985; Strobino & Sirageldin, 1981; Darity, 1980; Miller, 1991; Holzer, 2007; Willhelm, 1986; Curry, 2017, 2020; Hamilton et al., 2009; Amato, 2005; McLanahan & Sandefur, 1994; Seltzer, 1994; Geronimus & Korenman, 1992; Hoffman et al., 1993; Sampson, 1987; Chetty et al., 2018; Craigie et al., 2018; McLanahan & Booth, 1989; Fitzgerald & Ribar, 2004; Wilson, 1987; Lichter et al., 1991; South, 1996; Koball, 1998; Watson & McLanahan, 2011; Schneider, 2011; Kaplan et al., 2008; Landry, 1987; Alexis, 1998; Kearney & Levin, 2017; Darity et al., 2018; Pew Research Center, 2015; Wolfers et al., 2015; Stewart & Scott, 1978; Staples, 1985; Cho et al., 2021; Hagan & Dinovitzer, 1999; Pettit, 2012; Hampton, 1980; Blumstein & Beck, 1999; Noël, 2014.

7 Cox, 1940; Darity & Myers, 1983, 1984a, 1984b, 1989, 1995; Rodgers & Thornton, 1985; Strobino & Sirageldin, 1981; Darity, 1980; Miller, 1991; Holzer, 2007; Willhelm, 1986; Curry, 2017, 2020; Hamilton et al., 2009; Amato, 2005; McLanahan & Sandefur, 1994; Seltzer, 1994; Geronimus & Korenman, 1992; Hoffman et al., 1993; Sampson, 1987; Chetty et al., 2018; Craigie et al., 2018; McLanahan & Booth, 1989; Fitzgerald & Ribar, 2004; Wilson, 1987; Lichter et al., 1991; South, 1996; Koball, 1998; Watson & McLanahan, 2011; Schneider, 2011; Kaplan et al., 2008; Landry, 1987; Alexis, 1998; Kearney & Levin, 2017; Darity et al., 2018; Pew Research Center, 2015; Wolfers et al., 2015; Stewart & Scott, 1978; Staples, 1985; Cho et al., 2021; Hagan & Dinovitzer, 1999; Pettit, 2012; Hampton, 1980; Blumstein & Beck, 1999; Noël, 2014.

8 Woodson,1933;Frazier,1955,1962;Cruse,1967;Ferber,2007;Hamilton,2019;Tormala& Mc Kenzie, 2021; Sexton, 2008; Lemelle, 2001, 2010; Kaba, 2008; Moore, 2017, 2018a; Cooper, 2021; White, 2011; Ho, 2015; Baradaran, 2018; Ocampo, 2020; Gura, 2021; Wahba, 2021; Sidanius & Pratto, 1999.

9 Woodson,1933;Frazier,1955,1962;Cruse,1967;Ferber,2007;Hamilton,2019;Tormala& Mc Kenzie, 2021; Sexton, 2008; Lemelle, 2001, 2010; Kaba, 2008; Moore, 2017, 2018a; Cooper, 2021; White, 2011; Ho, 2015; Baradaran, 2018; Ocampo, 2020; Gura, 2021; Wahba, 2021; Sidanius & Pratto, 1999.

10 Woodson,1933;Frazier,1955,1962;Cruse,1967;Ferber,2007;Hamilton,2019;Tormala& Mc Kenzie, 2021; Sexton, 2008; Lemelle, 2001, 2010; Kaba, 2008; Moore, 2017, 2018a; Cooper, 2021; White, 2011; Ho, 2015; Baradaran, 2018; Ocampo, 2020; Gura, 2021; Wahba, 2021; Sidanius & Pratto, 1999; Powell, 2023.

11 Woodson,1933;Frazier,1955,1962;Cruse,1967;Ferber,2007;Hamilton,2019;Tormala& Mc Kenzie, 2021; Sexton, 2008; Lemelle, 2001, 2010; Kaba, 2008; Moore, 2017, 2018a; Cooper, 2021; White, 2011; Ho, 2015; Baradaran, 2018; Ocampo, 2020; Gura, 2021; Wahba, 2021; Sidanius & Pratto, 1999; Powell, 2023.

12 Woodson,1933;Frazier,1955,1962;Cruse,1967;Ferber,2007;Hamilton,2019;Tormala& Mc Kenzie, 2021; Sexton, 2008; Lemelle, 2001, 2010; Kaba, 2008; Moore, 2017, 2018a;

Cooper, 2021; White, 2011; Ho, 2015; Baradaran, 2018; Ocampo, 2020; Gura, 2021; Wahba, 2021; Sidanius & Pratto, 1999; Powell, 2023.

13 Rothstein,2017;Poe,2019;Nash,1988;Cell,1982;Williams&Collins,1995,2004;Massey& Denton, 1993; Jaynes & Williams, 1989; Wilson, 1987; Yinger, 1995; Oliver & Shapiro, 1997; Sampson & Wilson, 1995; Holzer, 2007; Fiscella & Williams, 2004; Massey, 2015; Lieberson, 1980; Massey & Denton, 1993; Rice, 1968; Helper, 1969; Philpott, 1978; Jackson, 1985; Bonastia, 2015; Katznelson, 2005; Massey et al., 2009; White, 1980; Hirsch, 1983; Bauman, 1987; Massey & Kanaiaupuni, 1993; Turner et al., 2002, 2003; Charles, 2003; Purnell et al., 1999; Massey & Lundy, 2001; Fischer & Massey, 2004; Squires & Chadwick, 2006; Cebul, 2020; Fullilove, 2001; Rothstein, 2017; Pudloski, 2020; Capps & Cannon, 2021; Hoffman et al., 2020; Leland, 2020, 2021; Stein, 2019; Craemer et al., 2020.

14 Rothstein,2017;Poe,2019;Nash,1988;Cell,1982;Williams&Collins,1995,2004;Massey& Denton, 1993; Jaynes & Williams, 1989; Wilson, 1987; Yinger, 1995; Oliver & Shapiro, 1997; Sampson & Wilson, 1995; Holzer, 2007; Fiscella & Williams, 2004; Massey, 2015; Lieberson, 1980; Massey & Denton, 1993; Rice, 1968; Helper, 1969; Philpott, 1978; Jackson, 1985; Bonastia, 2015; Katznelson, 2005; Massey et al., 2009; White, 1980; Hirsch, 1983; Bauman, 1987; Massey & Kanaiaupuni, 1993; Turner et al., 2002, 2003; Charles, 2003; Purnell et al., 1999; Massey & Lundy, 2001; Fischer & Massey, 2004; Squires & Chadwick, 2006; Cebul, 2020; Fullilove, 2001; Rothstein, 2017; Pudloski, 2020; Capps & Cannon, 2021; Hoffman et al., 2020; Leland, 2020, 2021; Stein, 2019; Craemer et al., 2020.

15 Rothstein,2017;Poe,2019;Nash,1988;Cell,1982;Williams&Collins,1995,2004;Massey& Denton, 1993; Jaynes & Williams, 1989; Wilson, 1987; Yinger, 1995; Oliver & Shapiro, 1997; Sampson & Wilson, 1995; Holzer, 2007; Fiscella & Williams, 2004; Massey, 2015; Lieberson, 1980; Massey & Denton, 1993; Rice, 1968; Helper, 1969; Philpott, 1978; Jackson, 1985; Bonastia, 2015; Katznelson, 2005; Massey et al., 2009; White, 1980; Hirsch, 1983; Bauman, 1987; Massey & Kanaiaupuni, 1993; Turner et al., 2002, 2003; Charles, 2003; Purnell et al., 1999; Massey & Lundy, 2001; Fischer & Massey, 2004; Squires & Chadwick, 2006; Cebul, 2020; Fullilove, 2001; Rothstein, 2017; Pudloski, 2020; Capps & Cannon, 2021; Hoffman et al., 2020; Leland, 2020, 2021; Stein, 2019; Craemer et al., 2020.

16 Rothstein,2017;Poe,2019;Nash,1988;Cell,1982;Williams&Collins,1995,2004;Massey& Denton, 1993; Jaynes & Williams, 1989; Wilson, 1987; Yinger, 1995; Oliver & Shapiro, 1997; Sampson & Wilson, 1995; Holzer, 2007; Fiscella & Williams, 2004; Massey, 2015; Lieberson, 1980; Massey & Denton, 1993; Rice, 1968; Helper, 1969; Philpott, 1978; Jackson, 1985; Bonastia, 2015; Katznelson, 2005; Massey et al., 2009; White, 1980; Hirsch, 1983; Bauman, 1987; Massey & Kanaiaupuni, 1993; Turner et al., 2002, 2003; Charles, 2003; Purnell et al., 1999; Massey & Lundy, 2001; Fischer & Massey, 2004; Squires & Chadwick, 2006; Cebul, 2020; Fullilove, 2001; Rothstein, 2017; Pudloski, 2020; Capps & Cannon, 2021; Hoffman et al., 2020; Leland, 2020, 2021; Stein, 2019; Craemer et al., 2020.

17 Rothstein, 2017; Poe, 2019; Nash, 1988; Cell, 1982; Williams & Collins, 1995, 2004; Massey & Denton, 1993; Jaynes & Williams, 1989; Wilson, 1987; Yinger, 1995; Oliver & Shapiro, 1997; Sampson & Wilson, 1995; Holzer, 2007; Fiscella & Williams, 2004; Massey, 2015; Lieberson, 1980; Massey & Denton, 1993; Rice, 1968; Helper, 1969; Philpott, 1978; Jackson, 1985; Bonastia, 2015; Katznelson, 2005; Massey et al., 2009; White, 1980; Hirsch, 1983; Bauman, 1987; Massey & Kanaiaupuni, 1993; Turner et al., 2002, 2003; Charles, 2003; Purnell et al., 1999; Massey & Lundy, 2001; Fischer &

Massey, 2004; Squires & Chadwick, 2006; Cebul, 2020; Fullilove, 2001; Rothstein, 2017; Pudloski, 2020; Capps & Cannon, 2021; Hoffman et al., 2020; Leland, 2020, 2021; Stein, 2019; Craemer et al., 2020.

18 Rothstein, 2017; Poe, 2019; Nash, 1988; Cell, 1982; Williams & Collins, 1995, 2004; Massey & Denton, 1993; Jaynes & Williams, 1989; Wilson, 1987; Yinger, 1995; Oliver & Shapiro, 1997; Sampson & Wilson, 1995; Holzer, 2007; Fiscella & Williams, 2004; Massey, 2015; Lieberson, 1980; Massey & Denton, 1993; Rice, 1968; Helper, 1969; Philpott, 1978; Jackson, 1985; Bonastia, 2015; Katznelson, 2005; Massey et al., 2009; White, 1980; Hirsch, 1983; Bauman, 1987; Massey & Kanaiaupuni, 1993; Turner et al., 2002, 2003; Charles, 2003; Purnell et al., 1999; Massey & Lundy, 2001; Fischer & Massey, 2004; Squires & Chadwick, 2006; Cebul, 2020; Fullilove, 2001; Rothstein, 2017; Pudloski, 2020; Capps & Cannon, 2021; Hoffman et al., 2020; Leland, 2020, 2021; Stein, 2019; Craemer et al., 2020.

19 Rothstein, 2017; Poe, 2019; Nash, 1988; Cell, 1982; Williams & Collins, 1995, 2004; Massey & Denton, 1993; Jaynes & Williams, 1989; Wilson, 1987; Yinger, 1995; Oliver & Shapiro, 1997; Sampson & Wilson, 1995; Holzer, 2007; Fiscella & Williams, 2004; Massey, 2015; Lieberson, 1980; Massey & Denton, 1993; Rice, 1968; Helper, 1969; Philpott, 1978; Jackson, 1985; Bonastia, 2015; Katznelson, 2005; Massey et al., 2009; White, 1980; Hirsch, 1983; Bauman, 1987; Massey & Kanaiaupuni, 1993; Turner et al., 2002, 2003; Charles, 2003; Purnell et al., 1999; Massey & Lundy, 2001; Fischer & Massey, 2004; Squires & Chadwick, 2006; Cebul, 2020; Fullilove, 2001; Rothstein, 2017; Pudloski, 2020; Capps & Cannon, 2021; Hoffman et al., 2020; Leland, 2020, 2021; Stein, 2019; Craemer et al., 2020.

20 Rothstein, 2017; Poe, 2019; Nash, 1988; Cell, 1982; Williams & Collins, 1995, 2004; Massey & Denton, 1993; Jaynes & Williams, 1989; Wilson, 1987; Yinger, 1995; Oliver & Shapiro, 1997; Sampson & Wilson, 1995; Holzer, 2007; Fiscella & Williams, 2004; Massey, 2015; Lieberson, 1980; Massey & Denton, 1993; Rice, 1968; Helper, 1969; Philpott, 1978; Jackson, 1985; Bonastia, 2015; Katznelson, 2005; Massey et al., 2009; White, 1980; Hirsch, 1983; Bauman, 1987; Massey & Kanaiaupuni, 1993; Turner et al., 2002, 2003; Charles, 2003; Purnell et al., 1999; Massey & Lundy, 2001; Fischer & Massey, 2004; Squires & Chadwick, 2006; Cebul, 2020; Fullilove, 2001; Rothstein, 2017; Pudloski, 2020; Capps & Cannon, 2021; Hoffman et al., 2020; Leland, 2020, 2021; Stein, 2019; Craemer et al., 2020.

21 Rothstein, 2017; Poe, 2019; Nash, 1988; Cell, 1982; Williams & Collins, 1995, 2004; Massey & Denton, 1993; Jaynes & Williams, 1989; Wilson, 1987; Yinger, 1995; Oliver & Shapiro, 1997; Sampson & Wilson, 1995; Holzer, 2007; Fiscella & Williams, 2004; Massey, 2015; Lieberson, 1980; Massey & Denton, 1993; Rice, 1968; Helper, 1969; Philpott, 1978; Jackson, 1985; Bonastia, 2015; Katznelson, 2005; Massey et al., 2009; White, 1980; Hirsch, 1983; Bauman, 1987; Massey & Kanaiaupuni, 1993; Turner et al., 2002, 2003; Charles, 2003; Purnell et al., 1999; Massey & Lundy, 2001; Fischer & Massey, 2004; Squires & Chadwick, 2006; Cebul, 2020; Fullilove, 2001; Rothstein, 2017; Pudloski, 2020; Capps & Cannon, 2021; Hoffman et al., 2020; Leland, 2020, 2021; Stein, 2019; Craemer et al., 2020.

22 Rothstein, 2017; Poe, 2019; Nash, 1988; Cell, 1982; Williams & Collins, 1995, 2004; Massey & Denton, 1993; Jaynes & Williams, 1989; Wilson, 1987; Yinger, 1995; Oliver & Shapiro, 1997; Sampson & Wilson, 1995; Holzer, 2007; Fiscella & Williams, 2004; Massey, 2015; Lieberson, 1980; Massey & Denton, 1993; Rice, 1968; Helper, 1969; Philpott, 1978; Jackson, 1985; Bonastia, 2015; Katznelson, 2005; Massey et al., 2009; White, 1980; Hirsch, 1983; Bauman, 1987; Massey & Kanaiaupuni, 1993; Turner et al., 2002, 2003; Charles, 2003; Purnell et al., 1999; Massey & Lundy, 2001; Fischer & Massey, 2004;

Squires & Chadwick, 2006; Cebul, 2020; Fullilove, 2001; Rothstein, 2017; Pudloski, 2020; Capps & Cannon, 2021; Hoffman et al., 2020; Leland, 2020, 2021; Stein, 2019; Craemer et al., 2020.

23 Rothstein,2017;Poe,2019;Nash,1988;Cell,1982;Williams&Collins,1995,2004;Massey& Denton, 1993; Jaynes & Williams, 1989; Wilson, 1987; Yinger, 1995; Oliver & Shapiro, 1997; Sampson & Wilson, 1995; Holzer, 2007; Fiscella & Williams, 2004; Massey, 2015; Lieberson, 1980; Massey & Denton, 1993; Rice, 1968; Helper, 1969; Philpott, 1978; Jackson, 1985; Bonastia, 2015; Katznelson, 2005; Massey et al., 2009; White, 1980; Hirsch, 1983; Bauman, 1987; Massey & Kanaiaupuni, 1993; Turner et al., 2002, 2003; Charles, 2003; Purnell et al., 1999; Massey & Lundy, 2001; Fischer & Massey, 2004; Squires & Chadwick, 2006; Cebul, 2020; Fullilove, 2001; Rothstein, 2017; Pudloski, 2020; Capps & Cannon, 2021; Hoffman et al., 2020; Leland, 2020, 2021; Stein, 2019; Craemer et al., 2020.

24 Stein, 2019; Fitch, 1993; O'Connor, 1973; Roy, 2009; Cebul, 2020; Berman et al., 2016; Callimachi, 2020.

25 Stein, 2019; Fitch, 1993; O'Connor, 1973; Roy, 2009; Cebul, 2020; Berman et al., 2016; Callimachi, 2020.

26 Stein, 2019; Fitch, 1993; O'Connor, 1973; Roy, 2009; Cebul, 2020; Berman et al., 2016; Callimachi, 2020.

27 Feagin, 2004; Pager, 2007; Goldsmith et al., 1996, 1997, 2000; Miller & Seligman, 1973; Brehm, 1966; Wortman & Brehm, 1975; Darity, 1999, 2003; Sen, 1997; Sibrava et al., 2019; Winkelmann & Winkelmann, 1998; Blustein, 2008; Gary et al., 1983; Staples, 1985, 1987; Stewart & Scott, 1978; Lemelle, 2001.

28 Feagin, 2004; Pager, 2007; Goldsmith et al., 1996, 1997, 2000; Miller & Seligman, 1973; Brehm, 1966; Wortman & Brehm, 1975; Darity, 1999, 2003; Sen, 1997; Sibrava et al., 2019; Winkelmann & Winkelmann, 1998; Blustein, 2008; Gary et al., 1983; Staples, 1985, 1987; Stewart & Scott, 1978; Lemelle, 2001.

29 Feagin, 2004; Pager, 2007; Goldsmith et al., 1996, 1997, 2000; Miller & Seligman, 1973; Brehm, 1966; Wortman & Brehm, 1975; Darity, 1999, 2003; Sen, 1997; Sibrava et al., 2019; Winkelmann & Winkelmann, 1998; Blustein, 2008; Gary et al., 1983; Staples, 1985, 1987; Stewart & Scott, 1978; Lemelle, 2001.

30 Feagin, 2004; Pager, 2007; Goldsmith et al., 1996, 1997, 2000; Miller & Seligman, 1973; Brehm, 1966; Wortman & Brehm, 1975; Darity, 1999, 2003; Sen, 1997; Sibrava et al., 2019; Winkelmann & Winkelmann, 1998; Blustein, 2008; Gary et al., 1983; Staples, 1985, 1987; Stewart & Scott, 1978; Lemelle, 2001.

31 Feagin, 2004; Pager, 2007; Goldsmith et al., 1996, 1997, 2000; Miller & Seligman, 1973; Brehm, 1966; Wortman & Brehm, 1975; Darity, 1999, 2003; Sen, 1997; Sibrava et al., 2019; Winkelmann & Winkelmann, 1998; Blustein, 2008; Gary et al., 1983; Staples, 1985, 1987; Stewart & Scott, 1978; Lemelle, 2001.

32 Feagin, 2004; Pager, 2007; Goldsmith et al., 1996, 1997, 2000; Miller & Seligman, 1973; Brehm, 1966; Wortman & Brehm, 1975; Darity, 1999, 2003; Sen, 1997; Sibrava et al., 2019; Winkelmann & Winkelmann, 1998; Blustein, 2008; Gary et al., 1983; Staples, 1985, 1987; Stewart & Scott, 1978; Lemelle, 2001.

CHAPTER 7

THE BLACK MESSIAH

PART I

Prevent the rise of a "messiah" who could unify, and electrify, the militant Black nationalist movement. Malcolm X might have been such a "messiah;" he is the martyr of the movement today. Martin Luther King, Stokely Carmichael and Elijah Muhammed all aspire to this position. Elijah Muhammed is less of a threat because of his age. King could be a very real contender for this position should he abandon his supposed "obedience" to "white, liberal doctrines" (nonviolence) and embrace Black nationalism. Carmichael has the necessary charisma to be a real threat in this way.

– J. Edgar Hoover, Director of the FBI

The marginalization of Black males is widely ignored, and their vulnerability remains invisible. The traumatizing effects of their marginalization and vulnerability rarely receives critical engagement that is empirically informed beyond theories and ideologies of masculinity, feminism, and superficial articulations of racism. The marginalization and vulnerability of Black males is critically analyzed through Black masculinity, Black male negation (BMN), anti-Blackness (anti-Black misandric aggression), patriarchy, feminist and intersectional framing of Black males, Black male death and dying, Black male suicide, No Humans Involved (N.H.I.)/dehumanization, genocide/gendercide, sexual victimization, phallicism, and intimate partner violence (IPV)/intimate partner homicide (IPH).

BLACK MASCULINITY (MANHOOD)

Masculinity encompasses the socially constructed characteristics that society expects of the male sex. Moreover, masculinity is performative and based on social context. Societal expectations of normative (i.e., heterosexual white male) masculinity includes the three notable markers of birth, marriage, and death. There is a societal expectation that males will accomplish education, athletic achievement, stable careers, marriage, and family. The construct of race differs from sex in that sex includes a biogenetically determined anatomical differential that is anchored and correlates with each culture's system of gendered oppositions. Black men don't just experience anti-Black racism because they are Black but because they are Black men (i.e., anti-Black misandry). Staples (1978) refers to this as the dual dilemma of being Black and male. Black males were not considered men but subhumans, and lesser men and boys. This maintained the social hierarchies and white power structure that sustained white male and female social, political, and economic dominance that preserved white totalitarianism. White paternalism and patriarchy have incessantly attacked the sense of self, value, worth, and humanity of Black men. Further, Black men were not considered men until the 1960s as a result of their self-determination that was manifested during the civil rights and Black Power movements.[1]

Studies of Black women emphasize how they were able to forge an identity of womanhood out of oppression that demonstrated their strengths (resilience) in spite of adversity. But Black men are not conceptualized in this manner and instead are thought of to be in crisis and walking pathologies (i.e., the *nigger*) who are broken and need to be fixed by *reclaiming/reimagining* a new masculinity or manhood or attempting to compensate for their

DOI: 10.4324/9781003430551-8

deficiency in manhood (i.e., compensatory masculinity) or attempting to emulate white masculinity (i.e., mimetic masculinity). These ideas are deficit frameworks that descend from such theories as the culture of poverty, and criminology problematize poor Black males as culturally pathological (e.g., the Cool Pose thesis-unique problematic cultural style). According to Lemelle (2010), Black masculinity is a major U.S. industry where service agents receive significant financial rewards in immeasurable ways by identifying and working on Black males as a social problem. Black males are often thought of as a mere variance of European American, middle-class, heterosexual men where they are at the margins of theories of masculinity that ultimately reproduce and perpetuate Eurocentrism. In addition, Black men are continually marginalized and compared to a norm by which they are deemed to be lacking when they are the subjects (i.e., objects of other people's projections and fantasies) of social, educational, and medical study. Often their personhood is only allowed to be constituted through a Black feminist framework. Their strength and resilience in spite of the incomprehensible deliberate violence and atrocities they have suffered are often an afterthought to their supposed deficits as Black males.[2]

Black families are egalitarian (e.g., authority, housekeeping, childcare, and employment) in family structure as a result of the harsh economic conditions that they were subjected to in the late 19th century, which is in sharp contrast to white family structure. Black men are not advantaged (e.g., education, labor market, income, housing, criminal justice system, health and healthcare, and retail sales market) compared to any group in the U.S. but are theorized and conceptualized as a privileged group. But Black men are routinely told they should not speak about their experience as they are centering their perspectives and their male privilege while taking up too much space. Black men are silenced from speaking about their oppression, vulnerability, or death and told it is patriarchal and centers their experience over women's oppression. This anti-Black misandry is not supported by research and actually censors Black men so that their positionality/experiences are erased and remain invisible while other groups capitalize on their oppression and deaths. Further, racial stereotypes about Black men are permissible and accepted as theory when coded as a sex/gender proposition. The discourse is moved from empirical data to ideology along with continued mechanisms of oppression and reinforces sex/gender-based hierarchy. There was no historical social scientific research or theory on Black (male) patriarchy until the late 1970s and early 1980s, which came from Black feminist reactions to the prominence of Eldridge Cleaver during the Black Power era. Black men have historically been anti-patriarchal (i.e., apatriarchal) while not identifying with feminist ideology and the analytic impositions imposed by feminist understanding and interpretations of sex/gender such as there being a worldwide hierarchy of male dominance of women within and throughout every society.[3]

Cazenave (1979) found that working-class Black men endorsed the following roles in order of importance: provider, husband, father, and worker. Hunter and Davis (1992, 1994) explored the meaning of manhood articulated by Black men and found that manhood emerged as a multidimensional construct where being a man was defined in terms of the self (e.g., self-determinism and accountability, pride), a man's relationship and responsibility to family (e.g., protecting family, child oriented), and a worldview or existential philosophy (e.g., spirituality and humanism). Four significant domains were identified: self-determinism, family, pride, and spirituality and humanism. Moreover, the domains included 15 distinct clusters of ideas. Discussions of masculinity were absent from their conceptions and definitions of manhood. Manhood was articulated as relational and interconnected meaning that relationships with others were instrumental in defining manhood. Therefore, it is questionable and problematic to conceptualize Black males within masculinity theories when they don't identify with these constructs. Research from Hammond and Mattis (2005) revealed that Black men define manhood within four distinct themes that included manhood as an interconnected state of being (e.g., meaning-making through the interconnection with God, self, family, community, and others), a fluid developmental process (e.g., manhood as being and becoming), a redemptive process (e.g., rectifying past behavior and recouping one's humanity through active family and civic participation), and a proactive course (e.g., anticipating potential barriers or threats to one's identity as well as ensuring its maintenance by initiating a set of positive life actions). These research studies determined that manhood among Black men is relationally constructed and multidimensional in nature.

Cazenave (1983) discovered that middle-class Black men have more progressive sex/gender attitudes than white men, support nontraditional roles for women, women's issues, egalitarian marital relationships, and believe that men can learn significantly from the way women act (i.e., show up in presence) that can be integrated into their own behavior. Gooley (1989) found similar levels of race and sex/gender consciousness among Black women and men. Research from Blee and Tickamyer (1995) continued to build upon prior research and confirmed that Black men and white men differ in their attitudes regarding women's sex/gender roles, where Black men were more progressive in their attitudes. Hunter and Seller's (1998) study on feminist attitudes among Black women and men found that Black men's experiences with unemployment may influence the acknowledgment of the importance of women and men inside and outside the home especially during difficult times. Simien's (2007) research discovered that the attitudes of Black men are overall more liberal and progressive than the attitudes of Black women. Black men in some instances were more likely to support Black feminist tenets (e.g., the interconnection of racism, poverty, and sexual discrimination, etc.) than Black women. This is attributed to an attitudinal shift by Black men that has persisted and widened over time.

Harnois (2010) found that Black men and women equally embrace many of the core ideas associated with Black feminist theory (i.e., Black women's standpoint), while Black men were more likely to support core themes (e.g., the interconnection of race, class, and sex/gender), which confirmed prior research. Harnois (2014) confirmed her previous research during a follow-up study which indicated that Black men have historically and continue to be significant supporters of sex/gender equality and are supportive of Black women's leadership roles in politics. The progressiveness of Black men is supported by research that spans over four decades and indicates that Black men are more sex/gender progressive than white men and women and on some measures exceeds the sex/gender consciousness of Black women.

Research from Jones and Mosher (2013) revealed that Black fathers are more involved with their children than white or Latino fathers. This was measured with residential and nonresidential fathers and separately for children aged 0–4 years old and aged 5–18 years old. Fathers were defined by whether they had biological or adopted children or if a step- or partner's children were living in the household. Black fathers fed or ate meals with their children, bathed, diapered, dressed, or helped them use the toilet, played with them, took them to or from activities, talked with them about things that happened during the day, and helped them with homework or checked completed homework more often than white or Latino fathers. McDougal and George's (2016) study on Black social fathers (i.e., residential and nonresidential stepfathers, mother's romantic partners, grandfathers, uncles, and other family associates who demonstrated parental behavior as fathers or father figures to a child) discovered that the package deal concept (i.e., in order to develop a healthy relationship with the mother, an equally fulfilling and healthy relationship needed to be developed with her offspring), the need for a male role model (e.g., Black children's need for a positive Black male role model), passing on a blessing (e.g., they themselves had one or more social fathers growing up), and biological father inadequacy were the reasons identified for becoming involved in non-biological children's lives. They were influenced by a sense of responsibility (i.e., social fathering taught them to be more responsible) and self-conscious role modeling (i.e., engaging in self-conscious monitoring of their own thoughts and behaviors to have a positive influence on the children). In addition, they identified influencing the children's lives through providing love and care, emphasizing education, and providing discipline. The phenomenon of social fathering has occurred due to changes in family structure (see Chapter 6 under "Black Relationships and Families" for details) and is also a part of Black culture and the concept of extended family, which came about as an adaptive strategy to maintain kinship beyond blood ties (i.e., fictive kin, informal adoption) due to the brutalizing effects of Black families being separated (i.e., assault on Black family relationships) during slavery. Enslaved Black Americans would informally adopt (i.e., "take in") children whose parents were sold away. Thus, family members receive needed instrumental (i.e., material needs) and expressive (i.e., socioemotional) support.

Black men are more sex/gender progressive than white men and women and have surpassed the sex/gender consciousness of Black women in many regards, are more involved with their children than white or Latino fathers, and have the most liberal sexual attitudes of all sex-race groups in the U.S. Black males have consistently demonstrated and embodied the essence of humanity and provided a template of an integrated whole human being. The development of a humane social and political consciousness by Black males (e.g., Martin Luther King Jr., Malcolm X, Huey P. Newton) emphasizes collective uplift, sexual egalitarianism, the significance of Black fatherhood within the Black community, and resistance to white racism (including their own sex/gender oppression). But their humanist orientation that creates and exhibits endless possibilities is not considered, and their experiences and embodiment are not viewed as a source of knowledge (i.e., knowledge production) that can advance humanity.[4]

BLACK MALE NEGATION (BMN)

Black men often discuss manhood and not masculinity in their self-conceptualizations. Therefore, concepts of masculinity are not applicable to Black men. Manhood for Black men often entails life-sustaining employment and the ability to support a family. Life-sustaining employment and the ability to support a family is deliberately elusive to Black men, which makes manhood unobtainable and controlled by the white power structure. Thus, Black men are not societally recognized as men and are thrust into a perpetual state of survival. Black males suffer disproportionate rates of intimate partner violence (IPV), intimate partner homicide (IPH), and child abuse (physical and sexual) compared to other groups of men, but their suffering is thought to be inconsequential. Black males in America are targeted for homicide, incarceration, unemployment, and an undercaste status. Black maleness is positioned as depositories of phobias (What Fanon (1952) refers to as a phobogenic object) and negativity. Black males continue to be theorized and described as hypermasculine, hypersexual, aggressive, immoral, and dangerous. Hypermasculinity was originally a term used to describe a female personality disorder that Black men acquired in female-headed households due to the absence of Black fathers, and now this pathological framework has been expanded to describe any and all behaviors (i.e., the pathological ontological beliefs about the Black male body) performed by Black males that one deems as problematic.[5]

Black men are a subordinated group and have the highest rates of victimization and are the primary targets of lethal violence by the state as they are thought of as living terrors. Moreover, they have the lowest life expectancy, the highest rates of mortality, and the greatest economic downward mobility of any race/sex group in the U.S. In academia, they are the most underrepresented group of professors and students next to brown men. The demonization and criminalization of young Black men in response to the Watts rebellions and others that followed as well as Black freedom struggle (civil rights and Black Power movements) generated a specific response from the white power structure that included incarceration and mechanisms of death and dying. The deployment and trafficking of constructed caricatures and mythology of Black males provided currency and the justification for their institutional decimation. Curry's (2017) theory of the *Man-Not* builds upon Wynter's (2001, 2003, 2006; Scott, 2000; Thomas, 2006) theory of genre where the Black male represents a specific genre category (i.e., kind of human/man that provides different articulations of the male body and psyche) and posits that Blackness negates or transfigures the political classifications of sex/gender or sexual orientation (i.e., markers of identity or one's claiming of identity). Further, all sexualities (e.g., heterosexual, homosexual, etc.) are defined by the imposition of (white) phobias (i.e., what social dominance theory (SDT) refers to as legitimizing myths) concerning the Black body and not by one's agency or claiming of sexual practice.[6]

Black male sexuality has been configured as pathological (e.g., the literal spreading of pathogens and disease) from slavery to present day. Black male heterosexuality is stigmatized as hypersexual and associated with rape, the procreation of "bastard" children, poverty, and superpredators, while Black male homosexuality is stigmatized as abnormal, diseased, and deviant. No identity is fixed in either case but fungible. Historically (slavery and Jim/Jane Crow), Black male bodies were configured by the desires of white men and women. Black men live in a world where they are the reflection of white society's fear. The neurosis of the white mind is activated by mere contact with the Blackened body that triggers the fleeing of the white mind from reality because of the physical proximity the white observer has to the Black male body. Frazier (1927) refers to this neurosis as *the pathology of race prejudice* where whites use mechanisms of rationalization (e.g., pro-slavery literature denying the humanity of Black Americans, opinion supporting lynching and oppression, justification for police killings, support for hypercriminalization/incarceration, etc.) to support their delusions.[7]

White fear is imposed upon Black males forcing them to struggle against white delusion to achieve social recognition. Black men are not simply othered but made nonexistent and reconfigured in the white imaginary for the justification of their subjugation and extermination. Western patriarchal societies are created through simultaneous negation and caricature of the Black male which renders him a *Man-Not*. The Black male is essentialized as a caricature of which he is not (i.e., the Man-Not) but what gender theory desires Black males to be. Caricatures are utilized to represent Black men (Black male bodies) as subhumans among humans and is deployed to animate the logics of dehumanization. Black males are thought to represent the pathological excess of white (bourgeois) masculinity in gender theories such as intersectionality.[8]

Building upon Curry's (2017, 2018) theories (Man-Not & Phallicism), Sidanius and Pratto's (1999) SDT subordinate male target hypothesis (SMTH), Miller's (1991, 2004), theory of patriarchy, and Jones' (2000) theory of gendercide, this author presents a comprehensive theory of *Black male negation* (BMN) that includes the interconnected mechanisms of caricature, dehumanization, gendercide, death/disposability, and sexual victimization/phallicism that operate to negate the experiences and existence of Black males. BMN encompasses the legitimizing myths of Black male pathology and deviance, the framing of

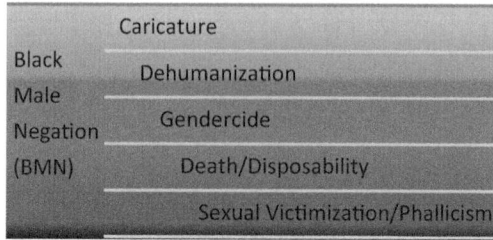

Figure 7.1 Black Male Negation (BMN)

Black males as patriarchs, the belief and behavior that Black males are nonhumans, geno-cidal logics that justify their disposability and deaths, and their positioning as subordinate out-group racialized males. The components of BMN are discussed in detail throughout Chapters 7 and 8.

ANTI-BLACKNESS (ANTI-BLACK MISANDRIC AGGRESSION)

The FBI 2020 Hate Crime Statistics indicated that approximately 62 percent of hate crimes were based on race/ethnicity/ancestry, 20 percent were based on sexual orientation, 13 per-cent were based on religion, approximately 3 percent were based on gender identity, 1 per-cent were based on disability, and approximately 1 percent were based on gender. Single-bias incidents totaled 8,052 and involved 11,126 victims while 211 were multiple-bias incidents that involved 346 victims. Anti-Black bias was the largest category of race-based hate with 2,871 incidents (a 49 percent increase from 2019), which indicates that 56 percent of race-based hate crimes are motivated by anti-Black bias. Moreover, there were 517 anti-Hispanic (Latino/a) incidents and 279 anti-Asian incidents.

According to Vargas (2018), anti-Blackness is fundamentally gendered as sex/gender modulates how Blackness is perceived and experienced (e.g., violence against Black males is related to violence against Black females but is also quantitatively and symbolically significantly distinct), and Blackness configures the ways in which sex/gender is perceived and experienced that does not translate to normative Western (i.e., non-Black) assumptions regarding femaleness being associated with subordination and maleness being associated with domination which do not apply to Black Americans. As previously emphasized, the research study of English et al. (2014) revealed that 89 percent of Black men reported experiencing racial discrimination. Black men report the highest rates of racial discrimination (e.g., job discrimination, police encounters, seeking employment, fair wages, getting a quality education, engaging with the healthcare system) than any group in the U.S. This includes racial discrimination and unfair treatment while shopping, while dining out, while at work, with the police, and while using public transportation. In addition, Black men report more experiences of racial discrimination and in more settings than women (e.g., seeking employment, working at their jobs, applying for bank loans, and interfacing with the justice system). A Gallup survey (2020) on Black adults and racial microaggressions found that Black men reported significantly higher rates of being feared, being treated with less courtesy, and mistrusted compared to Black women.[9]

Research from March et al. (2021) determined that white Americans automatically asso-ciate Black men with physical threat while Trawalter et al. (2008) found that the fear of young Black men as threatening and dangerous activates attentional resources in a similar manner to more evolutionary significantly threatening stimuli such as snakes and spiders. Holbrook et al. (2016) discovered that Black male-sounding names activate whites to envision that the imagined Black male is larger (i.e., bigger and taller) than their actual size and more aggressive independent of the actual size of the Black men in a white person's immediate vicinity, including Black men who were comparable in size to the white men. Wilson et al. (2017) examined racial bias in judgements of physical size and formidability and found that due to racial bias, people perceive young Black men to be bigger (i.e., taller, heavier, more muscular) and more physically threatening (i.e., stronger, more capable of harm) than young white men, thus believing that young Black men must be controlled using more aggressive measures. The research of Cobbina et al. (2019) revealed that when Black men challenged the police (i.e., verbal resistance through questioning their authority out of suspicion of being targeted), it proved to be harmful and resulted in the threat of or actual use of force where Black males were more likely to be handcuffed/arrested, experience police violence (i.e., assaulted), or jailed. When Black women challenged the police, they were often let go without adverse outcome or at the very worse received a traffic ticket. In addition, they found Black males to be more compliant than Black females, who were more likely to question the police. This supports Dollard's (1937) research that indicated that perceptions of aggression from Black men and Black women were qualitatively different where expressed resistance (identified as aggression, expressed resentment, or antagonism) is tolerated from Black women without penalty but not tolerated from Black men. He speculated that the aggression of Black women is tolerated due to Black women not posing a sexual threat (i.e., a sexual attack) and the chivalry (i.e., benevolent sexism) expected of men in society toward women but noted that there are limits to what is acceptable of Black women, but these limits are not as narrow as they are for Black men. Research from Gilliam et al. (2016) found that white and Black majority female (approximately 94 percent) teachers expecting "challenging behavior" looked (surveilled) at Black boys more often than Black girls and white children, which elucidated an implicit bias directed toward Black boys. Further, research from Owens (2023) revealed that Black boys are viewed as being more "blameworthy" among teachers than white boys for identical misbehavior. Quinn (2020) discovered that white and female teachers who evaluated the same second-grade writing sample graded it more harshly when it appeared to be written by a Black boy than when it appeared to be written by a white boy. Teachers were more likely to consider the writing to be at or above "grade level" if written by a white boy than an identical writing from a Black boy. Thompson (2023) established that Black girls experience a persistent advantage in educational attainment compared to Black boys due to Black boys experiencing higher levels of exposure to exclusionary school discipline and the criminal justice system. Goff et al. (2014) found that Black boys are viewed by most whites and non-whites as older and less innocent than their same-age white peers. In addition, dehumanization (i.e., the Black/ape association; *see N.H.I. No Humans Involved/Dehumanization section for details*) predicted police violence against Black boys. Todd et al. (2016) discovered that Black male faces whether adults or children (5-year-old Black boys) elicited race-based threat associations. Thiem et al. (2019) examined whether stereotypes that connect Black men and boys with violence and criminality generalize to Black women and girls. They found Black Americans are viewed as more dangerous than whites; whereas Black males were more strongly associated with danger than their female counterparts; and Black adults were more strongly associated with danger than were children. Moreover, research from March (2023) revealed that Black Americans may also perceive Black men as a physical threat.

McConnaughy and White (2011) found that whites view Black men as uniquely violent, where over 35 percent of respondents in their study believed that many or almost all Black men were violent. Consequently, approximately 15 percent thought of white men as violent, while 9 percent thought of Black women as violent, and 3 percent considered white women as violent. Moreover, 46 percent deemed Black men as promiscuous. Whites who characterize Blacks as a group as violent or promiscuous (42 and 42 percent respectively) are significantly more likely to describe Black men (35 and 46 percent) in this manner than Black women (9 and 23 percent). Respondents significantly positively evaluated Black women more frequently than Black men and viewed Black women more similarly to white women with the likelihood of both being equally deemed as violent or promiscuous. Therefore, the racial category of "Black" captures stereotypical attributions of Black men.

The stereotypes of Blacks as a violent and promiscuous group are driven by the views that whites have of Black men compared to other race-sex/gender sub-categories. Therefore, the meta-category of "Black" references to a differentiation regarding Black men. The negative evaluations of Black men affect assessments of Blacks as a group, where whites' cognitive schemas of Black men become accessible and dominant when thinking of Black people. Racial cues prime sex/gendered racial subgroup information that white Americans have stored in their implicit memory (e.g., crime primes the notion of Black male violence). This is further supported by the research of Navarrete et al. (2009) on fear extinction bias (i.e., fear-conditioning) and exposure to white and Black male and female faces who found that only Black males (out-group) prompted the fear response in white Americans (in-group), and further research (Navarrete et al., 2010) found that racial bias is targeted primarily toward Black males (out-group) by white men and women (in-group). Consequently, Black men are subjected to the most lethal forms of aggression and violence. In addition, the data supports SDT's SMTH that posits that the racial discrimination that Black women experience is a result of their proximity to Black men. This is further supported by Coles and Pasek (2020), who found that Black men and women are masculinized (identified as more masculine) by the dominant white group with Black men being significantly more masculinized than Black women. Consequently, masculinity is a necessary mechanism for dehumanization. The research of Ghavami and Peplau (2012) revealed that stereotypes associated with Black Americans ("Blacks") overlapped with a significant number of stereotypes associated with Black men than with Black women. Thus, Black men auto-populate the cognitions of people thinking about Blacks/Black Americans.

Blackness is attributed to Black maleness in the white racial imaginary. Veenstra's (2012) research on sex/gender discrimination by race, class, and sexuality compared intersectionality and the SMTH and found no evidence to empirically support intersectionality as a relevant framework but found evidence in support of the SMTH. In addition, research from Ifatunji and Harnois (2016) utilized intersectionality and examined sex/gender bias in the measure in perceptions of discrimination among Black Americans and found Black men report more personal experiences with discrimination than Black women in measures of everyday (i.e., racial microaggressions), major life (i.e., discrimination that could potentially block social mobility), and major life discrimination attributed to race (i.e., racial discrimination that could potentially block social mobility). The most significant items with sex/gender differences were "people act as if they are afraid of you" and "people act as if you are dishonest" (this aligns with the findings from a Gallup survey (2020) on Black adults and racial microaggressions). The most significant differences for items assessing major life discrimination that were racialized involved experiences with the police and in the labor market. Their research failed to empirically validate intersectionality but found evidence that supported the SMTH. Connor et al. (2023) evaluated intersectional implicit bias across race, gender, social class, and age and found no evidence to support the multiplicative interaction effects suggested by intersectional theorists. But they found a pro-women/anti-men bias followed by a pro-upper-class/anti-lower-class bias that was stronger among women than men. Blackness is primarily associated with Black maleness and anti-Black racism in the form of social mobility and lethal violence is primarily directed towards Black males. Moreover, Curry (2021c) refers to racism as misandric (i.e., anti-Black misandric aggression) due to the overwhelming evidence that racist violence disproportionately targets Black males for death and dehumanization.

PATRIARCHY

Patriarchy is routinely conceptualized by feminists as solely male domination of women. This includes the expropriation of household labor, workplace discrimination, use of violence such as rape, sexual assault, IPV, workplace sexual harassment, and child sexual abuse. The ideology of sex/gender inequality promotes the inferiority of women and the normalization of the socially constructed institution of heterosexuality. Further, patriarchy is characterized by many feminists as primarily a misogynist (i.e., hostile sexism) structure motivated by male hatred and contempt for women, but research indicates that the system of patriarchy in relation to women primarily consists of paternalism/benevolent sexism (i.e., chivalrous ideology that is favorable and approving of women who enact conventional sex/gender roles and the relationship between discriminatory intent and positive affect) and control of the sexual and social prerogatives of women rather than misogyny, hostility, and aggression. This correlates with attempts to control women along with the motivation and maintenance of positive intimate relationships (e.g., romantic relationships, friendships) with women. Therefore, sexism is an act of control, not an act of aggression, where patriarchal oppression against women is enacted through paternalism and coercion, while patriarchal oppression against Black males is enacted through violent, lethal, and exterminatory mechanisms. Sexism is routinely erroneously presented as a form of racism even though it is a distinctly different system of hierarchy that is designed to serve markedly different purposes.[10]

McMahon and Kahn (2017) found that protective paternalism (i.e., part of benevolent sexism that endorses the belief that men should protect and care for women) was related to anti-Black bias among whites only. Perceived threats among male participants such as reading about recent increases in violent crime increased endorsement of protective paternalism. Among white men this was associated with less support for policies that benefit racial groups and greater denial of racial bias in policing. A desire to protect women due to news of crime and danger increased racial bias.

While anti-Black racism is predominantly a project of usurpation and social predation that is primarily directed towards Black men who are routinely subjected to discrimination, violence, and acts of subjugation. Sex/gender analysis erroneously assumes solidarity between men and women who belong to different groups in society. Further, the brutality and terror that Black men are subjected to in the U.S. patriarchal system typically far exceeds patriarchal sex/gender hierarchies in both intensity and scope. What's missing from this analysis is how some men dominate other men and in a U.S. context how white women promote patriarchy. White women have economic and political power over Black men, and the domination and antagonism of Black men by white men and white women is completely ignored along with supporting empirical data. Ignoring this data is an anti-Black misandric mechanism that allows feminists and other groups to provide an ahistorical and revisionist account of history.[11]

Patriarchy is a system of dominance that is executed by both in-group men and women. Since antiquity, patriarchy has had an inherent problem with out-group men who are not covered by the bonds of kinship or culture and has historically sought to marginalize them. Weber (1947) defined patriarchy as the domination of younger men and women by older men. According to Miller (1991, 2004), the defining characteristics of patriarchy are kinship/genealogy, age (generation), and sex/gender. The sex/gender and generation elements of patriarchy relate primarily to the internal relations of the collective in-group, while the element of genealogy/kinship demarcates its external boundaries and relations. The patriarchal rank within the dominant in-group determines greatest access and first preference opportunities that are afforded to older men, while younger women are afforded the last choice and least preferences.[12]

Female marginalization within the in-group signifies an internal disagreement and quarrel. Kinship is extended by genealogy outside of the immediate household or family through the establishment of connections with other collectives through the notion of common ancestry. In the context of the U.S., kinship is signified by race where Black men as racialized out-group men are viewed as a threat and are the primary targets of patriarchy. Patriarchy does not only involve asymmetry in power between men and women but includes shared identity, group solidarity, common bonds, and mutual obligations. Patriarchy determines how a society is organized, and white men and women have vested interests in the perpetuation of patriarchy. Age and sex/gender are the basis of allocating power and social organization based on white lineage which enhances the survival of the group (white race). This includes relationships between women, children, younger men, and older men that adhere to a set of mutual and reciprocal rights (e.g., sexual division of power within the group), duties, and obligations which are encoded in culture, beliefs, rituals, economic relationships, status, and hierarchical power. It also sustains the codependency between men and women for reproduction and survival. Therefore, patriarchy is a system of social relationships and not simply male power. Issues of race, ethnicity, caste, and lineage are aspects of patriarchy.[13]

The in-group mobilizes in-group women to assist in the maximization of its appropriation of available opportunities. Therefore, in-group men and women cooperate and collaborate to advance or defend their group interests or position against others. Their cooperation and collaboration include exploitation or the denial of opportunities to other groups. The primary mission is to marginalize other groups in society and retain dominance not to marginalize in-group women; therefore, sex/gender is never the primary axis of solidarity. In-group men and women are partners who advance their group interests with men acting as senior partners and women acting as junior partners. Dominant in-group women exercise power over subordinate out-group men. The internal quarrel within the in-group between men and women does not obscure their solidarity in external subordinate group relations.[14]

A historical practice of patriarchy is to kill all the members of a defeated kinship group (i.e., men, women, and children), which is considered a double death, this includes death of individual members and death of the entire group (genocide). This permanently eliminates the possibility of the dead group from challenging the patriarchal group's power. Another tactic would be to kill the out-group men and capture the women and children while holding them captive. Killing the men not only prevented the disruption of the power structure but also produced genealogical death. The domination of out-group men is more severe and brutal than the domination of in-group or out-group women. The out-group men are routinely dehumanized and are conceptualized as nonhumans, and those that cannot be controlled are destroyed. Genocide entailed killing out-group males, castration of male captives (which prevented them from being able to reproduce), and nearly permanent enslavement of men. Out-group women were routinely integrated into the patriarchal societal structure.

Out-group men are not protected by the covenant of kinship and are always at risk of being killed, mutilated, emasculated, and permanently marginalized where they remain in a state of powerlessness. Kinship is the basis of social solidarity, while family is the unit of social organization, and patriarchy is the basis of the determination and exercise of power in and by the collective in-group.[15]

Out-group men who challenge the hegemony of the dominant group are subdued and severely punished by limiting their access to goods, services, capital, and status symbols of material progress, thus resulting in their elimination or marginalization. Therefore, their access to the material means and symbols that societally define and sustain manhood are limited. This includes the manipulation of opportunities for education, employment, income, and status symbols of material progress (e.g., lifestyles). This prevents out-group men from gaining access in numbers that would overturn the status quo. The dominant in-group will also punish the out-group men and defend their groups' interests from challenges by the out-group men by providing in-group and out-group women most of the opportunities for upward social mobility (e.g., education, employment, earnings, and status symbols). Some segments of the subordinate out-group will accept this socially engineered arrangement of upward social mobility within the opportunity structure created by the dominant in-group. Out-group males are excluded from employment opportunities in favor of out-group females. Out-group members who willingly accept these socially engineered conditions of sponsored mobility are participants in these sex/gendered outcomes.[16]

Subordinate out-group men pose a threat to the dominant in-group's political, social, economic, ideological, and cultural existence, which warrants their deliberate exclusion. This process entails dominant in-group men establishing alliances with subordinated out-group women, where out-group women are dependent upon in-group men to maintain their upward mobility into mid-level and intermediate positions within private and public bureaucracies. These out-group women operate as lieutenants to the in-group men who occupy the top positions (e.g., leaders of political parties, trade unions, colleges, schools, corporations, religious organizations, civil service, etc.) and are subject to the glass ceiling imposed by the in-group men but are in a significantly advantageous position in comparison to out-group men (subordinate out-group women who are not bestowed with sponsored mobility are continually marginalized). This fractures solidarity within the subordinated out-group, where the men are blamed for their lack of socioeconomic advancement. These partnerships with in-group and out-group women and deliberate exclusion contribute to out-group male marginalization through indirectly diverting opportunities to women along with a preference for women. This serves a dual purpose of keeping the out-group men in their traditional position (i.e., institutional decimation and the political economy of niggerdom) and defusing any challenge by dividing the social organization of the family (e.g., collapse of the Black family). This subversive tactic creates a rupture in the family structure where the idea proliferates that if the out-group woman can succeed in education, employment, income, and public recognition, why can't the men, and what is inherently wrong with them? Thus, the capacity of the out-group to continue to challenge the in-group is severely weakened.[17]

Out-group women are used as pawns by the in-group's conflict with out-group men. The out-group women are not considered a threat by the dominant group. An illusion of fundamental change is formed while patriarchy remains relatively unchanged. Dollard's (1937) research on racial caste in the South described this deliberate process that entailed the social, economic, and cultural isolation of Black men, which gave white men direct sexual access to Black women. Black Americans challenged the white holders of power for a greater share of the American Dream during the civil rights and Black Power movements of the 1960s and 1970s. Black women played a significant role, but this challenge was mainly led by Black men. The punishment for Black men has been downward social mobility and death. The challenge to the white totalitarian regime was stabilized through the penal apparatus in order to maintain domination of Black males.[18]

America's patriarchal treatment of subordinate out-group racialized males is supported by the theorization and research of SDT and SMTH. Other groups have followed suit and utilized the civil rights movement and Black freedom struggle as a blueprint to mount similar challenges with Asians being the only group to not have challenged white hegemony over opportunities.[19]

Patriarchy functions as a system of white dominance that utilizes racism, capitalism, militarism, hypercriminalization/incarceration, racialized policing, and sexual violence to subjugate and kill Black males who challenge or are viewed as a threat to the white power structure (i.e., the in-group). Connell (2005) defines hegemonic masculinity (i.e., authoritative masculinity) as the masculinity that occupies the hegemonic position within a specific context of sex/gender relations. Hegemonic masculinity is always positioned in relation to various subordinated masculinities (e.g., Black males within masculinities theory) and women.[20]

Hegemonic masculinity is the embodied configuration of sex/gender practice that legitimizes patriarchy and is interconnected with racist ideology and social dominance. Hegemony is established through collective cultural ideals and institutional power (e.g., business/corporate, military, and government) and deployed in structural interactions that function to legitimize patriarchal relations that guarantees social dominance. Hegemonic masculinity is the ruling class and includes both men and women. Schmitt and Wirth (2009) found the sex/gender difference within group identity in social dominance orientation (SDO) was mediated by sex/gender differences in feminine self-stereotyping (i.e., benevolence) and group interested responses to patriarchy (i.e., hostile sexism (misogyny) and benevolent sexism). Benevolent sexism was a powerful predictor of SDO among women, thus they posit that it offers advantages to women such as protection and admiration. Therefore, ruling class women (i.e., white women) are expected to endorse and legitimize patriarchal norms through emphasized femininity (i.e., vulnerability and acquiescence). Femininity or femaleness neutralizes some of the kinds of violence directed towards Black males.[21]

Research from Bracic et al. (2019) examined the 2016 presidential election of Donald Trump and sexism (politically defined as the belief that men are better suited emotionally for politics than women). They found that sexism was strongest and most consistent among white voters but not among non-white voters. Further, white women significantly endorsed sexist beliefs compared to white men (higher average levels of sexism) thus were more likely to vote for Trump and perceive him more favorably than presidential candidate Hilary Clinton. While 52 percent of the white female majority voted for Trump in 2016 and again in 2020, white women as a majority have only voted for Democratic candidates twice since 1952 [Lyndon B. Johnson (1964) and Bill Clinton (1996)]. Strolovitch et al. (2017) found that heteropatriarchy was of significant importance to white women specifically among married white women in the 2016 election. This is further supported by research from Project Implicit which discovered that women regardless of political ideology had higher levels of implicit gender bias than men.[22]

White men and women together operate within a heterarchy (non-hierarchical power structure) in relation to how they govern Black men within patriarchy, which Dollard (1937) referred to as the patriarchal caste. Jones-Rogers (2019) interrogates this relationship in her scholarship on white women as enslavers in the South. Racial bias is targeted primarily toward out-group racialized males by in-group men and women. Consequently, racialized out-group men are subjected to the most lethal forms of aggression and violence. According to McDonald et al. (2011), men and women are both agents of prejudice, but the character and underlying motivations of this prejudice differ among men and women, which is a function of different adaptive challenges (e.g., intergroup violence) that were confronted by men and women over evolutionary time. Prejudice held by in-group men is motivated by aggression against and dominance over out-group men, while in-group women's prejudice is characterized by wariness or fearfulness of out-group men. Men are more motivated to out-compete out-group men who are viewed as sexual rivals, while women are more motivated by perceived threats to their reproductive choice by out-group men. Schulman (1974) found that Black males are viewed as sexually threatening by white males and that the response to the sexual threat of Black men is potential racial violence. Black men are viewed as an out-group sexual competitor. According to Schulman (1974), the sexual threat of the Black male is much more prevalent than accepted in sociology. Men's out-group prejudice typically will be expressed through approach-oriented strategies that are characterized by aggression, violence, dominance, and social predation, while women's prejudice will be expressed through an avoidance strategy that is characterized by fear. Therefore, white men's racial prejudice manifests through aggressive and dominance-oriented prejudice (e.g., endorsement of white superiority and Black inferiority) primarily directed towards Black men, while white women's prejudice manifests through various forms of in-group favoritism and social distance from Black men. Recently, white women and white LGBTQ+ identified individuals have attempted to create symbolic distance from white men by verbally castigating (performative behavior) white men while retaining their mutual symbiotic relationship with white men. This smoke and mirrors tactic is part of the patriarchal apparatus where white women and white LGTBTQ+ individuals attempt to invoke a progressive and humane whiteness that ultimately preserves white dominance and Black subordination. This positioning is reminiscent of arguments made by white suffragettes and feminists in the late 19th and early 20th century, where they asserted that they were the best qualified to rule the so-called primitive groups (Native Americans, Black Americans, Chinese, and Filipinos). In addition, the "opposing" and antithetical embodiments of Black men and white women have consistently been weaponized in the American discourse of race as a marker of who is threatening to white patriarchal interests and who represents the greatest "good" of the in-group. Protection of white women is considered paramount as they are deemed to be the conservators of the white race. Research by Navarrete et al. (2009) on fear extinction bias (fear-conditioning) and exposure to white and Black male and female faces found that only Black males (out-group) prompted the fear response in white Americans (in-group).[23]

Wealth is primarily calcified in whiteness where in the patriarchal capitalist U.S., white men and white women maintain that wealth within their families (assortative mating) and the white kinship group ensuring an economic surplus in their families and white America. In addition, white women thrive on the inherited wealth (widowocracy) of white male patriarchy. America's patriarchal regime includes the long-standing practices of demonization, social marginalization, and extermination of Black males. Black men are disposable, and their oppression is linked to extermination, while Black women are exploitable, and their oppression is linked to coercion and control. Black men are viewed as cultural and biological threats to whites, thus becoming targets of the most extreme forms of lethal violence and discrimination (e.g., housing market, incarceration, employment, and policing). Black males are thought to be a threat to the futurity of the white kinship group, which includes its societal dominance and demographic prosperity. Throughout the 19th and 20th centuries, Black men were targeted by ethnologists, anthropologists, sociologists, sexologists, physicians, and politicians. Black men and boys are primarily framed as deviants and criminals, which deems their deaths as necessary for the survival of the dominant white group in the U.S. Lethal violence against Black males is not simply the product of fear or aversion but a program within the U.S. patriarchal capitalist society to ensure numerical majority, resources, and cultural influence of the dominant white group that derives a cumulative benefit from Black male death.[24]

FEMINIST AND INTERSECTIONAL (INTERSECTIONALITY) FRAMING OF BLACK MALES

Curry (2021b) found that intersectionality shares its conceptual foundation with subculture of violence theory. Feminist and intersectional (intersectionality) ideology harms Black males as it perpetuates racist myths and caricatures about Black males that are not based on empiricism but intuitive analytic projections. These projections justify and contribute to the marginalization (e.g., economic) of Black males, including the justification for their disposability and death. Gender represents a set of ideas or ideologies that describes and explains differences between individuals and differently sexed bodies (male and female). It is a normalized system of categorical social differentiation. The current configuration of gender is almost exclusively understood as the marking of difference between the female body and feminine kind in contrast to maleness. This construct was created by white women who sought to redefine themselves in contrast to the 19th century concept of woman as family.

The body and experience of the Black male was the template appropriated by white women to achieve their goal of conceptualizing themselves as an actual *minority group* despite the power and violence that white women inflicted upon racial and ethnic groups such as Black Americans and Jews. The gender construct was developed from the Black male's societal position within a caste system and is responsible for the disappearance of kinship within contemporary feminist gender theory. According to Thomas (2007), the neo-colonial context that has produced the commercialized gender and sexuality discourse in Western academia over the last several decades remains uninterrogated and mirrors COINTEL-PRO (FBI-Counter Intelligence Program) and U.S. imperialism in its effort to negate Black "nationalism" or militancy and Black popular culture. Further, according to Oyewùmí (1997) the construction of the social category of gender in Western society (Euro-American) invents biologies of difference (ideology of biological determinism) that are marked upon the body that is interpreted as universal. The effect is legitimacy and power derived from the supposed biology. The Black male body is the site of pathology and justification for the maintenance of social hierarchy. Oyewùmí's research on pre-colonial Yorùbá society indicated the absence of gender conceptions. Yorùbá society was based on social relations (not the body) and socially organized around seniority. Therefore, Oyewùmí critiques the universal Western hegemonic essentialist gender construct founded in biological determinism that is ethnocentric and imperialistic.[25]

Blackness ruptures Western ideas of gender but the complex lives of Black people who don't fit into the universalist accounts and narratives of grand theories such as Black feminism, queer theory, or Marxism are censored in order for these theories to remain legitimate. There is no empirical evidence to support the idea that race, class, and gender are defining aspects of interactions between groups. Data is not disaggregated regarding specific behavior groups impose on other groups among the grand theories of oppression. Race-sex/gender groups are described by abstractions that don't represent group dynamics but the ideological worldviews and politically motivated depictions of groups. Race, class, and gender as discourse is not a divestment from that which is positioned as natural (i.e., whiteness) but only reifies the cultural inventions of white supremacist taxonomies and identity abstractions that imagine disadvantage separate from actual empirical evidence. Until the 20th century, patriarchy was consistently conceptualized as a racialized system of domination. White women exploited the societal position of Black Americans, specifically the defining stigmas of the Black man's social location as the foundation for their formulation of the *woman*. The origin of this analysis of patriarchy in the U.S. is attributed to Alva Myrdal (1944/*A Parallel to the Negro Problem*), who proposed that women and children were suppressed classes. Thus, Black Americans, white women, and children all were subjugated by white male paternalism. Previous scholarship has focused on her conceptualization of the white woman's relationship to the slave as the foundation of gender along with influencing Simone De Beauvoir's (1949) *The Second Sex*. According to Myrdal, the paternal force of the white family similarly disadvantaged the woman and Negro. Female inferiority like Black inferiority was developed by white men. This argument would become adopted as accurate within current academic disciplines among researchers who have proclaimed that race and sex/gender are co-equal systems of oppression even though race and sex/gender has historically functioned quite differently.[26]

White women who owned enslaved Black Americans and declared patriarchy as the invention of their womb that manifested God's providence were now claiming in the mid-twentieth century to be disadvantaged by this patriarchy due to thwarted opportunities for wages and independence by the very same paternalistic system that was designed to protect them from external racial threats. The white woman was believed to be lesser than white men but part of the moral community of white civilization and not an outside animal (i.e., nonhuman/savage race of a different kind) like Black Americans. The Black male has always been thought of as a type of *being* that could not make any claims based on his humanity. Gunnar Myrdal (1944/*An American Dilemma: The Negro Problem and Modern Democracy*) described Black Americans as "undeveloped" and "childish." This was a register of inferiority that defined Black subordination to all white people and not solely social inferiority in relation to the white man. Myrdal's argument was justification for the racial caste system of the South and race relations in the North. The Black man and Black Americans whom he was thought to represent were to be governed through violence and intimidation which was not the case of the white woman who was fundamental to the caste superiority of the white race.[27]

Helen Hacker's essay (1951) "Women as a Minority Group" represents the dependency modern gender construct has on race. There was no account in the sociological literature of women being a minority group up to that point. The white woman's affinity towards group membership was based on race not gender. The *American Journal of Sociology* referenced racial and ethnic groups, but there was no reference to women. According to Hacker, the woman does not experience herself as the object of significant societal discrimination because of her group membership unlike the Negro and the Jew. Hacker theorizes that women endure the same social stigmas of the Black male due to the shared experience of subordination. Hacker appropriates the violence used to sustain subordination of the minority racial group to substantiate the idea of a hostile male class or the idea of men as a dominant group harboring hostility against women as a class and forgoes historical examples of horrific atrocities committed by white men against white women.[28]

White women invented the idea that all men have power over all women after observing the conditions of Black men under Western colonialism and the U.S. patriarchal caste system. Prior to the 1950s, white women were understood as primary members of the dominant race. This began to change in the 1950s when white women began to claim an oppressed status in a manner analogous to Black men who were stratified in a social system rooted in sharp caste distinctions. It was important for the kinship theory of patriarchy to be discarded and replaced in order for feminist ideology to obtain legitimacy with the conceptualization of white women as an oppressed class. This ahistorical and reconfigured current understanding of patriarchy has been particularly dangerous for Black men where they have become linked to patriarchy through claims of violence and savagery made by feminists. Moreover, white women being classified as a *minority group* has impacted affirmative action policy where white women are the primary beneficiaries.[29]

Feminist organizations routinely made attempts to obstruct singular concessions for Black Civil Rights that lacked specific provisions that advocated for increasing political opportunities for white women. The National Women's Party was a wealthy and exclusively white feminist organization that was committed to the political and economic interests of white women who developed a strategy to have *sex* added to Title VII legislation despite the barrier that it created to passing of the legislation. The National Women's Party approached Congressman Howard C. Smith, who was an 81-year-old conservative Democrat from Virginia with a history of opposition against Black Civil Rights initiatives and equal pay. Adding *sex* to the anti-discrimination laws had the effect of ensuring that white women captured the majority of the jobs and employment initiatives that were initially meant to address the racist distribution of labor participation and economic wealth. Smith had intended on obstructing the passage of Title VII since it was intended to protect Black Civil Rights and safeguard Black labor participation that would exceed beyond the 20th century. The scope of the legislation was radically altered with the addition of *sex* and the passage of the bill where remedying Black racial injustice was no longer a priority of the legislation which can be argued that remedying Black racial injustice through labor participation and economic wealth never was a priority of the legislation. The rights of white women were deliberately prioritized over Black Americans by adding the *sex* category. The precarious political vulnerability of Black Americans coupled with anti-Black sentiment left their economic prosperity to be determined by white lawmakers. The addition of *sex* to Title VII positioned the discrimination of white women equally alongside that of historically disadvantaged racial groups that had suffered enslavement and genocide. Employment practices were radically altered, and the political hiring initiatives associated with affirmative action permitted white women to substantially benefit more than the Black men and women who marched and died for racial equality, thus reinforcing white patriarchal dominance.[30]

Suffragettes were actively involved in the expansion of white patriarchal power through the utilization of ethnological tropes against Black males to assault their right to vote as well as issuing a rallying cry for mass lynching. White suffragettes demonized Black males as rapists and advocated for their destruction in order to achieve civilization. According to Terborg-Penn (1998), only 3 out of 83 Black men were opposed to women's suffrage. Therefore, 80 out of the 83 Black men who commented upon suffrage publicly supported and advocated for pro-women's rights organizations as well as participated in these organizations. Suffragettes attempted to convince white legislators and policymakers that Black men were too savage to obtain the right to vote, while the right to vote was being denied to more civilized white women. Elizabeth Cady Stanton and Susan B. Anthony created racist organizations that advocated for the barring of Negro men from the ballot. Suffragettes argued that the Black male did not deserve the ballot as he was a Negro rapist and a savage who would doom Western civilization. They circulated racist propaganda that claimed Black men were against women's rights and sought to destroy white womanhood through rape and called upon white men to protect them from the bestial lusts of Black men.[31]

It had not been more than 20 days that Black people had been granted citizenship when Elizabeth Cady Stanton and Susan B. Anthony began their campaign against Black men. Stanton was not only invested in white supremacy but white women ruling the world (i.e., imperialism) alongside white men. She espoused that womanhood perfected patriarchal power by making it less violent and more civilized. White feminist Charlotte Gilman claimed that patriarchy was rightfully theirs (white women) and that white women gifted patriarchy to white men. Suffrage literature would depict Black men as misogynists and hostile toward women's fight for voting rights. In addition, they trafficked the popular ethnological view that Black males were less evolved than white men, and as a result, Black men were crueler to Black women compared to white men. The trope of the Black male savage who beat their wives and abused their children was weaponized to demonstrate to the white world that Black men were uncivilized and underserving of the right to rule over others. They were to still be feared even though they were recently freed from slavery. These anti-Black misandric caricatures and tropes from the legacy of white feminism has endured and influenced 21st century sex/gender analyses. The political activity of Black men is still positioned as a threat and ideas about patriarchy remain framed around the idea that Black men impart violence upon women and children using domestic violence and rape. Suffragettes understood that venerated white womanhood in opposition to the vilified Black male was a powerful political identity tool for influencing public support and shaping public opposition. The ideological currency of Black male pathology and sexual violence proliferated discourses initiated by white women for white women to gain political power and standing in their white suprem-acist society.[32]

Intersectionality is a framework that posits that social identities (race, class, gender, etc.) interact simultaneously to influence the experience of discrimination but has not been able to provide empirical data on just how precisely these social identities interact. The under-lying assumption of intersectionality is that all previous theories only accounted for one dimension ("single-axis") of oppression at a time. Intersectional theorists posit that people with multiple identities routinely navigate privilege and oppression based on their multiple identities and multiple marginalized identities have an additive, interactive, or multiplica-tive effect where multiple forms of oppression are experienced, but emerging research has contradicted[33] these reductive propositions. The research of Macrae et al. (1995) found that people rely on a single category (i.e., Black males) that guides their perception when encoun-tering multiple categorizable targets. A specific category becoming dominant is contingent upon the situation or chronic salience of various categories, the perceiver's goals, or their prejudices. The activation of the dominant category becomes more cognitively accessible which inhibits the activation of competing categories. This allows the perceiver to categorize others quickly and automatically with minimal cognitive expenditure. The essentialism of intersectionality has become shorthand rhetoric used to describe complex social processes. This prevents legitimate rigorous research analyzing the relationship between the historical and political causes of continuous violence against Black males. Intersectionality recon-stitutes Black female identity around sameness and difference with Black men and white women while requiring that Black males be primarily theorized around sameness with white men as patriarchs. The intersectional reformulations afforded to Black females are denied to Black males. The primary thesis of intersectionality theorists is that Black men are oppressed

by racism and white supremacy but privileged (empowered) by their masculinity in a
Western patriarchal society. Moreover, the dominant view presented by intersectional and
Black feminist theories throughout American universities of Black masculinity is an assertion that Black men are less powerful than white men (hegemonic masculinity) and desire
power (male privilege) and endorse social hierarchy in order to dominate Black women and
other marginalized Black groups (LGBTQ+) in the Black community even though there
is no research to confirm these ideas, and the available research actually contradicts such
assertions.[34]

These theories and myths reduce the study of Black males to mimetic caricaturiza-
tion that has proliferated gender studies over the past several decades. According to this
scholarship, Black males imitate white masculinity out of their desire for completeness and
manhood. The caricatures and myths of Black males frame them as child-like creatures who
are dependent on white societal norms for the architecture of Black manhood. Further, this
ideology asserts that Black men use violence to compensate for centuries of racial discrimination and injuries as a result of being lesser men due to racism. These theories and myths
are primarily applied to Black men and boys with very little effort of empirical verification
to substantiate such claims.[35]

Intersectionality operates as an analytic dictum rather than an explanatory theory
where it requires the subordination of women to be a structural feature as well as a replicative function in every analysis of racial groups in order for it to hold historical relevance.
Absent from these theories are the disproportionate numbers of Black men who experience
lethal violence, rape, and IPV. These theories have their foundations in criminology's subculture of violence theories of the 1960s and feminist theories of the 1970s and 1980s who
constructed Black men as violent sexual predators who took pleasure in the murder and rape
of others. The premise of mimeticism has become the foundation and starting point for all
work on Black males in the academic arena that has become part of pop culture and everyday civilian life. Therefore, theoretical research (e.g., throughout various fields) on Black
men either attempts to affirm or refute the ideology of Black male deviance. Pathology is
the central origin and position in thinking about the Black male in either attempts to affirm
or refute Black male deviance (e.g., criminality, hypermasculinity, hypersexuality, misogyny,
violence). These anti-Black misandric caricatures of Black men frame them as the negative
element of the Black community. There is an apparent need by feminist theorists to proxi-
mally locate Black males within regimes of privilege and power due to their maleness even
though Black men have no privileges or institutional power in the U.S.[36]

An intersectional analysis relies on the deployment of the gender category that intui-
tively asserts Black men and boys are privileged compared to Black women and girls. Social
asymmetries between Black men and women are viewed by intersectionality theorists as
ontological with the effect of Black male privilege being assigned to Black male existence,
which completely ignores the economic, political, and educational advantage of Black
women over their male counterparts. The empiricism and sociological contextualization
that continues to demonstrate greater Black male disadvantage in health, education, economic (downward) mobility, mortality, police homicide, and imprisonment is completely
ignored. When empirical arguments have been made demonstrating the peculiar and peril-
ous condition of being Black and male in the U.S., intersectional theorists deploy distorted
and grotesque explanations (e.g., Black males are an endangered species and therefore fall
outside the scope of an intersectional analysis or the significant numbers of Black males
who are the primary targets of lethal violence and patriarchal oppression in the U.S. does
not alter their privileged and dominant position) that are genocidal logics. This legitimizes

the death and dying of Black males as it reinforces the myth that Black males are dangerous brutes that have to be controlled primarily through death and dying.[37]

Black males do not have structural power over Black women in American society. The analyses provided regarding ideas of Black male privilege and Black patriarchy routinely emphasize interpersonal physical threats Black males are thought to pose to female, queer, and trans-bodies, while systemic advantages in employment, economic mobility, or wealth is nonexistent in these analyses. The idea of Black male privilege lacks sociological or empirical evidence but provides ideological currency and is a tool to justify the mistreatment and absence of Black men throughout various American institutions. Black men are conceptualized as toxic perpetrators who are boogeyman. This gender schema interprets/positions Black males as distorted and pathological in their responses to anti-Black racism and white supremacy, while Black women are interpreted and positioned within group-based identities as opposed to patriarchy and committed to liberation. Black men are allowed to be publicly hated under the guise of progressive politics which makes anti-Black misandry permissible. Black men do not benefit from patriarchy but are primary targets for institutional decimation and the political economy of niggerdom in the U.S. patriarchal capitalist society. Historically, Black men have defined themselves in opposition to the imperialistic construct of sex/gender and patriarchy. Black men are not socialized with the expectation that the behavior or ideals of white masculinity will apply to them. Black male youth are aware of the high rate of Black male unemployment, lack of Black men in high-paying/high-prestige occupations, and the general inferior status of Black males in America. Framing Black men as dangerous, criminal, and as rapists has historically been identified as racist, but now the very same ideas can be repackaged and made acceptable with gender theories of Black (toxic) masculinity. It is important to note that the term toxic masculinity is a media term that is not empirically supported with adoption among conservative policymakers, therapists, feminists, and others that historically have targeted marginalized men. The politics of intersectionality requires the prioritization of other identity groups above the empirical disadvantage and suffering of specific racial and ethnic minorities. Intersectionality is invested in the predetermined deployment of categorical oppression that is absolute (Black and female) instead of a system of analysis in which comparisons between subjects of differing race, class, and gender positions can be empirically tested.[38]

The seemingly fixed perspective/position of intersectional analyses on the sexual pathology and social deviance of Black men and boys has its origins in the criminological formulation of Black maleness as a threat to women. The initial formulation of intersectional analysis by Kimberlé Crenshaw (1991) is contingent upon an understanding of racial patriarchy that is inextricably attached to dominance feminism's emphasis on physical violence and the criminological construct of the intra-racial rapist. Crenshaw (1991, 2010; Cho et al., 2013) cites Joyce Williams and Karen Holmes' work *The Second Assault: Rape and Public Attitudes* (1981) and has routinely cited MacKinnon's (1989) dominance feminism and its influence on her theory of intersectionality. Mackinnon's theory contends that women are a class that are defined by their subordination in a patriarchal world that is ruled by men. Therefore, the susceptibility to rape and sexual violence is what defines womanhood. MacKinnon's thesis indicates that the entity of "woman" is forced to engage the world not only through asymmetrical relationships with men but primarily defined by their susceptibility to violence from men. MacKinnon's (1989) work has been deemed gender essentialist whose conceptualization of womanhood is centered on white women's experience. Nonetheless, this idea of "woman" that equates to subordination has been consistently deployed throughout Crenshaw's work on intersectional subordination in relation to Black Americans and specifically regarding issues of domestic abuse and rape among Black women in the Black community and women of color generally. Crenshaw's intersectional explanations relies on theories that position the subordination of women within the Black community upon racist theories of Black male savagery and criminality. Crenshaw has relied on literature that has depicted Black males as brutish sexual predators and deviants. Crenshaw's (1991) work included unfounded claims that rape was used to control and discipline the Black community which comes out of subculture of violence theory. Citing and integrating the work of white feminists, intersectionality posits as fact that Black men rape simply for patriarchal power while simultaneously describing the sexual vulnerability of women and girls in the Black community in order to affirm the theory. This reproduces a mimetic theory of Black manhood where Black males aspire to imitate white masculinity (norms and power) with an attempt to replicate white patriarchy in response to their negation as a result of anti-Black racism.[39]

The deployment of various caricatures of Black men and boys by intersectionality theorists are based on speculative accounts of deviance and fail to be reconciled with existing empirical literature. bell hooks provides mimetic theorization of Black men in *We Real Cool: Black Men and Masculinity* (2004), where she claims that the history of racism and Jim Crow segregation caused Black hypersexuality, and Black men were forced to create a compensatory phallic identity. Thus, sexuality for Black men became a compensatory trait. According to hooks, Black males exaggerate the most deleterious characteristics of white masculinity because they have not had positive psychical or cultural resources of resistance to provide a foundation of Black manhood. Black masculinity is framed as vacuous that integrates white masculinity for substance. Further, Black masculinity developed an obsession with patriarchal sex to cope with racist oppression. hooks underscores the pathological nature of Black maleness and deemphasizes the oppressive conditions confining Black males. In contrast to subculture of violence theories that focus specifically on poor young Black males, hooks proposes that all Black masculinity is sexually coercive and the origin of Black male sexual pathology and aggression. Therefore, Black male resistance to white supremacy and social marginalization is understood by hooks as the internalization of racist tropes offered by white society regarding Black masculinity. hooks contends that the societal negation of Black men influences them to embrace the racialized caricature of the beast. hooks asserts in *Killing Rage: Ending Racism* (1995) that Black males are driven by rage and motivated by violence and in referencing the Central Park Five case states that the gang rape of the Central Park jogger (white woman) by the Central Park Five (Black and Latino boys) as teens is indicative of the use of Black rage as justification for despicable behavior enacted by Black men. Not only is such an assertion simply ludicrous and if it had been uttered by a white person would potentially be condemned as pure racist rhetoric directed at Black boys and men, but the Central Park Five were eventually exonerated in this case. hooks does not rely on empirical evidence or ethnographic accounts to reach her conclusions but instead seems to rely on an intuitive analysis.[40]

During Jim/Jane Crow, Black males were not considered men, they were conceptualized to be feminine and in search of their manhood. As the struggle for civil rights began to be realized, Black men were demonized for their aspiration to achieve manhood and political equality by white criminologists and white feminists. White feminists by the 1970s launched significant academic and political campaigns to frame Black militancy as a terroristic threat to white womanhood, and poor Black men were positioned as violent rapists that were a danger to American society who needed to be responded to with criminalization/incarceration. The pathological descriptions of Black manhood proposed by Martin Wolfgang and Franco Ferracuti (1967) as evidence of the Black subculture of violence is replicated by hooks in her descriptions of Black masculinity. According to Wolfgang and Ferracuti (1967/*The Subculture of Violence: Towards an Integrated Theory in Criminology*), subcultures are distinct and separate from the dominant culture and are characterized by violence, and subordinated groups such as Black Americans had a distinct culture that was separate from the mainstream white culture. Therefore, the supposed pathological self-destructive behavior of Black men and women was caused by Black subculture.[41]

The psychological traits and specific worldview that is distant from the dominant or parent culture is reflected in the use of force or violence whether interpersonally or in a group is normative within a subcultural grouping. Wolfgang and Ferracuti's theory primarily focused on homicide. They took a particular interest in why there was a disproportionate routine use of lethal violence and aggression by Black men and Black women within their communities. Wolfgang's student Menachem Amir's *Patterns in Forcible Rape* (1971) contributed a subculture of violence theory that claimed to provide an explanation as to why poor Black men became habituated to committing rape and how these values were transmitted from childhood and adulthood by Black women as mothers and partners. According to Amir, Black culture was pathological, and the Black family structure was improper, thus causing Black men to become rapists. Black mothers were unfit, which resulted in Black fathers being absent, and Black culture prioritized sensual pleasures over civilized ones, causing Black men to develop a psychological need to overcompensate for their feminized self-images, thus causing them to become rapists. His theory was an extension of Wolfgang and Feracutti's work in which he believed that the same subcultural values that produced criminality could elucidate the occurrence of rape. Amir's theory became the most prominent 20th century cultural explanation of Black male sexual aggression. According to Amir, Black male rapists were produced from the deviant racial norms (values) of Black Americans. Black masculinity was disfigured and more feminine because of absent Black fathers and the lack of a patriarchal structure. This theory presents Black masculinity as a distorted racial prototype of white patriarchal culture. Significant utility was found among American feminists in Amir's racialists accounts of rape. Amir asserted that sociology and criminology demonstrate that rape is primarily an intra-racial phenomenon, and the peculiar notions of masculinity found within the Black subculture produces rape. Subculture of violence explanations for rape in the Black community were enthusiastically supported by Susan Brownmiller, who took a particular interest in Amir's study of rape patterns in Philadelphia. Amir's work disproved the long-standing racist trope of the Black male rapist of white women but provided feminists with the construct of the intra-racial rapist, which motivated feminist theorization in the U.S. for the next several decades.[42]

Lynn A. Curtis sought to reformulate the deviant model of the Black male rapist offered by subculture of violence theorists Amir (1971) and Brownmiller (1975/*Against Our Will: Men, Women, and Rape*) into a theory of Black male pathology. According to Curtis (1975/*Violence, Race, and Culture*), the higher rates of rape perpetration by Black males were a result of their distortion of white patriarchy (i.e., emulation of white male patriarchy and its relationship with sexual violence). The patriarchy that Black males had been excluded from left them desperately attempting to join. Shulamith Firestone (1970/*The Dialectics of Sex*) makes a similar argument that in their attempts to emulate white men (i.e., white patriarchy), Black men substitute powerlessness with a distortion of white culture and pathology. While the subculture of violence theories (e.g., Wolfgang and Ferracuti, and Amir) framed the Black male rapist as a product of socialization that included the transmission of Black subcultural values that emphasized aggression and violence that were imparted upon young Black men by their mothers and the sexual behaviors of Black women, Curtis declared that the Black male rapist was a distinctive trait of poor Black male culture and removed the role attributed to Black women in maintaining subcultures of violence. Therefore, the analysis shifted from subcultural values shared by all members of poor Black communities to the sexual aggression and violence of Black males which represented the internalization of white patriarchal norms. Black women were recast as innocent victims of the brutality of pathological Black males instead of participants in violence. Curtis speculated that it was poor Black masculinity (race, class, and gender) that produced the most virulent form of rape culture in the U.S. Moreover, Black males altered and degraded white patriarchy, which became more savage and violent. According to Curtis (1975), Black male sexuality compared to white masculinity was compensatory and more exploitative of women. Therefore, a more brutish sexism directed towards women was possessed by Black males than white male patriarchy, which was more sophisticated. Black masculinity was more criminogenic in nature with the sole motivation of deviance, sexual aggression, and the rape of women, while white patriarchy encompassed paternalistic elements that were motivated to protect and care for women. Curtis conceptualized Black males as sexually insatiable, whose predatory conquests of women was central to their identity. Thus, Black males were socialized to be criminals and rapists.[43]

Joyce Williams and Karen Holmes (1981/ *The Second Assault: Rape and Public Attitudes*) theorized that the act of rape determined all relationships between men and women of white dominant racial groups, including the relationships within subordinate Black and brown minority groups. They cited Curtis and found his analysis to be in alignment with their feminist anti-rape ideology, thus further expanding his work. All women were under the constant threat of rape from all men due to patriarchy. White and Black masculinity were theorized as indistinguishable and the origin of rape and sexual assault. Black females were theorized to be victims, while Black males were theorized to be victimizers. Greater levels of sexual violence, homicide, and deviance in Black communities were attributed to sex/gender instead of racism and poverty. This feminist analysis positioned Black masculinity in a hierarchically fixed positionality within the Black race that contained mimetic tendencies of the white race. Black men become rapists because they imitate the patterns of white male patriarchy. This gave birth to the idea that Black men were patriarchal oppressors of Black women. White society created the sexual mania of the Black male who rejected the white master's civility. Williams and Holmes insist that white male patriarchy is a national and global concern, but they frame the Black male as the most pertinent social threat to women as well as a political problem for them. Williams and Holmes (1981) admitted that there was no empirical evidence for either the myth of Black male sexuality or sex as compensatory behavior. Black males' alleged proclivity to rape Black women was supposedly motivated by these claims (myths and caricatures) and remain the foundation of intersectional feminist thought. Crenshaw (1991) cites Williams and Holmes with the claim that rape is used to control and discipline the Black community as evidence of historical scholarship on rape and race, thus she relies on and perpetuates white supremacist theories of Black life and the Black male rapist caricature to provide credibility to her theory/assertions and this remains relatively unchallenged. Crenshaw's "gender" analysis is not grounded in historical and sociological evidence but racist scholarship that was motivated by the political needs of elite white women. Decades of social science scholarship was disregarded in order to provide these ideas with legitimacy.[44]

Intersectionality is inapplicable to Black males as it does not consider the suffering, sexual discrimination, and death of Black males. Advocates of intersectionality ideology are routinely unaware of its history/origins and how to perform an "intersectional analysis."

Moreover, spewing the word "intersectionality" or "intersectional" has become a marker of the right moral orientation and politics (liberal/progressive) through the deployment of baseless platitudes to signal/perform a certain consciousness (wokeness) and supposed opposition to racism, sexism, etc. Therefore, intersectionality amounts to a zombie ideology with a cult-like following that endorses specific political projects. Numerous research studies have contradicted the propositions set forth by intersectional theorists regarding the cumulative effect of oppression on multiple identities (double jeopardy hypothesis, i.e., race, class, and gender, etc.) in which race (particularly Blackness but applicable to other racialized groups) creates a rupture in these Western identity conceptualizations (i.e., white taxonomies or middle-class variants) of humanity. But despite this, the dogma of this framework remains as it provides the bourgeois elite and their followers symbolic and material rewards. Intersectionality also provides the ideological currency for individuals/groups to traffic an idealized personhood (virtual intersectional self) through the construction of a personal phantasm of victimhood. Haiphong (2022) refers to this apparatus as intersectional imperialism that reached a pinnacle during the Obama administration and was led by the Democratic Party and involved the elevation of a tiny fraction of those who supposedly related to multiple experiences of oppression and were committed to imperialism. Intersectional theorists' (e.g., Black academics), including activists' appropriate Black male death for symbolic and material rewards.[45]

Intersectionality theory continues the historical anti-Black misandric analyses of racist criminologists and white feminists who constructed Black manhood as imitative and a deviant mimetic imaginary of white masculinity while currently theorizing that Black male existence is primarily compensatory. These gender theories/ideologies of compensatory Black masculinity are not supported by empirical evidence but have endured for the last several decades and reflect the misandry targeted towards Black men throughout society. These theories are routinely deployed through feminist and intersectional theory in the academic arena, which reinforce common racist myths regarding Black males as inferior and violent. Hatred, fear, and the negation of Black males is acceptable under intersectional and feminist declarations, while empirical evidence countering such assertions are completely ignored. Horrific racial violence against Black men and institutional marginalization is endorsed and legitimized from these feminist analyses that bolster racist criminological and carceral logics of American empire. Therefore, the extremely negative and dangerous views (i.e., stigmas) of Black males endorsed by whites and white liberals are acceptable and not understood to be racist. These pathological presumptions about Black males permits theorists to frame them as tragic figures who obtain their humanity through enacting violence against other groups and reflects a speculative psychology of Black male criminality.[46]

The literature produced by intersectional theorists over the past 30 years has not deviated from subculture of violence theory, while compensatory Black masculinity and racial-sexual stratification remain as defining aspects of intersectionality and Black feminist thought since the 1980s. These enduring ideologies are abstractions that attempt to explain and frame the deviant behavior and the disproportionate rates of violence among a small number of Black males as the character traits of all Black males as a group. The non-patriarchal (i.e., apatriarchal) masculinity of Black males is a culturally viable alternative to white masculine and feminine patriarchal forms but is viewed as a sign of weakness and defect. Feminism in the U.S. has consistently targeted Black men and established its identity in comparison to Black men. An identity formed on the basis of caricatures and the mythology of Black male deviance. It is documented that white feminist Gloria Steinem was a CIA agent during the 1950s and 1960s. She received CIA funding during this time, and it is rumored that she continued her

CIA ties beyond this period while receiving funding. The funding allowed her to disseminate her feminist theses in the U.S. and globally. Steinem has described the CIA as "liberal, nonviolent and honorable" during her tenure. Interestingly, the CIA was involved in assassinations and assassination attempts of world leaders (e.g., Patrice Lumumba, Fidel Castro) while promoting political instability in decolonized countries during this time. In addition, the CIA had infiltrated and placed under surveillance the Black Panther Party (BPP). Meanwhile, feminist groups have depicted Black nationalist groups as being motivated by a desire for white patriarchal power. Oddly enough, Steinem was a founder of the National Black Feminist Organization (NBFO). It is well documented that the FBI (COINTELPRO) and CIA attempted and ultimately succeeded in halting Black freedom struggle (civil rights and Black Power movements) and disrupting and destroying Black militant groups (e.g., BPP) with some of the tactics including surveillance, police attacks and murder, incarceration, exhausting of financial resources through protracted court battles, infiltration, and disinformation (i.e., state terrorism). Espionage and professional intimidation were used to silence voices of dissent. There has not been any critical engagement in academia or scholarship that seriously analyzes these connections. An ideology that is supposed to be motivated by the liberation of women has been invested in imperialism and white supremacist patriarchy since its inception in the U.S.[47]

NOTES

1 Staples, 1982; Lemelle, 1995, 2001, 2010; Sidanius & Pratto, 1999; Curry, 2017a, 2017b, 2018, 2021; Utley, 2016; Flaherty, 2017; Fanon, 1952; Curtis, 2014; Hare, 1971; Allen, 1969, 2005, 2010; Curry & Utley, 2020; Pass et al., 2014; Franklin, 1982, 1986, 1994; Oluwayomi, 2020; Ogungbure, 2019a, 2019b; Quijano, 2000; Wynter, 2003; Hunter & Davis, 1994; Frazier, 1927; Gary, 1995; Forman et al., 1997; Broman et al., 2000; Broman, 1996; Weitzer & Tuch, 1999; Welch et al., 2001; Hausmann et al., 2008; Taylor & Turner, 2002; Barnes et al., 2004; Brown, 2001; Din-Dzietham et al., 2004; Herring et al., 1998; Ifatunji & Forman, 2006; Sigelman & Welch, 1991; Ifatunji & Harnois, 2016; Saint-Aubin, 1994; English et al., 2014; Bonilla-Silva et al., 2006; Pieterse & Carter, 2007; Hudson et al., 2012.

2 Staples, 1982; Lemelle, 1995, 2001, 2010; Sidanius & Pratto, 1999; Curry, 2017a, 2017b, 2018, 2021; Utley, 2016; Flaherty, 2017; Fanon, 1952; Curtis, 2014; Hare, 1971; Allen, 1969, 2005, 2010; Curry & Utley, 2020; Pass et al., 2014; Franklin, 1982, 1986, 1994; Oluwayomi, 2020; Ogungbure, 2019a, 2019b; Quijano, 2000; Wynter, 2003; Hunter & Davis, 1994; Frazier, 1927; Gary, 1995; Forman et al., 1997; Broman et al., 2000; Broman, 1996; Weitzer & Tuch, 1999; Welch et al., 2001; Hausmann et al., 2008; Taylor & Turner, 2002; Barnes et al., 2004; Brown, 2001; Din-Dzietham et al., 2004; Herring et al., 1998; Ifatunji & Forman, 2006; Sigelman & Welch, 1991; Ifatunji & Harnois, 2016; Saint-Aubin, 1994; English et al., 2014; Bonilla-Silva et al., 2006; Pieterse & Carter, 2007; Hudson et al., 2012; Majors & Billson, 1993.

3 Staples, 1982; Lemelle, 1995, 2001, 2010; Sidanius & Pratto, 1999; Curry, 2017a, 2017b, 2018, 2021; Utley, 2016; Flaherty, 2017; Fanon, 1952; Curtis, 2014; Hare, 1971; Allen, 1969, 2005, 2010; Curry & Utley, 2020; Pass et al., 2014; Franklin, 1982, 1986, 1994; Oluwayomi, 2020; Ogungbure, 2019a, 2019b; Quijano, 2000; Wynter, 2003; Hunter & Davis, 1994; Frazier, 1927; Gary, 1995; Forman et al., 1997; Broman et al., 2000; Broman, 1996; Weitzer & Tuch, 1999; Welch et al., 2001;

Hausmann et al., 2008; Taylor & Turner, 2002; Barnes et al., 2004; Brown, 2001; Din-Dzietham et al., 2004; Herring et al., 1998; Ifatunji & Forman, 2006; Sigelman & Welch, 1991; Ifatunji & Harnois, 2016; Saint-Aubin, 1994; English et al., 2014; Bonilla-Silva et al., 2006; Pieterse & Carter, 2007; Hudson et al., 2012.

4 Staples, 1982; Lemelle, 1995, 2001, 2010; Sidanius & Pratto, 1999; Curry, 2017a, 2017b, 2018, 2021; Utley, 2016; Flaherty, 2017; Fanon, 1952; Curtis, 2014; Hare, 1971; Allen, 1969, 2005, 2010; Curry & Utley, 2020; Pass et al., 2014; Franklin, 1982, 1986, 1994; Oluwayomi, 2020; Ogungbure, 2019a, 2019b; Quijano, 2000; Wynter, 2003; Hunter & Davis, 1994; Frazier, 1927; Gary, 1995; Forman et al., 1997; Broman et al., 2000; Broman, 1996; Weitzer & Tuch, 1999; Welch et al., 2001; Hausmann et al., 2008; Taylor & Turner, 2002; Barnes et al., 2004; Brown, 2001; Din-Dzietham et al., 2004; Herring et al., 1998; Ifatunji & Forman, 2006; Sigelman & Welch, 1991; Ifatunji & Harnois, 2016; Saint-Aubin, 1994; English et al., 2014; Bonilla-Silva et al., 2006; Pieterse & Carter, 2007; Hudson et al., 2012.

5 Staples, 1978, 1982; Lemelle, 1995, 2001, 2010; Sidanius & Pratto, 1999; Curry, 2017a, 2017b, 2018, 2021; Utley, 2016; Flaherty, 2017; Fanon, 1952; Curtis, 2014; Hare, 1971; Allen, 1969, 2005, 2010; Curry & Utley, 2020; Pass et al., 2014; Franklin, 1982, 1986, 1994; Oluwayomi, 2020; Ogungbure, 2019a, 2019b; Quijano, 2000; Wynter, 2003; Hunter & Davis, 1994; Frazier, 1927; Gary, 1995; Forman et al., 1997; Broman et al., 2000; Broman, 1996; Weitzer & Tuch, 1999; Welch et al., 2001; Hausmann et al., 2008; Taylor & Turner, 2002; Barnes et al., 2004; Brown, 2001; Din-Dzietham et al., 2004; Herring et al., 1998; Ifatunji & Forman, 2006; Sigelman & Welch, 1991; Ifatunji & Harnois, 2016; Pieterse & Carter, 2007; Hudson et al., 2012; Saint-Aubin, 1994; English et al., 2014; Barclay & Cusumano, 1967.

6 Staples, 1978, 1982; Lemelle, 1995, 2001, 2010; Sidanius & Pratto, 1999; Curry, 2017a, 2017b, 2018, 2021; Utley, 2016; Flaherty, 2017; Fanon, 1952; Curtis, 2014; Hare, 1971; Allen, 1969, 2005, 2010; Curry & Utley, 2020; Pass et al., 2014; Franklin, 1982, 1986, 1994; Oluwayomi, 2020; Ogungbure, 2019a, 2019b; Quijano, 2000; Wynter, 2003; Hunter & Davis, 1994; Frazier, 1927; Gary, 1995; Forman et al., 1997; Broman et al., 2000; Broman, 1996; Weitzer & Tuch, 1999; Welch et al., 2001; Hausmann et al., 2008; Taylor & Turner, 2002; Barnes et al., 2004; Brown, 2001; Din-Dzietham et al., 2004; Herring et al., 1998; Ifatunji & Forman, 2006; Sigelman & Welch, 1991; Ifatunji & Harnois, 2016; Pieterse & Carter, 2007; Hudson et al., 2012; Saint-Aubin, 1994; English et al., 2014; Barclay & Cusumano, 1967.

7 Staples, 1978, 1982; Lemelle, 1995, 2001, 2010; Sidanius & Pratto, 1999; Curry, 2017a, 2017b, 2018, 2021; Utley, 2016; Flaherty, 2017; Fanon, 1952; Curtis, 2014; Hare, 1971; Allen, 1969, 2005, 2010; Curry & Utley, 2020; Pass et al., 2014; Franklin, 1982, 1986, 1994; Oluwayomi, 2020; Ogungbure, 2019a, 2019b; Quijano, 2000; Wynter, 2003; Hunter & Davis, 1994; Frazier, 1927; Gary, 1995; Forman et al., 1997; Broman et al., 2000; Broman, 1996; Weitzer & Tuch, 1999; Welch et al., 2001; Hausmann et al., 2008; Taylor & Turner, 2002; Barnes et al., 2004; Brown, 2001; Din-Dzietham et al., 2004; Herring et al., 1998; Ifatunji & Forman, 2006; Sigelman & Welch, 1991; Ifatunji & Harnois, 2016; Pieterse & Carter, 2007; Hudson et al., 2012; Saint-Aubin, 1994; English et al., 2014; Barclay & Cusumano, 1967.

8 Staples, 1978, 1982; Lemelle, 1995, 2001, 2010; Sidanius & Pratto, 1999; Curry, 2017a, 2017b, 2018, 2021; Utley, 2016; Flaherty, 2017; Fanon, 1952; Curtis, 2014; Hare, 1971; Allen, 1969, 2005, 2010; Curry & Utley, 2020; Pass et al., 2014; Franklin, 1982, 1986, 1994; Oluwayomi, 2020; Ogungbure, 2019a, 2019b; Quijano, 2000; Wynter, 2003;

Hunter & Davis, 1994; Frazier, 1927; Gary, 1995; Forman et al., 1997; Broman et al., 2000; Broman, 1996; Weitzer & Tuch, 1999; Welch et al., 2001; Hausmann et al., 2008; Taylor & Turner, 2002; Barnes et al., 2004; Brown, 2001; Din-Dzietham et al., 2004; Herring et al., 1998; Ifatunji & Forman, 2006; Sigelman & Welch, 1991; Ifatunji & Harnois, 2016; Pieterse & Carter, 2007; Hudson et al., 2012; Saint-Aubin, 1994; English et al., 2014; Barclay & Cusumano, 1967.

9   Staples, 1978, 1982; Lemelle, 1995, 2001, 2010; Sidanius & Pratto, 1999; Curry, 2017a, 2017b, 2018, 2021; Utley, 2016; Flaherty, 2017; Fanon, 1952; Curtis, 2014; Hare, 1971; Allen, 1969, 2005, 2010; Curry & Utley, 2020; Pass et al., 2014; Franklin, 1982, 1986, 1994; Oluwayomi, 2020; Ogungbure, 2019a, 2019b; Quijano, 2000; Wynter, 2003; Hunter & Davis, 1994; Frazier, 1927; Gary, 1995; Forman et al., 1997; Broman et al., 2000; Broman, 1996; Weitzer & Tuch, 1999; Welch et al., 2001; Hausmann et al., 2008; Taylor & Turner, 2002; Barnes et al., 2004; Brown, 2001; Din-Dzietham et al., 2004; Herring et al., 1998; Ifatunji & Forman, 2006; Sigelman & Welch, 1991; Ifatunji & Harnois, 2016; Saint-Aubin, 1994; Eagly & Kite, 1987; Pieterse & Carter, 2007; Hudson et al., 2012; Lloyd, 2020.

10   Miller, 1991, 2004; Sidanius et al., 2018; Sidanius & Veniegas, 2000; Sidanius & Pratto, 1999; Jackman, 1994; Levin et al., 2002; Dworkin, 1974; Mies et al., 1988; Fiske & Stevens, 1993; Glick & Fiske, 1996, 1997; Gul & Kupfer, 2019; Jones-Rogers, 2019; Lemelle, 1995, 2001, 2010; Curry, 2017, 2018, 2021; Flaherty, 2017; Connell, 1987, 2005; McConnaughy, 2017; Navarrete et al., 2010; Hills & Vanatta, 2019; Ogungbure, 2018, 2019a, 2019b; Morgan, 1975; Wacquant, 2005; Blee, 2008; Junn, 2017; Newman, 1999.

11   Miller, 1991, 2004; Sidanius et al., 2018; Sidanius & Veniegas, 2000; Sidanius & Pratto, 1999; Jackman, 1994; Levin et al., 2002; Dworkin, 1974; Mies et al., 1988; Fiske & Stevens, 1993; Glick & Fiske, 1996, 1997; Gul & Kupfer, 2019; Jones-Rogers, 2019; Lemelle, 1995, 2001, 2010; Curry, 2017, 2018, 2021; Flaherty, 2017; Connell, 1987, 2005; McConnaughy, 2017; Navarrete et al., 2010; Hills & Vanatta, 2019; Ogungbure, 2018, 2019a, 2019b; Morgan, 1975; Wacquant, 2005; Blee, 2008; Junn, 2017; Newman, 1999.

12   Miller, 1991, 2004; Sidanius et al., 2018; Sidanius & Veniegas, 2000; Sidanius & Pratto, 1999; Jackman, 1994; Levin et al., 2002; Dworkin, 1974; Mies et al., 1988; Fiske & Stevens, 1993; Glick & Fiske, 1996, 1997; Gul & Kupfer, 2019; Jones-Rogers, 2019; Lemelle, 1995, 2001, 2010; Curry, 2017, 2018, 2021; Flaherty, 2017; Connell, 1987, 2005; McConnaughy, 2017; Navarrete et al., 2010; Hills & Vanatta, 2019; Ogungbure, 2018, 2019a, 2019b; Morgan, 1975; Wacquant, 2005; Blee, 2008; Junn, 2017; Newman, 1999.

13   Miller, 1991, 2004; Sidanius et al., 2018; Sidanius & Veniegas, 2000; Sidanius & Pratto, 1999; Jackman, 1994; Levin et al., 2002; Dworkin, 1974; Mies et al., 1988; Fiske & Stevens, 1993; Glick & Fiske, 1996, 1997; Gul & Kupfer, 2019; Jones-Rogers, 2019; Lemelle, 1995, 2001, 2010; Curry, 2017, 2018, 2021; Flaherty, 2017; Connell, 1987, 2005; McConnaughy, 2017; Navarrete et al., 2010; Hills & Vanatta, 2019; Ogungbure, 2018, 2019a, 2019b; Morgan, 1975; Wacquant, 2005; Blee, 2008; Junn, 2017; Newman, 1999.

14   Miller, 1991, 2004; Sidanius et al., 2018; Sidanius & Veniegas, 2000; Sidanius & Pratto, 1999; Jackman, 1994; Levin et al., 2002; Dworkin, 1974; Mies et al., 1988; Fiske & Stevens, 1993; Glick & Fiske, 1996, 1997; Gul & Kupfer, 2019; Jones-Rogers, 2019; Lemelle, 1995, 2001, 2010; Curry, 2017, 2018, 2021; Flaherty, 2017; Connell, 1987, 2005; McConnaughy, 2017; Navarrete et al., 2010; Hills & Vanatta, 2019; Ogungbure, 2018, 2019a, 2019b; Morgan, 1975; Wacquant, 2005; Blee, 2008; Junn, 2017; Newman, 1999.

15 Miller, 1991, 2004; Sidanius et al., 2018; Sidanius & Veniegas, 2000; Sidanius & Pratto, 1999; Jackman, 1994; Levin et al., 2002; Dworkin, 1974; Mies et al., 1988; Fiske & Stevens, 1993; Glick & Fiske, 1996, 1997; Gul & Kupfer, 2019; Jones-Rogers, 2019; Lemelle, 1995, 2001, 2010; Curry, 2017, 2018, 2021; Flaherty, 2017; Connell, 1987, 2005; McConnaughy, 2017; Navarrete et al., 2010; Hills & Vanatta, 2019; Ogungbure, 2018, 2019a, 2019b; Morgan, 1975; Wacquant, 2005; Blee, 2008; Junn, 2017; Newman, 1999.

16 Miller, 1991, 2004; Sidanius et al., 2018; Sidanius & Veniegas, 2000; Sidanius & Pratto, 1999; Jackman, 1994; Levin et al., 2002; Dworkin, 1974; Mies et al., 1988; Fiske & Stevens, 1993; Glick & Fiske, 1996, 1997; Gul & Kupfer, 2019; Jones-Rogers, 2019; Lemelle, 1995, 2001, 2010; Curry, 2017, 2018, 2021; Flaherty, 2017; Connell, 1987, 2005; McConnaughy, 2017; Navarrete et al., 2010; Hills & Vanatta, 2019; Ogungbure, 2018, 2019a, 2019b; Morgan, 1975; Wacquant, 2005; Blee, 2008; Junn, 2017; Newman, 1999.

17 Miller, 1991, 2004; Sidanius et al., 2018; Sidanius & Veniegas, 2000; Sidanius & Pratto, 1999; Jackman, 1994; Levin et al., 2002; Dworkin, 1974; Mies et al., 1988; Fiske & Stevens, 1993; Glick & Fiske, 1996, 1997; Gul & Kupfer, 2019; Jones-Rogers, 2019; Lemelle, 1995, 2001, 2010; Curry, 2017, 2018, 2021; Flaherty, 2017; Connell, 1987, 2005; McConnaughy, 2017; Navarrete et al., 2010; Hills & Vanatta, 2019; Ogungbure, 2018, 2019a, 2019b; Morgan, 1975; Wacquant, 2005; Blee, 2008; Junn, 2017; Newman, 1999.

18 Miller, 1991, 2004; Sidanius et al., 2018; Sidanius & Veniegas, 2000; Sidanius & Pratto, 1999; Jackman, 1994; Levin et al., 2002; Dworkin, 1974; Mies et al., 1988; Fiske & Stevens, 1993; Glick & Fiske, 1996, 1997; Gul & Kupfer, 2019; Jones-Rogers, 2019; Lemelle, 1995, 2001, 2010; Curry, 2017, 2018, 2021; Flaherty, 2017; Connell, 1987, 2005; McConnaughy, 2017; Navarrete et al., 2010; Hills & Vanatta, 2019; Ogungbure, 2018, 2019a, 2019b; Morgan, 1975; Wacquant, 2005; Blee, 2008; Junn, 2017; Newman, 1999.

19 Miller, 1991, 2004; Sidanius et al., 2018; Sidanius & Veniegas, 2000; Sidanius & Pratto, 1999; Jackman, 1994; Levin et al., 2002; Dworkin, 1974; Mies et al., 1988; Fiske & Stevens, 1993; Glick & Fiske, 1996, 1997; Gul & Kupfer, 2019; Jones-Rogers, 2019; Lemelle, 1995, 2001, 2010; Curry, 2017, 2018, 2021; Flaherty, 2017; Connell, 1987, 2005; McConnaughy, 2017; Navarrete et al., 2010; Hills & Vanatta, 2019; Ogungbure, 2018, 2019a, 2019b; Morgan, 1975; Wacquant, 2005; Blee, 2008; Junn, 2017; Newman, 1999.

20 Miller, 1991, 2004; Sidanius et al., 2018; Sidanius & Veniegas, 2000; Sidanius & Pratto, 1999; Jackman, 1994; Levin et al., 2002; Dworkin, 1974; Mies et al., 1988; Fiske & Stevens, 1993; Glick & Fiske, 1996, 1997; Gul & Kupfer, 2019; Jones-Rogers, 2019; Lemelle, 1995, 2001, 2010; Curry, 2017, 2018, 2021; Flaherty, 2017; Connell, 1987, 2005; McConnaughy, 2017; Navarrete et al., 2010; Hills & Vanatta, 2019; Ogungbure, 2018, 2019a, 2019b; Morgan, 1975; Wacquant, 2005; Blee, 2008; Junn, 2017; Newman, 1999.

21 Miller, 1991, 2004; Sidanius et al., 2018; Sidanius & Veniegas, 2000; Sidanius & Pratto, 1999; Jackman, 1994; Levin et al., 2002; Dworkin, 1974; Mies et al., 1988; Fiske & Stevens, 1993; Glick & Fiske, 1996, 1997; Gul & Kupfer, 2019; Jones-Rogers, 2019; Lemelle, 1995, 2001, 2010; Curry, 2017, 2018, 2021; Flaherty, 2017; Connell, 1987, 2005; McConnaughy, 2017; Navarrete et al., 2010; Hills & Vanatta, 2019; Ogungbure, 2018, 2019a, 2019b; Morgan, 1975; Wacquant, 2005; Blee, 2008; Junn, 2017; Newman, 1999.

22 Bialik, 2017.

23 Miller, 1991, 2004; Sidanius et al., 2018; Sidanius & Veniegas, 2000; Sidanius & Pratto, 1999; Jackman, 1994; Levin et al., 2002; Dworkin, 1974; Mies et al., 1988; Fiske &

Stevens, 1993; Glick & Fiske, 1996, 1997; Gul & Kupfer, 2019; Jones-Rogers, 2019; Lemelle, 1995, 2001, 2010; Curry, 2017, 2018, 2021; Flaherty, 2017; Connell, 1987, 2005; McConnaughy, 2017; Navarrete et al., 2010; Hills & Vanatta, 2019; Ogungbure, 2018, 2019a, 2019b; Morgan, 1975; Wacquant, 2005; Blee, 2008; Junn, 2017; Newman, 1999.

24 Miller, 1991, 2004; Sidanius et al., 2018; Sidanius & Veniegas, 2000; Sidanius & Pratto, 1999; Jackman, 1994; Levin et al., 2002; Dworkin, 1974; Mies et al., 1988; Fiske & Stevens, 1993; Glick & Fiske, 1996, 1997; Gul & Kupfer, 2019; Jones-Rogers, 2019; Lemelle, 1995, 2001, 2010; Curry, 2017, 2018, 2021; Flaherty, 2017; Connell, 1987, 2005; McConnaughy, 2017; Navarrete et al., 2010; Hills & Vanatta, 2019; Ogungbure, 2018, 2019a, 2019b; Morgan, 1975; Wacquant, 2005; Blee, 2008; Junn, 2017; Newman, 1999.

25 Curry, 2014, 2017, 2018, 2021a, 2021b, 2021c, 2021d, 2021e, 2022b, 2023a; Oyewùmí, 1997; Oluwayomi, 2020; Rhode, 1989; Bird, 1968; Hu-DeHart, 1997; Goodwin, 2013; Massie, 2016; Crenshaw, 1989, 1991; Sidanius et al., 2018; Sidanius & Veniegas, 2000; Levin et al., 2002; Pedulla, 2014; Curry & Curry, 2018; Cooper, 2005, 2020; White, 2008; Hunter & Davis, 1994; Hunter & Sellers, 1998; Hammond & Mattis, 2005; Wolfgang & Ferracuti, 1967; Amir, 1971; Brownmiller, 1975; Williams & Holmes, 1981; Staples, 1978, 1982; Johnson, 2018; Franklin, 1982, 1984; McDaniel et al., 2011; Mutua, 2012; Kaba, 2005a, 2005b, 2008, 2011; Butler, 2013; Carbado et al., 2013; Purdie-Vaughns & Eibach, 2008; Lemell, 2010; Harris, 1990, 1999; Brody, 1961; Anderson, 2021; Broeck, 2011; Massie, 2016; Oyewùmí, 1997; Newman, 1999, 2007; Sawyer, 2018; McConnaughy & White, 2011; McConnaughy, 2017; Oluwayomi, 2020; Scott, 2000; Sherman, 2018; Kounalakis, 2015; Kaplan, 2021; MacAskill, 2017; Hersh, 1978; Newton, 1980; Allen, 1969, 2005, 2010, 2014; Bhattacharyya, 2009; Feimster, 2009; McRae, 2018; Alexander, 2022; Bumiller, 2008; Reed, 2021; Perry, 2021; Campbell, 2022.

26 Curry, 2014, 2017, 2018, 2021a, 2021b, 2021c, 2021d, 2021e, 2022b, 2023a; Oyewùmí, 1997; Oluwayomi, 2020; Rhode, 1989; Bird, 1968; Hu-DeHart, 1997; Goodwin, 2013; Massie, 2016; Crenshaw, 1989, 1991; Sidanius et al., 2018; Sidanius & Veniegas, 2000; Levin et al., 2002; Pedulla, 2014; Curry & Curry, 2018; Cooper, 2005, 2020; White, 2008; Hunter & Davis, 1994; Hunter & Sellers, 1998; Hammond & Mattis, 2005; Wolfgang & Ferracuti, 1967; Amir, 1971; Brownmiller, 1975; Williams & Holmes, 1981; Staples, 1978, 1982; Johnson, 2018; Franklin, 1982, 1984; McDaniel et al., 2011; Mutua, 2012; Kaba, 2005a, 2005b, 2008, 2011; Butler, 2013; Carbado et al., 2013; Purdie-Vaughns & Eibach, 2008; Lemell, 2010; Harris, 1990, 1999; Brody, 1961; Anderson, 2021; Broeck, 2011; Massie, 2016; Oyewùmí, 1997; Newman, 1999, 2007; Sawyer, 2018; McConnaughy & White, 2011; McConnaughy, 2017; Oluwayomi, 2020; Scott, 2000; Sherman, 2018; Kounalakis, 2015; Kaplan, 2021; MacAskill, 2017; Hersh, 1978; Newton, 1980; Allen, 1969, 2005, 2010, 2014; Bhattacharyya, 2009; Feimster, 2009; McRae, 2018; Alexander, 2022; Bumiller, 2008; Reed, 2021; Perry, 2021; Campbell, 2022.

27 Curry, 2014, 2017, 2018, 2021a, 2021b, 2021c, 2021d, 2021e, 2022b, 2023a; Oyewùmí, 1997; Oluwayomi, 2020; Rhode, 1989; Bird, 1968; Hu-DeHart, 1997; Goodwin, 2013; Massie, 2016; Crenshaw, 1989, 1991; Sidanius et al., 2018; Sidanius & Veniegas, 2000; Levin et al., 2002; Pedulla, 2014; Curry & Curry, 2018; Cooper, 2005, 2020; White, 2008; Hunter & Davis, 1994; Hunter & Sellers, 1998; Hammond & Mattis, 2005; Wolfgang & Ferracuti, 1967; Amir, 1971; Brownmiller, 1975; Williams & Holmes, 1981; Staples, 1978, 1982; Johnson, 2018; Franklin, 1982, 1984; McDaniel et al., 2011; Mutua, 2012; Kaba, 2005a, 2005b, 2008, 2011; Butler, 2013; Carbado et al., 2013; Purdie-Vaughns & Eibach, 2008; Lemell, 2010; Harris, 1990, 1999; Brody, 1961; Anderson, 2021; Broeck, 2011; Massie, 2016; Oyewùmí, 1997; Newman, 1999, 2007; Sawyer, 2018; McConnaughy &

White, 2011; McConnaughy, 2017; Oluwayomi, 2020; Scott, 2000; Sherman, 2018; Kounalakis, 2015; Kaplan, 2021; MacAskill, 2017; Hersh, 1978; Newton, 1980; Allen, 1969, 2005, 2010, 2014; Bhattacharyya, 2009; Feimster, 2009; McRae, 2018; Alexander, 2022; Bumiller, 2008; Reed, 2021; Perry, 2021; Campbell, 2022.

28 Curry, 2014, 2017, 2018, 2021a, 2021b, 2021c, 2021d, 2021e, 2022b, 2023a; Oyewùmí, 1997; Oluwayomi, 2020; Rhode, 1989; Bird, 1968; Hu-DeHart, 1997; Goodwin, 2013; Massie, 2016; Crenshaw, 1989, 1991; Sidanius et al., 2018; Sidanius & Veniegas, 2000; Levin et al., 2002; Pedulla, 2014; Curry & Curry, 2018; Cooper, 2005, 2020; White, 2008; Hunter & Davis, 1994; Hunter & Sellers, 1998; Hammond & Mattis, 2005; Wolfgang & Ferracuti, 1967; Amir, 1971; Brownmiller, 1975; Williams & Holmes, 1981; Staples, 1978, 1982; Johnson, 2018; Franklin, 1982, 1984; McDaniel et al., 2011; Mutua, 2012; Kaba, 2005a, 2005b, 2008, 2011; Butler, 2013; Carbado et al., 2013; Purdie-Vaughns & Eibach, 2008; Lemell, 2010; Harris, 1990, 1999; Brody, 1961; Anderson, 2021; Broeck, 2011; Massie, 2016; Oyewùmí, 1997; Newman, 1999, 2007; Sawyer, 2018; McConnaughy & White, 2011; McConnaughy, 2017; Oluwayomi, 2020; Scott, 2000; Sherman, 2018; Kounalakis, 2015; Kaplan, 2021; MacAskill, 2017; Hersh, 1978; Newton, 1980; Allen, 1969, 2005, 2010, 2014; Bhattacharyya, 2009; Feimster, 2009; McRae, 2018; Alexander, 2022; Bumiller, 2008; Reed, 2021; Perry, 2021; Campbell, 2022.

29 Curry, 2014, 2017, 2018, 2021a, 2021b, 2021c, 2021d, 2021e, 2022b, 2023a; Oyewùmí, 1997; Oluwayomi, 2020; Rhode, 1989; Bird, 1968; Hu-DeHart, 1997; Goodwin, 2013; Massie, 2016; Crenshaw, 1989, 1991; Sidanius et al., 2018; Sidanius & Veniegas, 2000; Levin et al., 2002; Pedulla, 2014; Curry & Curry, 2018; Cooper, 2005, 2020; White, 2008; Hunter & Davis, 1994; Hunter & Sellers, 1998; Hammond & Mattis, 2005; Wolfgang & Ferracuti, 1967; Amir, 1971; Brownmiller, 1975; Williams & Holmes, 1981; Staples, 1978, 1982; Johnson, 2018; Franklin, 1982, 1984; McDaniel et al., 2011; Mutua, 2012; Kaba, 2005a, 2005b, 2008, 2011; Butler, 2013; Carbado et al., 2013; Purdie-Vaughns & Eibach, 2008; Lemell, 2010; Harris, 1990, 1999; Brody, 1961; Anderson, 2021; Broeck, 2011; Massie, 2016; Oyewùmí, 1997; Newman, 1999, 2007; Sawyer, 2018; McConnaughy & White, 2011; McConnaughy, 2017; Oluwayomi, 2020; Scott, 2000; Sherman, 2018; Kounalakis, 2015; Kaplan, 2021; MacAskill, 2017; Hersh, 1978; Newton, 1980; Allen, 1969, 2005, 2010, 2014; Bhattacharyya, 2009; Feimster, 2009; McRae, 2018; Alexander, 2022; Bumiller, 2008; Reed, 2021; Perry, 2021; Campbell, 2022.

30 Curry, 2014, 2017, 2018, 2021a, 2021b, 2021c, 2021d, 2021e, 2022b, 2023a; Oyewùmí, 1997; Oluwayomi, 2020; Rhode, 1989; Bird, 1968; Hu-DeHart, 1997; Goodwin, 2013; Massie, 2016; Crenshaw, 1989, 1991; Sidanius et al., 2018; Sidanius & Veniegas, 2000; Levin et al., 2002; Pedulla, 2014; Curry & Curry, 2018; Cooper, 2005, 2020; White, 2008; Hunter & Davis, 1994; Hunter & Sellers, 1998; Hammond & Mattis, 2005; Wolfgang & Ferracuti, 1967; Amir, 1971; Brownmiller, 1975; Williams & Holmes, 1981; Staples, 1978, 1982; Johnson, 2018; Franklin, 1982, 1984; McDaniel et al., 2011; Mutua, 2012; Kaba, 2005a, 2005b, 2008, 2011; Butler, 2013; Carbado et al., 2013; Purdie-Vaughns & Eibach, 2008; Lemell, 2010; Harris, 1990, 1999; Brody, 1961; Anderson, 2021; Broeck, 2011; Massie, 2016; Oyewùmí, 1997; Newman, 1999, 2007; Sawyer, 2018; McConnaughy & White, 2011; McConnaughy, 2017; Oluwayomi, 2020; Scott, 2000; Sherman, 2018; Kounalakis, 2015; Kaplan, 2021; MacAskill, 2017; Hersh, 1978; Newton, 1980; Allen, 1969, 2005, 2010, 2014; Bhattacharyya, 2009; Feimster, 2009; McRae, 2018; Alexander, 2022; Bumiller, 2008; Reed, 2021; Perry, 2021; Campbell, 2022.

31 Curry, 2014, 2017, 2018, 2021a, 2021b, 2021c, 2021d, 2021e, 2022b, 2023a; Oyewùmí, 1997; Oluwayomi, 2020; Rhode, 1989; Bird, 1968; Hu-DeHart, 1997; Goodwin, 2013; Massie, 2016; Crenshaw, 1989, 1991; Sidanius et al., 2018; Sidanius & Veniegas, 2000;

Levin et al., 2002; Pedulla, 2014; Curry & Curry, 2018; Cooper, 2005, 2020; White, 2008; Hunter & Davis, 1994; Hunter & Sellers, 1998; Hammond & Mattis, 2005; Wolfgang & Ferracuti, 1967; Amir, 1971; Brownmiller, 1975; Williams & Holmes, 1981; Staples, 1978, 1982; Johnson, 2018; Franklin, 1982, 1984; McDaniel et al., 2011; Mutua, 2012; Kaba, 2005a, 2005b, 2008, 2011; Butler, 2013; Carbado et al., 2013; Purdie-Vaughns & Eibach, 2008; Lemell, 2010; Harris, 1990, 1999; Brody, 1961; Anderson, 2021; Broeck, 2011; Massie, 2016; Oyewùmí, 1997; Newman, 1999, 2007; Sawyer, 2018; McConnaughy & White, 2011; McConnaughy, 2017; Oluwayomi, 2020; Scott, 2000; Sherman, 2018; Kounalakis, 2015; Kaplan, 2021; MacAskill, 2017; Hersh, 1978; Newton, 1980; Allen, 1969, 2005, 2010, 2014; Bhattacharyya, 2009; Feimster, 2009; McRae, 2018; Alexander, 2022; Bumiller, 2008; Reed, 2021; Perry, 2021; Campbell, 2022.

32 Curry, 2014, 2017, 2018, 2021a, 2021b, 2021c, 2021d, 2021e, 2022b, 2023a; Oyewùmí, 1997; Oluwayomi, 2020; Rhode, 1989; Bird, 1968; Hu-DeHart, 1997; Goodwin, 2013; Massie, 2016; Crenshaw, 1989, 1991; Sidanius et al., 2018; Sidanius & Veniegas, 2000; Levin et al., 2002; Pedulla, 2014; Curry & Curry, 2018; Cooper, 2005, 2020; White, 2008; Hunter & Davis, 1994; Hunter & Sellers, 1998; Hammond & Mattis, 2005; Wolfgang & Ferracuti, 1967; Amir, 1971; Brownmiller, 1975; Williams & Holmes, 1981; Staples, 1978, 1982; Johnson, 2018; Franklin, 1982, 1984; McDaniel et al., 2011; Mutua, 2012; Kaba, 2005a, 2005b, 2008, 2011; Butler, 2013; Carbado et al., 2013; Purdie-Vaughns & Eibach, 2008; Lemell, 2010; Harris, 1990, 1999; Brody, 1961; Anderson, 2021; Broeck, 2011; Massie, 2016; Oyewùmí, 1997; Newman, 1999, 2007; Sawyer, 2018; McConnaughy & White, 2011; McConnaughy, 2017; Oluwayomi, 2020; Scott, 2000; Sherman, 2018; Kounalakis, 2015; Kaplan, 2021; MacAskill, 2017; Hersh, 1978; Newton, 1980; Allen, 1969, 2005, 2010, 2014; Bhattacharyya, 2009; Feimster, 2009; McRae, 2018; Alexander, 2022; Bumiller, 2008; Reed, 2021; Perry, 2021; Campbell, 2022.

33 Sidanius et al., 2018; Wilson et al., 2017; Ifatunji & Harnois, 2016; Pedulla, 2014; Veenstra, 2012; Navarrete et al., 2010; Navarrete et al., 2009; Levin et al., 2002; Sidanius & Veniegas, 2000; Sidanius & Pratto, 1999; Connor et al., 2023.

34 Curry, 2014, 2017, 2018, 2021a, 2021b, 2021c, 2021d, 2021e, 2022b, 2023a; Oyewùmí, 1997; Oluwayomi, 2020; Rhode, 1989; Bird, 1968; Hu-DeHart, 1997; Goodwin, 2013; Massie, 2016; Crenshaw, 1989, 1991; Sidanius et al., 2018; Sidanius & Veniegas, 2000; Levin et al., 2002; Pedulla, 2014; Curry & Curry, 2018; Cooper, 2005, 2020; White, 2008; Hunter & Davis, 1994; Hunter & Sellers, 1998; Hammond & Mattis, 2005; Wolfgang & Ferracuti, 1967; Amir, 1971; Brownmiller, 1975; Williams & Holmes, 1981; Staples, 1978, 1982; Johnson, 2018; Franklin, 1982, 1984; McDaniel et al., 2011; Mutua, 2012; Kaba, 2005a, 2005b, 2008, 2011; Butler, 2013; Carbado et al., 2013; Purdie-Vaughns & Eibach, 2008; Lemell, 2010; Harris, 1990, 1999; Brody, 1961; Anderson, 2021; Broeck, 2011; Massie, 2016; Oyewùmí, 1997; Newman, 1999, 2007; Sawyer, 2018; McConnaughy & White, 2011; McConnaughy, 2017; Oluwayomi, 2020; Scott, 2000; Sherman, 2018; Kounalakis, 2015; Kaplan, 2021; MacAskill, 2017; Hersh, 1978; Newton, 1980; Allen, 1969, 2005, 2010, 2014; Bhattacharyya, 2009; Feimster, 2009; McRae, 2018; Alexander, 2022; Bumiller, 2008; Reed, 2021; Perry, 2021; Campbell, 2022.

35 Curry, 2014, 2017, 2018, 2021a, 2021b, 2021c, 2021d, 2021e, 2022b, 2023a; Oyewùmí, 1997; Oluwayomi, 2020; Rhode, 1989; Bird, 1968; Hu-DeHart, 1997; Goodwin, 2013; Massie, 2016; Crenshaw, 1989, 1991; Sidanius et al., 2018; Sidanius & Veniegas, 2000; Levin et al., 2002; Pedulla, 2014; Curry & Curry, 2018; Cooper, 2005, 2020; White, 2008; Hunter & Davis, 1994; Hunter & Sellers, 1998; Hammond & Mattis, 2005; Wolfgang & Ferracuti, 1967; Amir, 1971; Brownmiller, 1975; Williams & Holmes, 1981; Staples, 1978, 1982; Johnson, 2018; Franklin, 1982, 1984; McDaniel et al., 2011; Mutua, 2012; Kaba,

2005a, 2005b, 2008, 2011; Butler, 2013; Carbado et al., 2013; Purdie-Vaughns & Eibach, 2008; Lemell, 2010; Harris, 1990, 1999; Brody, 1961; Anderson, 2021; Broeck, 2011; Massie, 2016; Oyewùmí, 1997; Newman, 1999, 2007; Sawyer, 2018; McConnaughy & White, 2011; McConnaughy, 2017; Oluwayomi, 2020; Scott, 2000; Sherman, 2018; Kounalakis, 2015; Kaplan, 2021; MacAskill, 2017; Hersh, 1978; Newton, 1980; Allen, 1969, 2005, 2010, 2014; Bhattacharyya, 2009; Feimster, 2009; McRae, 2018; Alexander, 2022; Bumiller, 2008; Reed, 2021; Perry, 2021; Campbell, 2022.

36 Curry, 2014, 2017, 2018, 2021a, 2021b, 2021c, 2021d, 2021e, 2022b, 2023a; Oyewùmí, 1997; Oluwayomi, 2020; Rhode, 1989; Bird, 1968; Hu-DeHart, 1997; Goodwin, 2013; Massie, 2016; Crenshaw, 1989, 1991; Sidanius et al., 2018; Sidanius & Veniegas, 2000; Levin et al., 2002; Pedulla, 2014; Curry & Curry, 2018; Cooper, 2005, 2020; White, 2008; Hunter & Davis, 1994; Hunter & Sellers, 1998; Hammond & Mattis, 2005; Wolfgang & Ferracuti, 1967; Amir, 1971; Brownmiller, 1975; Williams & Holmes, 1981; Staples, 1978, 1982; Johnson, 2018; Franklin, 1982, 1984; McDaniel et al., 2011; Mutua, 2012; Kaba, 2005a, 2005b, 2008, 2011; Butler, 2013; Carbado et al., 2013; Purdie-Vaughns & Eibach, 2008; Lemell, 2010; Harris, 1990, 1999; Brody, 1961; Anderson, 2021; Broeck, 2011; Massie, 2016; Oyewùmí, 1997; Newman, 1999, 2007; Sawyer, 2018; McConnaughy & White, 2011; McConnaughy, 2017; Oluwayomi, 2020; Scott, 2000; Sherman, 2018; Kounalakis, 2015; Kaplan, 2021; MacAskill, 2017; Hersh, 1978; Newton, 1980; Allen, 1969, 2005, 2010, 2014; Bhattacharyya, 2009; Feimster, 2009; McRae, 2018; Alexander, 2022; Bumiller, 2008; Reed, 2021; Perry, 2021; Campbell, 2022.

37 Curry, 2014, 2017, 2018, 2021a, 2021b, 2021c, 2021d, 2021e, 2022b, 2023a; Oyewùmí, 1997; Oluwayomi, 2020; Rhode, 1989; Bird, 1968; Hu-DeHart, 1997; Goodwin, 2013; Massie, 2016; Crenshaw, 1989, 1991; Sidanius et al., 2018; Sidanius & Veniegas, 2000; Levin et al., 2002; Pedulla, 2014; Curry & Curry, 2018; Cooper, 2005, 2020; White, 2008; Hunter & Davis, 1994; Hunter & Sellers, 1998; Hammond & Mattis, 2005; Wolfgang & Ferracuti, 1967; Amir, 1971; Brownmiller, 1975; Williams & Holmes, 1981; Staples, 1978, 1982; Johnson, 2018; Franklin, 1982, 1984; McDaniel et al., 2011; Mutua, 2012; Kaba, 2005a, 2005b, 2008, 2011; Butler, 2013; Carbado et al., 2013; Purdie-Vaughns & Eibach, 2008; Lemell, 2010; Harris, 1990, 1999; Brody, 1961; Anderson, 2021; Broeck, 2011; Massie, 2016; Oyewùmí, 1997; Newman, 1999, 2007; Sawyer, 2018; McConnaughy & White, 2011; McConnaughy, 2017; Oluwayomi, 2020; Scott, 2000; Sherman, 2018; Kounalakis, 2015; Kaplan, 2021; MacAskill, 2017; Hersh, 1978; Newton, 1980; Allen, 1969, 2005, 2010, 2014; Bhattacharyya, 2009; Feimster, 2009; McRae, 2018; Alexander, 2022; Bumiller, 2008; Reed, 2021; Perry, 2021; Campbell, 2022.

38 Curry, 2014, 2017, 2018, 2021a, 2021b, 2021c, 2021d, 2021e, 2022b, 2023a; Oyewùmí, 1997; Oluwayomi, 2020; Rhode, 1989; Bird, 1968; Hu-DeHart, 1997; Goodwin, 2013; Massie, 2016; Crenshaw, 1989, 1991; Sidanius et al., 2018; Sidanius & Veniegas, 2000; Levin et al., 2002; Pedulla, 2014; Curry & Curry, 2018; Cooper, 2005, 2020; White, 2008; Hunter & Davis, 1994; Hunter & Sellers, 1998; Hammond & Mattis, 2005; Wolfgang & Ferracuti, 1967; Amir, 1971; Brownmiller, 1975; Williams & Holmes, 1981; Staples, 1978, 1982; Johnson, 2018; Franklin, 1982, 1984; McDaniel et al., 2011; Mutua, 2012; Kaba, 2005a, 2005b, 2008, 2011; Butler, 2013; Carbado et al., 2013; Purdie-Vaughns & Eibach, 2008; Lemell, 2010; Harris, 1990, 1999; Brody, 1961; Anderson, 2021; Broeck, 2011; Massie, 2016; Oyewùmí, 1997; Newman, 1999, 2007; Sawyer, 2018; McConnaughy & White, 2011; McConnaughy, 2017; Oluwayomi, 2020; Scott, 2000; Sherman, 2018; Kounalakis, 2015; Kaplan, 2021; MacAskill, 2017; Hersh, 1978; Newton, 1980; Allen, 1969, 2005, 2010, 2014; Bhattacharyya, 2009; Feimster, 2009; McRae, 2018; Alexander, 2022; Bumiller, 2008; Reed, 2021; Perry, 2021; Campbell, 2022.

39 Curry, 2014, 2017, 2018, 2021a, 2021b, 2021c, 2021d, 2021e, 2022b, 2023a; Oyewùmí,
    1997; Oluwayomi, 2020; Rhode, 1989; Bird, 1968; Hu-DeHart, 1997; Goodwin, 2013;
    Massie, 2016; Crenshaw, 1989, 1991; Sidanius et al., 2018; Sidanius & Veniegas, 2000;
    Levin et al., 2002; Pedulla, 2014; Curry & Curry, 2018; Cooper, 2005, 2020; White, 2008;
    Hunter & Davis, 1994; Hunter & Sellers, 1998; Hammond & Mattis, 2005; Wolfgang &
    Ferracuti, 1967; Amir, 1971; Brownmiller, 1975; Williams & Holmes, 1981; Staples, 1978,
    1982; Johnson, 2018; Franklin, 1982, 1984; McDaniel et al., 2011; Mutua, 2012; Kaba,
    2005a, 2005b, 2008, 2011; Butler, 2013; Carbado et al., 2013; Purdie-Vaughns & Eibach,
    2008; Lemell, 2010; Harris, 1990, 1999; Brody, 1961; Anderson, 2021; Broeck, 2011;
    Massie, 2016; Oyewùmí, 1997; Newman, 1999, 2007; Sawyer, 2018; McConnaughy
    & White, 2011; McConnaughy, 2017; Oluwayomi, 2020; Scott, 2000; Sherman, 2018;
    Kounalakis, 2015; Kaplan, 2021; MacAskill, 2017; Hersh, 1978; Newton, 1980; Allen,
    1969, 2005, 2010, 2014; Bhattacharyya, 2009; Feimster, 2009; McRae, 2018; Alexander,
    2022; Bumiller, 2008; Reed, 2021; Perry, 2021; Campbell, 2022.
40 Curry, 2014, 2017, 2018, 2021a, 2021b, 2021c, 2021d, 2021e, 2022b, 2023a; Oyewùmí,
    1997; Oluwayomi, 2020; Rhode, 1989; Bird, 1968; Hu-DeHart, 1997; Goodwin, 2013;
    Massie, 2016; Crenshaw, 1989, 1991; Sidanius et al., 2018; Sidanius & Veniegas, 2000;
    Levin et al., 2002; Pedulla, 2014; Curry & Curry, 2018; Cooper, 2005, 2020; White, 2008;
    Hunter & Davis, 1994; Hunter & Sellers, 1998; Hammond & Mattis, 2005; Wolfgang &
    Ferracuti, 1967; Amir, 1971; Brownmiller, 1975; Williams & Holmes, 1981; Staples, 1978,
    1982; Johnson, 2018; Franklin, 1982, 1984; McDaniel et al., 2011; Mutua, 2012; Kaba,
    2005a, 2005b, 2008, 2011; Butler, 2013; Carbado et al., 2013; Purdie-Vaughns & Eibach,
    2008; Lemell, 2010; Harris, 1990, 1999; Brody, 1961; Anderson, 2021; Broeck, 2011;
    Massie, 2016; Oyewùmí, 1997; Newman, 1999, 2007; Sawyer, 2018; McConnaughy
    & White, 2011; McConnaughy, 2017; Oluwayomi, 2020; Scott, 2000; Sherman, 2018;
    Kounalakis, 2015; Kaplan, 2021; MacAskill, 2017; Hersh, 1978; Newton, 1980; Allen,
    1969, 2005, 2010, 2014; Bhattacharyya, 2009; Feimster, 2009; McRae, 2018; Alexander,
    2022; Bumiller, 2008; Reed, 2021; Perry, 2021; Campbell, 2022.
41 Curry, 2014, 2017, 2018, 2021a, 2021b, 2021c, 2021d, 2021e, 2022b, 2023a; Oyewùmí,
    1997; Oluwayomi, 2020; Rhode, 1989; Bird, 1968; Hu-DeHart, 1997; Goodwin, 2013;
    Massie, 2016; Crenshaw, 1989, 1991; Sidanius et al., 2018; Sidanius & Veniegas, 2000;
    Levin et al., 2002; Pedulla, 2014; Curry & Curry, 2018; Cooper, 2005, 2020; White, 2008;
    Hunter & Davis, 1994; Hunter & Sellers, 1998; Hammond & Mattis, 2005; Wolfgang &
    Ferracuti, 1967; Amir, 1971; Brownmiller, 1975; Williams & Holmes, 1981; Staples, 1978,
    1982; Johnson, 2018; Franklin, 1982, 1984; McDaniel et al., 2011; Mutua, 2012; Kaba,
    2005a, 2005b, 2008, 2011; Butler, 2013; Carbado et al., 2013; Purdie-Vaughns & Eibach,
    2008; Lemell, 2010; Harris, 1990, 1999; Brody, 1961; Anderson, 2021; Broeck, 2011;
    Massie, 2016; Oyewùmí, 1997; Newman, 1999, 2007; Sawyer, 2018; McConnaughy &
    White, 2011; McConnaughy, 2017; Oluwayomi, 2020; Scott, 2000; Sherman, 2018;
    Kounalakis, 2015; Kaplan, 2021; MacAskill, 2017; Hersh, 1978; Newton, 1980; Allen,
    1969, 2005, 2010, 2014; Bhattacharyya, 2009; Feimster, 2009; McRae, 2018; Alexander,
    2022; Bumiller, 2008; Reed, 2021; Perry, 2021; Campbell, 2022.
42 Curry, 2014, 2017, 2018, 2021a, 2021b, 2021c, 2021d, 2021e, 2022b, 2023a; Oyewùmí,
    1997; Oluwayomi, 2020; Rhode, 1989; Bird, 1968; Hu-DeHart, 1997; Goodwin, 2013;
    Massie, 2016; Crenshaw, 1989, 1991; Sidanius et al., 2018; Sidanius & Veniegas, 2000;
    Levin et al., 2002; Pedulla, 2014; Curry & Curry, 2018; Cooper, 2005, 2020; White, 2008;
    Hunter & Davis, 1994; Hunter & Sellers, 1998; Hammond & Mattis, 2005; Wolfgang &
    Ferracuti, 1967; Amir, 1971; Brownmiller, 1975; Williams & Holmes, 1981; Staples, 1978,
    1982; Johnson, 2018; Franklin, 1982, 1984; McDaniel et al., 2011; Mutua, 2012; Kaba,

2005a, 2005b, 2008, 2011; Butler, 2013; Carbado et al., 2013; Purdie-Vaughns & Eibach, 2008; Lemell, 2010; Harris, 1990, 1999; Brody, 1961; Anderson, 2021; Broeck, 2011; Massie, 2016; Oyewùmí, 1997; Newman, 1999, 2007; Sawyer, 2018; McConnaughy & White, 2011; McConnaughy, 2017; Oluwayomi, 2020; Scott, 2000; Sherman, 2018; Kounalakis, 2015; Kaplan, 2021; MacAskill, 2017; Hersh, 1978; Newton, 1980; Allen, 1969, 2005, 2010, 2014; Bhattacharyya, 2009; Feimster, 2009; McRae, 2018; Alexander, 2022; Bumiller, 2008; Reed, 2021; Perry, 2021; Campbell, 2022.

43 Curry, 2014, 2017, 2018, 2021a, 2021b, 2021c, 2021d, 2021e, 2022b, 2023a; Oyewùmí, 1997; Oluwayomi, 2020; Rhode, 1989; Bird, 1968; Hu-DeHart, 1997; Goodwin, 2013; Massie, 2016; Crenshaw, 1989, 1991; Sidanius et al., 2018; Sidanius & Veniegas, 2000; Levin et al., 2002; Pedulla, 2014; Curry & Curry, 2018; Cooper, 2005, 2020; White, 2008; Hunter & Davis, 1994; Hunter & Sellers, 1998; Hammond & Mattis, 2005; Wolfgang & Ferracuti, 1967; Amir, 1971; Brownmiller, 1975; Williams & Holmes, 1981; Staples, 1978, 1982; Johnson, 2018; Franklin, 1982, 1984; McDaniel et al., 2011; Mutua, 2012; Kaba, 2005a, 2005b, 2008, 2011; Butler, 2013; Carbado et al., 2013; Purdie-Vaughns & Eibach, 2008; Lemell, 2010; Harris, 1990, 1999; Brody, 1961; Anderson, 2021; Broeck, 2011; Massie, 2016; Oyewùmí, 1997; Newman, 1999, 2007; Sawyer, 2018; McConnaughy & White, 2011; McConnaughy, 2017; Oluwayomi, 2020; Scott, 2000; Sherman, 2018; Kounalakis, 2015; Kaplan, 2021; MacAskill, 2017; Hersh, 1978; Newton, 1980; Allen, 1969, 2005, 2010, 2014; Bhattacharyya, 2009; Feimster, 2009; McRae, 2018; Alexander, 2022; Bumiller, 2008; Reed, 2021; Perry, 2021; Campbell, 2022.

44 Curry, 2014, 2017, 2018, 2021a, 2021b, 2021c, 2021d, 2021e, 2022b, 2023a; Oyewùmí, 1997; Oluwayomi, 2020; Rhode, 1989; Bird, 1968; Hu-DeHart, 1997; Goodwin, 2013; Massie, 2016; Crenshaw, 1989, 1991; Sidanius et al., 2018; Sidanius & Veniegas, 2000; Levin et al., 2002; Pedulla, 2014; Curry & Curry, 2018; Cooper, 2005, 2020; White, 2008; Hunter & Davis, 1994; Hunter & Sellers, 1998; Hammond & Mattis, 2005; Wolfgang & Ferracuti, 1967; Amir, 1971; Brownmiller, 1975; Williams & Holmes, 1981; Staples, 1978, 1982; Johnson, 2018; Franklin, 1982, 1984; McDaniel et al., 2011; Mutua, 2012; Kaba, 2005a, 2005b, 2008, 2011; Butler, 2013; Carbado et al,, 2013; Purdie-Vaughns & Eibach, 2008; Lemell, 2010; Harris, 1990, 1999; Brody, 1961; Anderson, 2021; Broeck, 2011; Massie, 2016; Oyewùmí, 1997; Newman, 1999, 2007; Sawyer, 2018; McConnaughy & White, 2011; McConnaughy, 2017; Oluwayomi, 2020; Scott, 2000; Sherman, 2018; Kounalakis, 2015; Kaplan, 2021; MacAskill, 2017; Hersh, 1978; Newton, 1980; Allen, 1969, 2005, 2010, 2014; Bhattacharyya, 2009; Feimster, 2009; McRae, 2018; Alexander, 2022; Bumiller, 2008; Reed, 2021; Perry, 2021; Campbell, 2022.

45 Curry, 2014, 2017, 2018, 2021a, 2021b, 2021c, 2021d, 2021e, 2022b, 2023a; Oyewùmí, 1997; Oluwayomi, 2020; Rhode, 1989; Bird, 1968; Hu-DeHart, 1997; Goodwin, 2013; Massie, 2016; Crenshaw, 1989, 1991; Sidanius et al., 2018; Sidanius & Veniegas, 2000; Levin et al., 2002; Pedulla, 2014; Curry & Curry, 2018; Cooper, 2005, 2020; White, 2008; Hunter & Davis, 1994; Hunter & Sellers, 1998; Hammond & Mattis, 2005; Wolfgang & Ferracuti, 1967; Amir, 1971; Brownmiller, 1975; Williams & Holmes, 1981; Staples, 1978, 1982; Johnson, 2018; Franklin, 1982, 1984; McDaniel et al., 2011; Mutua, 2012; Kaba, 2005a, 2005b, 2008, 2011; Butler, 2013; Carbado et al., 2013; Purdie-Vaughns & Eibach, 2008; Lemell, 2010; Harris, 1990, 1999; Brody, 1961; Anderson, 2021; Broeck, 2011; Massie, 2016; Oyewùmí, 1997; Newman, 1999, 2007; Sawyer, 2018; McConnaughy & White, 2011; McConnaughy, 2017; Oluwayomi, 2020; Scott, 2000; Sherman, 2018; Kounalakis, 2015; Kaplan, 2021; MacAskill, 2017; Hersh, 1978; Newton, 1980; Allen,

1969, 2005, 2010, 2014; Bhattacharyya, 2009; Feimster, 2009; McRae, 2018; Alexander, 2022; Bumiller, 2008; Reed, 2021; Perry, 2021; Campbell, 2022.

46 Curry, 2014, 2017, 2018, 2021a, 2021b, 2021c, 2021d, 2021e, 2022b, 2023a; Oyewùmí, 1997; Oluwayomi, 2020; Rhode, 1989; Bird, 1968; Hu-DeHart, 1997; Goodwin, 2013; Massie, 2016; Crenshaw, 1989, 1991; Sidanius et al., 2018; Sidanius & Veniegas, 2000; Levin et al., 2002; Pedulla, 2014; Curry & Curry, 2018; Cooper, 2005, 2020; White, 2008; Hunter & Davis, 1994; Hunter & Sellers, 1998; Hammond & Mattis, 2005; Wolfgang & Ferracuti, 1967; Amir, 1971; Brownmiller, 1975; Williams & Holmes, 1981; Staples, 1978, 1982; Johnson, 2018; Franklin, 1982, 1984; McDaniel et al., 2011; Mutua, 2012; Kaba, 2005a, 2005b, 2008, 2011; Butler, 2013; Carbado et al., 2013; Purdie-Vaughns & Eibach, 2008; Lemell, 2010; Harris, 1990, 1999; Brody, 1961; Anderson, 2021; Broeck, 2011; Massie, 2016; Oyewùmí, 1997; Newman, 1999, 2007; Sawyer, 2018; McConnaughy & White, 2011; McConnaughy, 2017; Oluwayomi, 2020; Scott, 2000; Sherman, 2018; Kounalakis, 2015; Kaplan, 2021; MacAskill, 2017; Hersh, 1978; Newton, 1980; Allen, 1969, 2005, 2010, 2014; Bhattacharyya, 2009; Feimster, 2009; McRae, 2018; Alexander, 2022; Bumiller, 2008; Reed, 2021; Perry, 2021; Campbell, 2022.

47 Curry, 2014, 2017, 2018, 2021a, 2021b, 2021c, 2021d, 2021e, 2022b, 2023a; Oyewùmí, 1997; Oluwayomi, 2020; Rhode, 1989; Bird, 1968; Hu-DeHart, 1997; Goodwin, 2013; Massie, 2016; Crenshaw, 1989, 1991; Sidanius et al., 2018; Sidanius & Veniegas, 2000; Levin et al., 2002; Pedulla, 2014; Curry & Curry, 2018; Cooper, 2005, 2020; White, 2008; Hunter & Davis, 1994; Hunter & Sellers, 1998; Hammond & Mattis, 2005; Wolfgang & Ferracuti, 1967; Amir, 1971; Brownmiller, 1975; Williams & Holmes, 1981; Staples, 1978, 1982; Johnson, 2018; Franklin, 1982, 1984; McDaniel et al., 2011; Mutua, 2012; Kaba, 2005a, 2005b, 2008, 2011; Butler, 2013; Carbado et al., 2013; Purdie-Vaughns & Eibach, 2008; Lemell, 2010; Harris, 1990, 1999; Brody, 1961; Anderson, 2021; Broeck, 2011; Massie, 2016; Oyewùmí, 1997; Newman, 1999, 2007; Sawyer, 2018; McConnaughy & White, 2011; McConnaughy, 2017; Oluwayomi, 2020; Scott, 2000; Sherman, 2018; Kounalakis, 2015; Kaplan, 2021; MacAskill, 2017; Hersh, 1978; Newton, 1980; Allen, 1969, 2005, 2010, 2014; Bhattacharyya, 2009; Feimster, 2009; McRae, 2018; Alexander, 2022; Bumiller, 2008; Reed, 2021; Perry, 2021; Campbell, 2022.

CHAPTER 8

THE BLACK MESSIAH

PART II

BLACK MALE DEATH AND DYING

Black male vulnerability encompasses the conditions and disadvantages that Black males endure in comparison to other groups, the erasure of their actual lived experience from theory, and the violence and death they suffer in society as a consequence of being a Black male. The vulnerable condition that being Black and male engenders is captured through the sheer fungibility of the Black male as a living terror who at any given moment can be killed, raped, or dehumanized, which is contingent upon the disposition of those who encounter him. Black male vulnerability includes death and dying, genocide/gendercide, dehumanization, suicide, sexual victimization, and IPV.[1]

After Emancipation, it was expected and there was even hope that Black Americans would cease to exist. It was believed by the American Medical Association (AMA) president Hunter McGuire and his contemporaries that the Black race was dying out in the wake of Emancipation. The assault on Black life includes death and dying, which constitutes the core of racist organization through the apparatus of elimination and processes of eliminating Black Americans. Black humanity is negated in a white supremacist society like America which routinely leads to death. The Black male's existence within white empire is conditioned by death, and his body has been marked for destruction. Black men are simply disposable.[2]

The public lynching of George Floyd is an example where the life of a Black man was snuffed out over the course of eight minutes and 46 seconds, where his body was transformed into a corpse. The unabated murder of Black males in the U.S. has a long history. The long-standing tradition of killing Black males in the U.S. is not simply an act of racism but part of an apparatus of societal-level stigmatization that sanctions this repetition of death with attempts to remove them from American society. Black men are routinely thought of as a corpse, and their quotidian existence is almost nonexistent in theory. The routine display of the Black male corpse is normalized/ritualized evoking reactions of indifference and does not cause offense in America but moments of performative outrage. Black men are executed by police officers and white vigilantes and blamed for their own deaths. The legacies of slavery, lynching, and police brutality has continually organized Black life in America where 21st century policing operates as an instrument of racial terror and social control. According to Rodríguez (2006), the U.S. prison is a material prototype of organized punishment and death that includes social, civil, and biological death. The white imagination frames Black men as criminals and deviants deserving of death for the danger they pose to society and the fear they inspire. On the other end of the spectrum, there are activists who appropriate Black male death for symbolic and material rewards. Black Lives Matter (BLM) as an organization fronted by Black queer women is a prime example of this parasitic dynamic where they capitalized off of Black male deaths while minimizing their existence and became millionaires. The deaths of Black males by the police were not impacted by their supposed efforts, and this was the first time that the leaders of a Black Civil Rights movement became wealthy from a movement while pathologizing and disavowing Black male existence.[3]

DOI: 10.4324/9781003430551-9

Black male vulnerability is not investigated outside of the framing of Black feminism or other paradigms that frame Black males as culturally maladjusted and pathologically violent. Any attempts to study Black male vulnerability is positioned to be in opposition to Black female suffering. Moreover, Black male vulnerability is framed as invalidating or erasing Black female suffering.[4]

There is an insistence within the current political milieu that the examination of the deaths of Black men outside the scope of "racism" is unnecessary even though Black men are disproportionately affected by violence, incarceration, poverty, unemployment, and suicide. This reductive analysis represents an intellectual failure as the complexities and motivations implicated within the genocidal logics of American racism are absent and not fully understood, which could potentially indicate that over 50 percent of explanatory research on racism remains nonexistent. Thus, the lack of scientific rigor in critically analyzing anti-Black racism sociologically ensures that any effort to lessen police violence will fail. The 1.5 million Black men missing due to early death and hyperincarceration does not elicit any critical engagement or a public health response. Research from Bovell-Ammon et al. (2021) examined the association between incarceration and mortality risk and found that incarceration was associated with higher mortality among Black participants but not among non-Black participants. This indicated that incarceration which was prevalent and unevenly distributed may have contributed to the lower life expectancy of the Black population. Overexposure to incarceration is an instrumental mechanism in life expectancy between Black and other populations. Therefore, the carceral state is an apparatus of terror and anti-Black violence that produces a slow death (i.e., weathering) among Black males.[5]

Generations of young Black males in the U.S. between the ages of 15 to 24 are prematurely dying from homicide and suicide. They are dying five to six decades prior to their life expectancy. The average death rate of young Black males between 1950 and 2010 due to homicide was approximately 82 per 100,000, and suicide was approximately 12 per 100,000. The deaths of young Black males who are developmentally transitioning from adolescence into young adulthood creates collective trauma and ceases procreation prospects (e.g., birth rates, family history, generational prospects, and cultural demographics) that severely impacts the Black community. The killing of Black males is not viewed as an offense, but the effect of the deaths of Black males on Black mothers and their community is often more of a pressing concern. A void is created with the loss of fathers, brothers, uncles, sons, nephews, and cousins among Black families due to the premature deaths of Black males. Black family functioning is severely impacted due to the lifelong and traumatic effects of the loss of Black males. Black males experienced a sharp escalation of homicide deaths between 1970 and 2010 that is indicative of a birth to homicide death pipeline. The increase of the birth to homicide death pipeline began after the civil rights and Black liberation movement eras and during the presidencies of Nixon, Reagan, Bush, and Clinton where federal zero-tolerance criminal justice policies were enacted that targeted Black males (see Chapter 4: "The Carceral State and Black Men" for details).[6]

There is no place safe for Black males to exist in America as Black men and boys are killed at the grocery store, in the parking lot, on the street, inside their own cars, and inside their own homes. Lynching as a technology of murder that was sanctioned by America and motivated by negrophobia is driven by the white public's same anxiety and fear that now sanctions the murder of Black men and boys as "justifiable homicides." The institutional program that justifies police violence, ostracism, and incarceration is normalized/ritualized by the phobia of Black men. This fear is embodied in white America and shared among many racial and ethnic groups in the U.S. This consensus generates Black male vulnerability. Black males can be killed under this agreement, and the individual perpe-trators of these murders will be ideologically supported in their rationalizations and even financially rewarded. Therefore, the ideological currency of pathological Black masculinity is used as a justification for the murder of Black males in American society, thus obscuring the full scope of Black male oppression. The health of American democracy is contingent upon the deaths of Black men and boys. Racist caricatures and decadent tropes (e.g., rapist, criminal, deviant-thug) offered by white patriarchy of Black manhood saturate society and legitimate the fear Americans have of Black men. Dead Black men are no longer economic competition, and their political radicality against white society becomes an afterthought. Societal support for the imposition of death on Black male bodies is justified by the phobia of Black males and provides consent to the police state and the subsequent justifications for the execution of the Black-male beast/superpredator.[7]

Genocidal logics rationalize Black male death as necessary for the safety and secu-rity of American society. Disregarding the genocidal disposition of America toward Black males obscures the motivation that undergirds the levels of violence and sanctions enforced against Black communities (Black women and Black families) in order to regulate the lives of young Black males. Hetey and Eberhardt (2014) found that racial disparities in incarceration increase acceptance of punitive policies when the penal institution was represented as "more Black." This activated a concern about crime followed by the endorsement of punitive poli-cies compared to the penal institution being represented as "less Black" where there was less endorsement of punitive policies.[8]

Black males are death-bound due to the perception/construction that they are ter-rors (e.g., rapists, murderers, criminals, and sexual deviants) and the American consen-sus is to control and deter their propagation through death. The engineered societal program that orchestrates Black male death and dying obscures and denies the human-ity, vulnerability, and fragility of Black male existence. Black maleness is positioned as a constant state of deprivation. The process of dehumanization entails vacating the personality and character of Black men and boys and replacing them with white delu-sional fears. These delusional white fears create caricatures out of Black males and position them for extermination. The state and the white population benefit from the deaths of Black Americans. This necropolitical dynamic within the U.S. indicates that the republic thrives off of the deaths of Black Americans. Death for Black Americans is the norm in the U.S. and an omnipresent managerial strategy of Western democracy. This ensures that the population growth of Black Americans is managed and lessens competition with the dominant white population. The anti-Black misandry within the U.S. creates conditions of disposability of Black men who are conditioned for death. Black males are conditioned to suffer from premature death and illness as a part of their lives. Black Americans are particularly vulnerable to disease and health-related deaths due to economic and political segregation.[9]

Demographies of death and dying are a deliberate apparatus that is integrated into America's democratic infrastructure where Black Americans who are marked for death not only suffer direct violence but are conditioned for death due to living in segregated neigh-borhoods, suffering from poverty, chronic higher levels of stress, surviving on deficient diets, and coping with exposure to the extra-legal deaths of members from their racial group that results in earlier mortality than white Americans. A grim example of this can be seen with the slow governmental response to Hurricane Katrina, where the corpses of Black victims were left floating in the streets of New Orleans and over half (51 percent) of those who died were Black. This can be critically analyzed beyond ideas of benign neglect and thought of as a natural disaster that was utilized to hasten Black death and dying.[10]

It was revealed that the recent surge in U.S. drug overdose deaths has hit Black men the hardest. Black men have experienced the largest increase in overdose death rates among all demographic groups in the U.S. They have surpassed white men and are now on par with Native American or Alaska Native men who are the most likely to die from overdoses. As late as 2015, Black men were significantly less likely than white men and Native American or Alaska Native men to die from drug overdoses. But since then, the rate of drug overdose deaths among Black men has tripled increasing 213 percent. Black existence in the U.S. is a dynamic state of dying due to the premature death that results from the vulnerability and disadvantage of Black life.[11]

Black males have the highest lifetime risk of being killed by police. The deaths of Black Americans by police officers leaves an imprint upon the collective psyche of Black Americans that causes collective trauma potentially for generations and remembered through collective/ancestral memory. An exponential loss is produced from the public killings of Black Americans. Not only is the personal and political loss of Black Americans amplified due to their public murders, but an increase in allostatic load and a decrease in coping mechanisms in relation to death are magnified. Black men experience a persistent proximity to death while simultaneously managing and navigating traumatic loss and bereavement due to the loss of male family members and peers that conveys a sense of absence and nonexistence. Black Americans are continuously experiencing, enduring, and coping with death, which is experienced as an eschatological psychology and not simply only a biological stressor. Those who recognize and uplift Black people and fully articulate the humanity of Black males while attempting to end their annihilation may themselves be greeted with death. Black males are forced to engage in their own dying.[12]

Malcolm X, Martin Luther King Jr., and Huey P. Newton elucidated the existential dilemmas of eschatological psychology through their articulation of their death-bound experiences. Martin Luther King Jr.'s *I've Been to the Mountaintop* speech prior to his assassination speaks to his eschatological vision where he speaks of not fearing potential death. The trauma the Black community suffered as a result of the assassinations of Malcolm X and Martin Luther King Jr. have yet to be fully articulated but serves as examples to what happens to Black men who live beyond their subordinated space and dare to speak out against and challenge the U.S. patriarchal caste system. Not only was the momentum of Black liberation cut down, but a movement (civil rights and Black Power movements) of this magnitude has not been seen since in the Black community. Therefore, the Black community experienced the physical deaths of its beloved leaders and the symbolic death of a liberation movement that brought the possibility of an alternative existence.[13]

Black life is not only largely determined by the deaths of other Black Americans but the fear that death is a pervasive feature of Black existence that will claim its next victim. Routine police interactions with young Black males not only confirms their subordinate undercaste status but is a death grooming mechanism that exposes them to direct and indirect death. Black males are the primary targets and the majority among the Black population killed by police. As previously underscored, Black males (ages 18–24 years old) in Baltimore, Maryland, disclosed witnessing and experiencing police violence (e.g., racial profiling, harassment, physical injury (witnessing police beat up and injure older Black men), threats, and verbal aggression) that began in childhood and continued into emerging adulthood, which met the *DSM-5* criteria for trauma exposure and embodied theoretical conceptualizations of racial trauma. The exposures to police violence created distrust and fear of police among Black males and informed appraisals and understandings of their vulnerability (i.e., Black male vulnerability to physical, psychological, social, economic, or legal harm) to police violence (i.e., racial profiling, injury, and death) across the life course. Black males disclosed losing loved ones to police killings, which activated hypervigilance and grief. They were challenged to navigate morbidity, mortality, and traumatic loss as a function of community violence while concomitantly challenged to navigate the chronic risk of exposures to violence and premature death due to police encounters. As previously mentioned, Black males killed by police officers are more likely to be younger, and the documentation regarding their deaths is less likely to include public health worker (PHW) coded mental health or substance use histories, weapon use, or positive toxicology for alcohol or psychoactive drugs compared to white male decedents. Therefore, physical aggression or escalation is more likely to be attributed to white men than Black men. Moreover, the greater risk that Black males pose that warrants their deaths in greater numbers remains undetermined. Black victims of police killings have 60 percent lower odds of exhibiting signs of mental illness, 23 percent lower odds of being armed, and 28 percent higher odds of fleeing in comparison to whites. Therefore, the threshold for being perceived as dangerous which is related to lethal police violence is higher for white civilians.[14]

The regimes of racial violence directed towards Black males produces life-depleting effects that lead to the utter exhaustion of life. Living in a racist society increases race-related stress, which ages Black Americans and contributes to the early onset of gerontological illnesses (i.e., weathering). The Black body experiences profound harm as a result of being made to endure anti-Black racism, which forces Black Americans to merely exist (a walking dead sort of existence) while their white counterparts live and thrive. Thus, Black Americans are substantially more vulnerable than the white majority. Accordingly, Black males compared to their white male counterparts are more likely to have someone close to them murdered. The research of Umberson (2017) revealed that Black Americans experience the deaths of more friends and family members from childhood throughout later life than white Americans. Black Americans are at a greater risk of experiencing the death of a mother, father, sibling, spouse, and child compared to white Americans. Black Americans are at a greater risk of losing a mother during childhood through young adulthood, losing a father through mid-teens, and losing a child through late twenties compared to white Americans. The result is a cumulative exposure to family member deaths among Black Americans across generations.[15]

The bereavement and losses create a unique stressor for Black Americans through interconnected social, psychological, behavioral, and biological pathways that affects social ties, health, and well-being. The repeated relationship losses over the life course creates significant racial disadvantage in relationships along with the potential health and well-being benefits from social ties. Important Black social connections are obliterated, and other relationships and health are undermined over the life course due to a cascade of psychological, social, behavioral, and biological consequences that result from the premature deaths of friends and loved ones that leaves surviving children, adults, and families grappling with tremendous loss. The ever-present threat of premature death is a constant in the lives of Black Americans that occupies the conscious of every Black parent. These losses create a specific type of stress and adversity that produces health disparities among Black Americans. The loss of Black Americans directly impacts Black Americans in mourning and affect their mortality (i.e., slow death for those living in mourning). Therefore, living Black Americans are continually subjected to the pain of oppression, while their dying is accelerated due to the deaths of other Black Americans. Surviving family members not only experience a void but their life chances are lessened due to the distress caused by the deaths of relatives and close friends. These cumulative experiences contribute to the weathering (i.e., early health deterioration) of Black Americans. Further, the deaths and dying of Black Americans and Black men within America's patriarchal empire is a form of *necropolitics*, which is the demonstration of sovereignty (social and political) by dictating who may live and who must die where Black life is inconsequential. The commitment to Black male death is formed through the political and legal structures of social organization. These mass suicide-homicide killings, premature deaths, and death disparities among young Black males is a public health crisis.[16]

BLACK MALE SUICIDE

The overall suicide rate for Black youth (ages 15 to 24) from 1960 to 1984 more than doubled with Black males (between the ages 20 to 24) accounting for most of the increase. The suicide rate for Black youth (ages 15 to 24) doubled for Black females and nearly tripled for Black males. Hendin (1969) noted that suicide was a serious problem among Black Americans of both sexes between the ages of 20 to 35 in New York City but for Black men was double that of white men of the same age group. But most research on suicide in the Black community has focused primarily on Black women followed by Black adolescents or Black Americans in general, but there is a paucity of research that focuses on Black male adults even though suicide deaths among Black males have drastically risen over the past 20 years.[17]

The suicide rates of Black Americans has continued to increase year over year with Black men comprising the highest percentage of the attempts and deaths within this group. Black men also have the highest percentage increase in attempts compared to all other racial/ethnic and sex subgroups. From 1980 to 1995 the rate of suicide for Black males aged 15–19 increased 146 percent. From 1991 to 2019, Black males had the highest increase in suicide attempts (162 percent) compared to all other racial/ethnic and sex subgroups. From 1999 to 2020, approximately 29,735 Black males (between the ages of 10–44) died by suicide.[18]

According to Hendin (1969), suicidal patients are a barometer of the pressures felt by everyone in that culture. Therefore, Black suicide is indicative of the frustration and anger that culminates from the general pressures and conflicts of Black life for Black Americans in urban America who are at the bottom of the racial caste. Goodwill et al. (2021) found that race-based everyday discrimination (i.e., racial microaggressions) was the only type of discrimination that was significantly associated with both increased rates of depressive symptoms and death/suicide ideation among Black men. Moreover, they found race-based everyday discrimination had a significant indirect effect on suicide ideation. Therefore, the daily encounters with discrimination that this author would deem anti-Black misandry extends beyond depressive symptoms and is related to higher rates of suicide ideation. Everyday discrimination is not an overt form of discrimination but is harmful nonetheless and impacts the mental health of Black men. Black men are at greater risk for suicide ideation that is mediated by depressive symptoms due to racial discrimination (i.e., anti-Black misandry).

The research of Walker et al. (2017) discovered that race-based discrimination predicted higher rates of depression and suicide ideation among Black boys and girls two years after the initial racist incident. Racial discrimination had a direct and mediated effect on suicide ideation and was mediated by depressive symptoms. In addition, Hollingsworth et al. (2017) found the frequency of experiencing racial microaggressions and the increased likelihood of suicide ideation among Black college students was mediated by depressive symptoms.

Research from Oh et al. (2019) examined major discriminatory events as a social risk factor for suicidal thoughts and behaviors amongst Black Americans. They found police abuse, unfairly fired, denied a promotion, bad service, discouraged from education, neighborhood exclusion, and neighbor harassment were all associated with suicidal ideation. The major discriminatory events of being unfairly fired, police abuse, discouraged from education, neighborhood exclusion, and neighbor harassment were all associated with either suicide attempt, an increase in the reporting of suicidal ideation (upon adjustment for sociodemographic characteristics and psychiatric disorders), or an increase in reporting a suicide plan. Police abuse and discouraged from education were the only major discriminatory events that were associated with an increase in a suicide attempt.

NO HUMANS INVOLVED (N.H.I.)/DEHUMANIZATION

According to Harris and Fiske (2006), dehumanization is an extreme form of prejudice that is not equal to other forms of prejudice. Black Americans were at one point considered three-fifths of a human being as part of the Three-fifths Compromise (1787) and inferior beings by the Supreme Court as indicated within the Chief Justice Roger Taney issued decision regarding the *Dred Scott v. Sandford* (1857) case. This dehumanizing classification and nonbeing constitution are reflected in present-day biases in the majority of the U.S. population. N.H.I. (No Humans Involved) refers to the acronym used by the Los Angeles Police Department (LAPD) to describe young, jobless, Black males in L.A. in cases that entailed a breach of their rights. This was brought to light as a result of the Rodney King beating case. This classification positions Black males as nonhumans (i.e., a thing) or nonbeings (i.e., nothingness or an absence) and reinforces their systemic condemnation.[19]

Black males inhabit what Fanon (1952) refers to as the zone of nonbeing. This zone of nonbeing that is inhabited by Blackness is described by Warren (2018) as the metaphysical nothing that sustains anti-Blackness where Blacks experience existence (i.e., inhabitation) but not *Being*. *Human* is not a biological category but an ideological construct. Wynter (1992) interrogates this idea of the *human* being defined by whiteness along with optimal middle-class variants. Black males are shut out of humanity, which is reserved for whites as well as the moral obligation reserved for humans. The connection between humanism and whiteness and dehumanization and Blackness has historical and sociological implications. Humanism and colonialism are an interconnected construct that permeates the same cognitive-political universe where it structures Europe's discovery of its Self as human and the simultaneous discovery of its Others (i.e., the darker races) as nonhuman/nonbeing. This entailed the construction of the idea of *Man* as a biological concept and the systematic degradation of non-European men and women. White men and women experience the fullness of being human that is verified by the lack of humanity ascribed to Black men and women. In addition, Black men and women experience their existence and lack of humanity in relation to whiteness. Therefore, Blackness is positioned as the antithesis of humanity.[20]

Black identity is incessantly negated in the U.S., and Black men serve as a negation of *Man* in Western humanistic thought, thus rendering them non-relatable to other *human* beings. The *nigger* is a thing that is outside of the construction of the human and what Césaire (1955) refers to as *thingification*. Marriott (2000) asserts that Black males who had been lynched were reduced to something that visibly did not look human due to the destruction of their flesh and corpse, while whites simultaneously affirmed their white identity/humanity through the image of a dead Black male. Further, the genocide of Armenians and Jews was preceded by dehumanization that enabled them to be unrecognizable (i.e., deemed aliens/strangers due to the dominant group's alienation from them that was motivated by antipathy) outside of the category of human (i.e., a different species). The social effects of N.H.I. are indirectly genocidal and achieves similar results of direct genocide through the routinized incarceration and elimination of young Black males (i.e., institutional decimation; gendercide).[21]

Simianization is a specific form of the general phenomenon of dehumanization. Livingstone Smith and Panaitiu (2015) define dehumanization as the act of conceiving others as subhuman creatures (i.e., nonhuman kinds). A persistent dehumanizing trope has been the deployment of racialized minoritized groups as apes. At one point in time, Jewish, Irish, and Japanese people have been simianized, while Arab, Japanese, and Chinese people at one point have been perpetrators of simianization. Black people in the U.S. and globally have routinely been simianized by white people. African and people of African descent have been associated with nonhuman primates by white people beginning the modern era. Africans were dehumanized as apes (i.e., ape-like essence) and thought to be subhuman.[22]

In Europe during the later medieval period, Apes were associated with Satan (i.e., sinfulness, lust, and degeneracy) and imbued with evil, impurity, and sin, which eventually was attributed to Africans by Europeans. These associations routinely were made prior to enslavement of Africans to support colonial enterprise. The belief that Black people were kin to apes permeated the scholarship of the academic class (intelligentsia) and popular culture. Scientist during the early 20th century endorsed confident declarations regarding the atavistic character of Africans and Black Americans (e.g., prominent athletes and entertainers) were routinely depicted in racist cartoons in simian form. The dehumanization of Black Americans was utilized as justification for Jim/Jane Crow. Black people have been conceptualized as either pliable, amusing apes, or as brutal, demonic apes. Dehumanization historically has occurred in situations of intense intergroup conflict which creates the foundation for violence, oppression, extermination, or other types of harm. People who are dehumanized are imagined as appearing human but inwardly subhuman (a denial of their humanity). Thus, the dehumanized are conceptualized to be subhuman, humanoid, or the simulacra of humans instead of genuine human beings, which renders them to a peculiar metaphysical status where they lack human essence (that is shared among all human beings) and instead embody a subhuman essence that situates them within a lower-than-human rank on the Great Chain of Being. They are ultimately transformed into contradictory beings.[23]

The white human is encased by a body, but Black Americans are believed to be nonhumans or nonbeings that are devoid of a body and are just Black flesh. Moreover, the dehumanized are believed to be beneath human beings in a moral sense which renders them less morally considerable compared to humans. Therefore, it is morally permissible (no matter how heinous) to treat the dehumanized in ways that are considered appropriate for subhumans (i.e., nonhuman animals) but deemed inappropriate and unethical for human beings. Culturally enshrined metaphysical boundaries are transgressed by a being that possesses a subhuman essence coupled with a human appearance which evokes a different response than a being whose essence and appearance are congruent. Beings imagined in this manner are unsettling to those doing the imagining. They are imagined to be frightening, creepy, eerie, unsettling, horrifying, impure, fascinating, and monsters if they are framed as physically dangerous.[24]

The dehumanization of others disables the inhibitions of the perpetrators in harming the dehumanized. Dehumanized populations are segregated due to their supposed impure and contaminating (metaphysically) nature. The metaphysically contaminating nature of the dehumanized group can manifest in segregated drinking fountains and being spatially confined to ghettos, townships, reservations, etc. where interaction with the dominant group is heavily regulated to prevent cross-contamination. Black men are taught (explicitly and implicitly) that they are an inferior approximation of humanity (i.e., a thing, beast, or non-entity) in which they can be ignored or disposed of at any given moment.[25]

Dehumanized people who are considered physically dangerous are imagined having superhuman powers to do harm. Waytz et al. (2014) found that whites dehumanize Black people, which entails attributing powers beyond human capacity that they identify as *superhumanization* (i.e., supernatural, extrasensory, and magical mental and physical qualities). Black men have been characterized as superpredators with supernatural strength, insensitivity to pain, superhuman sexual appetites, etc., which has been embodied and immortalized within the racist historic image of King Kong.[26]

Black Americans were increasingly demonized after slavery was abolished. Black men were routinely characterized by white writers as fiends, wretched creatures, brutal and merciless, and a monstrous beast crazed with lust. Black men were described as embodying demoniacal ferocity who obsessively desired sex with white women and savagely raped them upon opportunity. The descriptions of the alleged assaults deployed demonizing language (e.g., beastly, diabolical persistence, malignant atrocity, bestial, ferocious animals and predatory apes). The depiction of Black men as murderous and sexually rampant apes created the justification for lynchings. Goff et al. (2008) found that majority whites and non-whites implicitly associate Black people (images of Black male faces were used in the experiments) with apes while exhibiting a white-ape inhibition effect. Thus, Black Americans are mentally represented as less evolved with a closer relationship to apes than whites, who are represented as more evolved and farthest removed from apes thus representing humanity. The Black-ape association was found to alter visual perception and attention and increase the endorsement of violence against Black suspects in criminal justice contexts. In addition, news articles written about Black Americans convicted of capital crimes were more likely to contain ape-relevant language compared to news articles written about white convicts. Moreover, those who were implicitly framed as more ape-like in the articles were more likely to be executed by the state compared to those who were not framed in this manner.[27]

Further, Goff et al. (2014) found that Black boys are viewed by the majority of whites and non-whites as older and less innocent than their same-age white peers. In addition, dehumanization (i.e., the Black/ape association) predicted police violence against Black boys. The simianization of Black males diminishes sympathy for their humanity and increases acceptance of greater levels of violence directed towards them. Dehumanization is a mechanism that is used to target individuals and social groups for cruelty, social degradation, and state-sanctioned violence and has been identified as a necessary precursor to genocide.[28]

GENOCIDE/GENDERCIDE

Jones (2000) defines genocide as the actualization of the intent to murder in whole or in substantial part any racial, national, ethnic, religious, political, social, sex/gender or economic group that is defined by the perpetrator. Staub (1989) defines genocide as an attempt to exterminate a racial, ethnic, religious, cultural, or political group directly (i.e., murder) or indirectly (i.e., systematic deprivation: socially engineered conditions that lead to the group's destruction). Physical extermination is not required as destruction of group cohesion and identity that includes bodily or mental harm can constitute genocide. Nonlethal techniques of destruction can be genocidal such as culturally destructive acts that are connected to a coordinated effort of eradicating a national group. The widespread destruction of human lives through the systematic degradation of a group that results in psychological and material impoverishment is a form of genocide. Twentieth-century genocides are a product of modernity's (it is important to note that the colonial/imperial foundation is still present through practices of domination and exploitation) defining features that includes the combining force of new technologies of warfare, enhanced state powers of surveillance through new administrative techniques, and the categorization of people along strict lines of nation and race through fairly new ideologies that have also made populations the choice object of state policies. Modern genocides include the seizure of state power while concomitantly getting rid of a specific population(s) and the recruitment and participation of ordinary civilians in the brutalities and killing of targeted groups. Women have not only been targets and victims of genocides but have participated in the mass mobilization of women as direct (i.e., violent aggressors) and indirect participants of genocide. They have aided in nation-building (e.g., motherhood) as well as acted in defense of the nation (e.g., supporting mass violence or actively engaging in atrocities). Another defining feature of modernity is the biologization of ethnicity, nationality, and race (still has ideological currency that is deployed to propagate racist ideas) combined with the centrality of women to genocidal violence through the ideology of women as mothers of the national/ethnic/racial collective.[29]

The slaughter of male bodies is a marker and evidence of war and genocide. Gendercide against men is a common form of genocide. Gendercide are sex/gender-selective mass killings that is a defining feature of human conflict and social organization that extends back to antiquity. Gendercide is a routine and ubiquitous feature of contemporary worldwide politico-military conflicts. Gendercide encompasses the deliberate extermination of persons of a specific sex/gender (i.e., male or female). *Non-combatant* men are the most frequent targets of mass killing and genocidal slaughter including lesser atrocities and abuses. Non-combatant males (i.e., civilians, prisoners-of-war, and former fighters) includes those who do not bear arms in a specific conflict or during a specific stage of a conflict. The history of conflict between human communities entails the mass killing of males, which includes *battle-age* men who are of reproductive age (approximately 15–55 years old). But the problem with this term (battle-age) is that it lends itself to genocidal logics that ascribes military combat to men of a certain age and male identity and falsely implicitly suggests that they are willing participants where an equivalency is generated between males and combatants. Patriarchal societies have had a fundamental problem with men who are not covered by the bonds of kinship or culture and has historically sought to marginalize and dominate them through various mechanisms. This has included killing all male captives, the castration of male captives who have been allowed to live, and reduced opportunities offered to men for manumission from slavery. The domination of the men outside the bonds of kinship and community has historically been more severe and brutal than that of the women who are within and outside the kin or ethnic group. Some of the gendercide/genocide is what is referred to as *root-and-branch* extermination where the men are targeted first followed by the women and children (i.e., wholesale annihilation of the targeted group). According to Jones (2000), the Stalinist purges of the 1930s and 1940s are an example of gendercide. The extermination of groups of men resulted in women significantly outnumbering men between 67 to 32 percent between the age ranges of 35 to 70+[30]

Pervasive features of contemporary conflict entail the sex/gender-selective mass killing and "disappearance" of males particularly battle-age males during warfare, state terrorism, mob violence, and paramilitary brigandage. Kosovo (1999), Jammu and Kashmir (1999), Columbia (1998), Rwanda (1997), Bosnia-Herzegovina (1992), Sri Lanka (1991), and Iraqi Kurdistan (1983) all provide examples of gendercide where men were targeted for extermination. Military logic undergirds the destruction of males (battle-age) of a targeted community which might be a sufficient measure in lieu of the root-and-branch extermination of the community. The scale of physical destruction of opposed populations has been limited by some highly warlike societies though mechanisms of enslavement, concubinage, or through the freeing of women and children. Historically and worldwide, non-combatant men of battle age are the most vulnerable and consistently targeted population group. They are the group universally perceived as posing the greatest danger to the conquering force and most likely to have oppressive mechanisms of the state directed against them. Non-combatant men are not armed and are without means to defend themselves and are subject to be detained and exterminated by the thousands or millions. This can extend beyond the ages of 15–55 years old.[31]

The systematic targeting of males is supported by institutional, material, political, and cultural interests. Part of the process of gendercide includes the physical separation of men from women as a prelude to consignment to death. The killing of unarmed men is normalized though genocidal logics (i.e., they are expendable as men), while the killing of women and children is considered revolting and egregious. Women and children are routinely framed as civilians while men are expunged from this framing and undefined in genocidal killing and analysis even though they are often the prime target of genocidal assault. Patriarchy and hegemonic masculinity inform military action that includes feminizing (emasculating) enemies who have been defeated by virtue of their defeat and includes castration (genocidal sexual violence) as a prelude to being killed where severed genitals are sometimes paraded as a token of victory as well as male rape and gendercidal mass murder (i.e., group annihilation). The sexual mutilation of males and male rape has a demasculinizing and feminizing component while simultaneously valorizing heterosexual virility. Not only are these men disempowered and feminized by male perpetrators, but their ethnic group is humiliated by this assertion of patriarchal hegemonic masculinity. The biological and social continuance of groups can be impeded by the rape and sexual torture of men in a similar fashion to women. Curry (2021) found that the rape of Jewish men and boys during the Holocaust was a common occurrence that was well-known among Jewish men in concentration camps. An uprising by a subordinate ethnic group can activate patriarchal hegemonic military action with the goal of suppression. In addition, the sex/gender-selective killing of male civilians that belong to a specific ethnic/racial/national group may be indicative that the more generalized destruction and mass murder of that population is soon to follow.[32]

Gendercide against Black males in the U.S. entails a long historical continuum of de facto war involving race and class. Poor Black males are subjected to numerous disabling conditions that restrict opportunity, inflict pain and suffering, and shorten lifespans. The systematic dismantling of kinship and cultural ties over time is central to this sociopolitical condition which has made the Black male vulnerable to various forms of gendercidal targeting. Black male gendercide evolved through a series of power-relation regimes that are embedded within the economic and sociopolitical order of the U.S. Initially Black male gendercide began with less sophisticated methods of domination and punishment informed by a slave-based agrarian economy (slaveocracy) that evolved into a more complex, indirect system of male selective genocide under ideologies of globalization. Del Zotto (2004) identifies various stages of control and punishment that includes ideologies, institutions, and disciplinary forms along with shared features that has been historically resilient. The features consist of a preoccupation by cultural and political elites with economic institutions and the identification of the Black male as an indirect threat to these institutions. This involves the preservation and expansion of socioeconomic interests through the implementation of various mechanisms of social engineering. Including the intent to impose harm (e.g., discursive, social, and physical) upon Black males as a primary feature of the social-engineering schema. The social-engineering schema is discussed in detail in previous chapters, but the following are pivotal aspects that are important to mention. It includes destroying the Black family and destroying Black men who became the focus of this project. Leadership and group cohesion within the enslaved Black population was discouraged through the public spectacle of ritual flogging, burning, castration, and the execution of enslaved Black males. Moreover, the plantation system's male-to-female ratio was carefully monitored, which included males being sold to other plantations or indirectly killed by being overworked as they began to reach adult age with the intent to break family bonds. These early historical and social practices informed discursive and symbolic cultural mechanisms that created bifurcated caricatures of Black Americans.[33]

The enduring caricature of Black men post-Emancipation has framed them as dangerous violent criminals and sexual deviants who are threats to white society which serves the function as a legitimizing myth (SDT) to justify their annihilation. The Black male criminal caricature is continually culturally constructed and reproduced through media, political, and academic discourse (see Chapter 4: "The Carceral State and Black Men" for details). Between 1882 and 1968, 3,220 Black men (approximately 72 percent of all lynching victims) were targeted and destroyed through lynchings by white communities. The Jim/Jane Crow era included sociospatial control and economic deprivation (see Chapters 4: "The Carceral State and Black Men" and 5 and 6: "Starving the Black Beast—Part I and II" for details). These mechanisms and practices are gendercidal in scope and nature and manifest through two interconnected forms, which are overt force (i.e., direct gendercide) and psychological coercion (i.e., indirect gendercide). The construction of the Black male criminal results in direct gendercide through overt force. The overt force of gendercide is what Williams-Myers (1995) refers to as the *destructive impulses* of white violence and rage that is part and parcel of the American democratic process and its socioeconomic and political structure. This includes disparities in hypercriminalization/incarceration as well as the disparate application of the death penalty to Black men. Further, police brutality and killings of Black men are forms of overt force.[34]

Black femaleness often provides a protective identity against police use of lethal violence compared to Black maleness. Research discovered that police in the U.S. killed an estimated 30,800 people between 1980 and 2018. This indicates 17,000 more deaths than reported by the National Vital Statistics System (NVSS), which is a misclassification rate of 55 percent. The deaths of Black Americans were the most likely to be undercounted with 5,670 deaths missing out of an estimated 9,540. Medical examiners in 47 documented cases falsely claimed that sickle cell trait (SCT) was the cause of death of Black men killed by police. As previously emphasized, there are 1.5 million Black men missing due to early death and hyperincarceration. This leaves 83 Black men for every 100 Black women not incarcerated.[35]

The death and dying (i.e., premature deaths) of Black males is either direct or indirect genocide (contingent on how the death(s) occurred). In addition, academic institutions along with supporting public and private sectors endorse direct gendercide through force. This is achieved through pseudoscience arguments by psychologists, sociologists, and political scientists who reinforce the image of the dangerous Black male. The preoccupation with Black males in U.S. society denotes a historical trend that informs how the perceived "problem" is addressed by important and diverse institutions that form a complex social, political, and economic nexus. Indirect gendercide can manifest through internalized oppression and suicide. The negative view of self (e.g., worthlessness) and other Black Americans from internal oppression can negatively impact health and contribute to health disparities (see Chapter 2: "Racial Discrimination and Health" for details) contributing to indirect gendercide.[36]

Gendercide in the U.S. is an ongoing historical program of controlling and eradicating Black males. The gendercide directed towards Black men in the U.S. is distinct from gendercide in other regions of the world (e.g., Kosovo, Rwanda, and Kashmir) as it is not bound by a limited time frame or constrained under specific conditions of war or political repression. Black men have expressed greater fears of genocide than Black women, which might indicate that they have a general sense of the deliberate practice of Black male gendercide. Further, every chapter in this volume provides detailed information on the mechanisms of Black male gendercide. The violence that Black males experience that causes or contributes to their deaths and dying is not theorized beyond their corpse.[37]

SEXUAL VICTIMIZATION

*The terms *sexual victimization* and *sexual assault* are used as more expansive terms than the narrow definitions of rape by the CDC and the FBI that perpetuates sex/gender and heterosexist bias and fails to fully capture male victimization: rape includes unwanted intercourse regardless of directionality.

Stemple and Meyer (2014) discovered that the high prevalence of sexual victimization among men was similar to the prevalence of sexual victimization among women. They found reliance on traditional sex/gender stereotypes, outdated and inconsistent definitions, and methodological sampling biases that excluded inmates were all factors that perpetuated misperceptions about men's sexual victimization. Research from Stemple et al. (2017) indicated that sexual victimization perpetrated by women is not uncommon.

The Centers for Disease Control and Prevention (CDC) National Intimate Partner and Sexual Violence Survey (NISVS/2017) revealed that men suffered higher rates of sexual violence compared to women in the U.S. According to Smith et al. (2017), 1,715,000 males were victims of made-to-penetrate violence while 1,473,000 females were victims of rape over a 12-month period. Moreover, 272,000 Black males reported being made to penetrate and 264,000 Black females reported being raped over a 12-month period. Black men reported 830,000 cases (approximately 7 percent), while Black women reported 849,000 cases (approximately 6 percent) of contact sexual violence over a 12-month period. The percentage is slightly lower among Black women, but this is in proportion to their larger population size. Black men reported higher rates of contact sexual violence (e.g., rape, being made to penetrate, sexual coercion, and unwanted sexual contact/approximately 7 percent) than white men (approximately 3 percent), white women (approximately 4 percent), Latino men (5 percent), Latina women (4 percent), and Black women (approximately 6 percent). In addition, the lifetime prevalence of contact sexual violence for Black males was 19 percent, which equates to approximately 2.5 million Black male victims. Approximately 49 percent of perpetrators of contact sexual violence of male victims were an acquaintance while 41 percent were a current or former intimate partner.

Male rape victims were primarily victimized by an acquaintance (47 percent) followed by a current or former intimate partner (approximately 21 percent) and approximately 87 percent of the perpetrators were male. Men who were made to penetrate reported being victimized by a current or former partner (approximately 51 percent) followed by an acquaintance (44 percent), and approximately 79 percent of the perpetrators were female.

Moreover, 24 percent of made-to-penetrate male victimization occurred before the age of 18. Male victims who experienced sexual coercion indicated being victimized by a current or former intimate partner (66 percent) followed by an acquaintance (approximately 33 percent), and approximately 82 percent of the perpetrators were female. Male victims of unwanted sexual contact reported being victimized by an acquaintance (approximately 53 percent) followed by a stranger (approximately 24 percent) and a current or former intimate partner (approximately 22 percent), while 53 percent of the perpetrators were female and approximately 37 percent were male.[38]

Men who reported non-contact unwanted sexual experiences were victimized by an acquaintance (45 percent) followed by a stranger (34 percent) and a current or former intimate partner (approximately 25 percent), while 48 percent of the perpetrators were male and approximately 38 percent were female. These figures are likely underestimates due to the stigma of sexual victimization among males, the fear of revenge, the perception of being gay, the desire of self-reliance or an attempt to maintain an internal locus of control, and the potential loss of independence after disclosure of their sexual victimization. The specific rates of Black male sexual victimization that is comparable and even surpasses women is considered inconceivable by many scholars, activists, and gender theorists and is rejected outright. These stats are ignored as they contradict ingrained sex/gender stereotypes regarding commonly held beliefs about rape and patriarchy that isolate sexual violence, assault, and coercion to the male sex. Black males are believed to be dangerous and in need of control, and their criminalization prevents them from being perceived as victims of violence perpetrated by other groups of men and women. Therefore, the formation of dangerous racist and sex/gendered caricatures of Black men as criminals, deviants, and sexual predators (i.e., the insatiable sexual savage) positions them as being invulnerable to sexual violence, which serves as the foundation of disciplinary method and gender theory. This makes it impossible to recognize Black male victims of sexual violence in the U.S. Further, the dehumanization of Black males converts them into entities who are capable of an endless array of imaginable atrocities against women, children, and society.[39]

Abram Kardiner is credited with defining PTSD as a result of authoring *The Traumatic Neuroses of War* (Kardiner, 1941) in which symptom description would later be used in the 1980 definition of PTSD by the APA. Kardiner and Ovesey authored *The Mark of Oppression* (1951) in which they mention their research on working-class Black boys' sexual debut (statutory rape) commonly occurring between the ages of 7–9 years old with much older girls or women. This is not examined or interrogated as Black boys being sexually victimized by older girls or women but framed as a marker of the sexual deviancy of Black boys. The research of Hernandez et al. (1993) explored the effects of child abuse and race on risk-taking in male adolescents. They found that more Black males reported experiencing incest, extrafamilial sexual abuse, and physical abuse (their average age of first intercourse was 13). Thus, Black males were more likely to engage in the following risk-taking behaviors: illegal substance use, run away, skip school, attempt suicide, force partners into sex, and commit violent acts; however, the racial effects decreased upon consideration of abuse histories. Duncan and Williams (1998) examined sex/gender role socialization and male-on-male vs. female-on-male child sexual abuse of boys who were primarily Black (89 percent). They found that Black men who were survivors of male-on-male and female-on-male child sexual abuse were more likely to report violence toward intimate partners, which indicates that physical aggression and violence is modeled for boys who are sexually victimized. Moreover, female-on-male child sexual victimization significantly increased the likelihood of adult sex offending. The IPV and adult sex offending perpetrated by those initially sexually victimized are trauma responses. The research of Reid and Piquero (2014) analyzed age-graded risks for commercial sexual exploitation (CSE)/prostitution of male and female youth and found that Black male youth were at a heightened risk for CSE/prostitution while female youth of all races/ethnicities were at a similar risk. Maternal substance use and earlier age of first sex were associated with early age of onset of CSE/prostitution for all youth, while experiencing rape and substance use dependency were associated with early age of onset for male youth.

French et al. (2015) examined sexual coercion and psychosocial correlates among diverse males who were adolescents and emerging adults in high school and college. Forty-three percent of the participants experienced sexual coercion (i.e., verbal, seduction, physical, and substance). The respondents reported that women were the primary perpetrators (95 percent) of sexual coercion.

Greater sexual risk-taking (e.g., multiple sex partners, unsafe sex practices) and alcohol use was associated with sexual coercion that resulted in sexual intercourse. Psychological distress was associated with verbal and substance coercion and sexual risk-taking was also associated with substance coercion. Black males reported a greater proportion of verbal coercion compared to Asians and Latinos and unwanted seduction compared to Asians. In addition, Black males reported a significantly greater proportion of coercion that involved kissing and fondling compared to Asians. Follow-up research from French et al. (2019) on male sexual victimization, risk-taking, and attitudes towards women and racially stereotyped attitudes towards women found that the more males were sexually victimized, the more they engaged in sexual risk-taking, which was associated with an increase in stereotypical sex/gender attitudes regarding dating and sex. They posit that hypersexual stereotypes of racialized women (e.g., the Jezebel trope of Black women) gets activated and reinforced when males are sexually victimized by females in their same racial group. The research of Curry and Utley (2018) examined the adult sexual violations of Black boys. The average age of the Black males in their study was 42 years old. The average age of the participant's first sexual experience was 9 years old, and their first sexual interaction with an adult was 13 years old. They found that Black males were uniquely at risk for sexual impropriety and statutory rape primarily perpetrated by older women and teenage girls as well as being at risk from same-sex sexual violations. Many of the research participants were violated by women who were family friends, caretakers, or older peers. This supports Kardiner and Ovesey's (1951) findings on the sexual debut of Black boys with older girls and women. The research of Lindberg et al. (2019) reviewed the prevalence of sexual initiation before the age of 13 years among male adolescents and young adults in the U.S., which revealed a significantly higher number of Black males reported having sexual intercourse before the age of 13 than other racial/ethnic groups.[40]

Black male celebrities DeRay Davis, Tech N9Ne, and Lil Wayne have revealed that they were sexually victimized by adult women as adolescents (between the ages of 11 and 14). In addition, R. Kelly's brother alleges that he and R. Kelly were sexually victimized by their older sister and that R. Kelly was also sexually victimized by an adult male neighbor as a child. Chris Brown disclosed being sexually victimized by a teenage girl as a child. Terry Crews had his genitals groped by a white male Hollywood executive in front of his wife, and Tyler Perry has spoken about being sexually victimized as a child by men and a woman. A *CNN* article highlighted that more than 1,000 people (90 percent were men and 40 percent were Black men) were sexually victimized by University of Michigan athletics doctor Robert Anderson. Black boys routinely experience unwantedness and are disproportionately sent to local or state facilities where they are raped or sexually assaulted. The violence of the sexual assaults often occurs in group home settings, foster homes, and rehabilitative centers.

During Jim/Jane Crow, Black boys and men were raped during convict leasing, and it can be argued, the convict leasing system orchestrated their sexual victimization. This has current application to Black males who are victims of hypercriminalization/incarceration who suffer sexual victimization within these institutionalized contexts.[41]

Frequent police contact is associated with trauma and anxiety symptoms where non-consensual encounters are experienced as intrusive contributing to a higher prevalence of PTSD among Black males. Black males are routinely sexually assaulted during police stops (e.g., stop-and-frisk) where their genitals are fondled and grabbed, which is not permissible on a female sexed body. In addition, Black males have had their genitals kicked, squeezed, and they have been sodomized by police officers with a plunger (e.g., Abner Louima), had their underwear pulled down exposing their genitals on a public street (e.g., Clarence Green and his brother who was a minor), had their pants and underwear pulled down followed by their genitals being fondled along with their testicles being grabbed/pulled or a finger inserted into their anus (e.g., Kevin Campbell and Deaundra Billingsley), and Officer Rachel Sorkow video recorded a Black man's exposed genitals without the victim's knowledge while referring to him as a nigger and shared the recording with friends. Foster's (2011, 2019) research exposed the sexual victimization of Black men under American slavery by white men and white women. Whites found Black male bodies sexually appealing. The sexual victimization of enslaved Black men included the fixation (both desire and horror) and exploitation of Black male bodies and genitals (i.e., Black male flesh). Their bodies were devalued, objectified, fetishized, degraded, and abused. The genitalia of enslaved Black males were groped, scrutinized, imagined, and tortured in an effort to possess or degrade them. Legal ownership enabled control of the enslaved Black male body in which various forms of sexual assault took place in a wide variety of contexts. Enslaved Black men and boys were raped by white male enslavers who would sodomize them as punishment for not completing assigned tasks or for their pleasure where Black male bodies were used to fulfill their sexual desires. Black men were forced (e.g., including at gunpoint) to rape Black women for the pleasure of white men, which not only sexually victimized Black women but also Black men (i.e., a multilayered sexual assault) and forced to engage in what is often referred to as slave breeding (i.e., forced reproduction) to produce more enslaved Black Americans, which is another form of this multilayered sexual assault of Black women and men. In addition, white women (including wives and daughters of planters) sexually assaulted and exploited enslaved Black men. This included sexual coercion that ranged from direct threats (e.g., threatening to sell them or claim rape), indirect manipulation, and subtle threats of violence. White women could use enslaved Black men as sexual objects for sexual experimentation or sexual release while retaining their appearance of puritanical virtue, passionlessness, and virginity.[42]

PHALLICISM

According to Fanon (1952), there is a fixation/obsession with the Black male phallus that motivates a fear/anxiety/disgust (i.e., negrophobia) response and an attraction/erotic (i.e., negrophilia) response from white men and women that is a primary function of anti-Black misandry. A *CNN* (2020) article titled "There's One Epidemic We May Never Find a Vaccine For: Fear of Black Men in Public Spaces" mentions white America's long-standing history of associating Black men with criminality and hypersexuality. Curry's (2017, 2018) theory of *phallicism* refers to the condition of a subordinated racialized or ethnicized group of males who are imagined to be a sexual threat and predatory while simultaneously sexually desired (e.g., libidinal fantasies and fetishes) by the dominant racial group. Phallicism is supported by Lemelle's (2010) theory of Black males being simultaneously constructed as hypersexual and feminized (i.e., emasculated). Foster (2019) questioned if the myth/fiction of the Black male rapist that was created after Emancipation was partly informed by white women to justify their actions during enslavement (i.e., the sexual victimization of Black males) and fear of retribution. This included the idea that Black males were a sexual menace and suffered from *furor sexualis* (i.e., hypersexuality), which was a biological imperative that drove them to rape white women. Journals routinely featured articles with scientific claims regarding the supposed enlarged genitalia and unrestrained sexual impulses of Black men.[43]

According to Frazier (1927), the white male experiences a psychosexual conflict where he demonstrates an exaggerated antagonism toward the desire that he projects upon the Black male. This sexual violence is a defense mechanism for unacceptable desires followed by compensatory reactions to their desires. Further, according to Saint-Aubin (1994), Black males are necessary products of white male fantasies and projections and the object of the white male, heterosexual gaze that is motivated by a desire to possess and appropriate Black male flesh. Baldwin (1963) refers to this as the white man's private fears and longings.

Black males are positioned as predatory (rapists) but in actuality are sexually vulnerable and raped within a patriarchal society. Phallicism exposes the contradiction in the depiction of Black males within repressive and murderous patriarchal regimes and the hyper-sexualization of Black males as objects of desire and possession. Black maleness is synonymous with rape (rapist) while concomitantly being subjugated to rape by both male and female members of the dominant white racial group who can displace their sexual violence through the deliberate hypervisibility of the constructed Black male rapist. The objectification and sexualization of Black men and boys are routinely dismissed due to their framing as predators by the dominant group. Thus, their sexual victimization is obscured.[44]

Phallicism is an apparatus of gendercide that is understudied. Historically, patriarchal imposition and imperial conquest (e.g., Africa, Asia, and Indigenous America) justified the disposability of male victims of genocide or conquest through the construction of the racialized male rapist while ridding the world of this apex predator (i.e., primitive and evil being) while simultaneously denigrating their flesh through sexual violence (e.g., castration during lynching, rape). The ritual of castration of Black males during lynchings served to emasculate them by removing their penis ("unsexing") and to take ownership of not only their penis (i.e., the Black phallus) but their sexuality and essence. Whites were able to enact their sexual inhibitions through the collective ritual of lynching and castration. The rape of Black men does not serve a reproductive purpose and is markedly different from the rape of Black women or other subordinated racialized women. Historically, the rape of Black women was intended to create intermediary populations between the white dominant group and the subordinated Black group throughout British populations as well as sexual arousal and satisfaction, while the rape of Black men primarily served as an expression of force, power, or coercion over Black male bodies as well as sexual arousal and satisfaction. According to Curry (2018), the violence against Black males is not simply rooted in their extermination but the simultaneous function of the Black male rapist (i.e., sexual threat) that legitimizes their death and the erotics (i.e., the fascination/fetishization that functions as a depository of white sexual excess) of the Black male body and phallus.[45]

Miller's (1991, 2004) theory of patriarchy, Jones' (2000) theory of gendercide, and Sidanius and Pratto's (1999) theory of SDT fails to fully account for this duality and seemingly contradictory apparatus. Thus, phallicism builds upon these theories. Black maleness creates a rupture in accepted and established modern gender hierarchies that are positioned as universal to all sexed bodies in Western patriarchal societies. In addition, a rupture is created within current configurations of heteronormativity, identity, and sexuality in that the attraction/objectification/sexualization to/of Black males/bodies by same-sex males is not necessarily a marker of a gay/queer/homosexual identity but denotes a homoerotic attraction (i.e., homoeroticism, same-sex desire/arousal). This is difficult for many to grasp due to the medicalization of sexual practice in the West that included the creation of identities around sexual practice, which serves as a historical heteronormative framing that obscures reality. Woodard (2014) examines and highlights the parasitic relationship between human consumption (i.e., cannibalism) by white males of enslaved Black males on U.S. plantations and homoeroticism. He describes the consumption of Nat Turner and the harvesting of his body parts as a ritual of sexual dominance and white male fixation on Black male virility. Therefore, white males hungered for Black male flesh where Black males were viewed as a delectable and desirous object of consumption. Nat Turner was hung, doctors skinned his corpse, boiled-down his flesh to grease, and dissected (included being beheaded) and distributed his body parts among white families. In addition, a money purse was made from his skin. It was reported that the boiled-down flesh was ingested by whites as a medical substance (an elixir referred to as *Nat's Grease*) that was saved and sold over a period of time. Whites were able to taste the terror, fascination, hatred, and death of Nat Turner. This represents a literal desire to possess his flesh and fetish and symbolic corporeal possession. His skull had long been missing and believed to be safeguarded as if it were a cherished family trophy or heirloom to recently have been given back to his family (awaiting DNA test results to confirm if it is indeed his skull). The lynching of Claude Neal (1934) entailed his penis and testicles being removed and placed in his mouth where he was forced to eat them. This gruesome act symbolizes white male oral fixations with Black male virility and reflects the deep-seated fear of Black men as a perceived sexual threat. Neal was made to consume the evidence of white desire and erotic fascination.[46]

The long-standing superstitious preoccupation with the Black male body and phallus in the U.S. has historical roots and present-day implications. Black men are rendered to being a walking phallus (i.e., the commodification of the Black phallus) that is disembodied where the magical Black phallus has the capacity to cause unusual and extreme levels of pleasure that are not humanly possible. But since Black males are not constituted as human but a phallus, this becomes not only a possibility but a reality in the imagination of others. Phallicism adds to the discourse of Black male victimization by the brute power of white patriarchy that encompasses a range of experiences from police killings of Black men and boys, hypercriminalization/incarceration, and the rape of Black male prisoners or suspects while justifying this brutality to supposedly protect women, society, and civility from the Black male primitive. The ruling-class white woman's social articulation of fear (i.e., continuous imposing danger) legitimizes the paranoia of Black males as sexual terrors. Murderous acts enacted upon Black male bodies are legitimized by anti-Black misandric stereotypes that are motivated by the lust or antipathy (both serve as forms of desire) of white male and white female sexual power.[47]

INTIMATE PARTNER VIOLENCE (IPV)/INTIMATE PARTNER HOMICIDE (IPH)

Johnson (1995, 2006) created a typology of IPV that includes two distinct types of IPV which includes *situational couple violence* (SCV) and *intimate terrorism* (IT). SCV is primarily population-based where women and men use IPV equally (bidirectional). This entails conflicts that "get out of hand" (i.e., escalating interactions) with men and women typically utilizing low levels of violence such as pushing, shoving, grabbing, or slapping one another. The primary characteristic of IT is a general pattern of control (coercion/e.g., not allowing to leave the house, monitoring time and whereabouts) and intimidation where violence is one tactic of control. The IPV is severe (e.g., punching, kicking, choking, beating up, using a knife or gun) and occurs frequently at least monthly; it is not bidirectional but unidirectional (asymmetrical) and commonly involves serious injury (e.g., broken bone, passing out) and emotional abuse (e.g., name-calling, humiliation). Women who perpetuate IT routinely use objects and weapons while assaulting their partners when they are asleep, drunk, or not pay- ing attention. Any size and strength differential a male may have in comparison to a female is neutralized by guns and knives, boiling water, fireplace pokers, bricks, and baseball bats. Female perpetrators of IPV are significantly more likely than men to throw something, slap, kick, bite, punch, or hit with an object. Assaulting a male's reproductive system (e.g., "being kicked in the balls") for reasons outside of physical self-defense is a form of sexual assault. Men compared to women are more likely to be stabbed with a knife (6 percent compared to 1 percent), hit by an object other than a gun (12 percent compared to 3 percent), hit by a thrown object (10 percent compared to 3 percent), and are more likely to be victims of an attempted attack with an object (2 percent compared to 1 percent). Women are more likely to use a non-firearm weapon than men in IPV, and men are disproportionately victimized with blunt objects and knives. In addition, *violent resistance* (VR) is defined by the victim's occasional reaction to their partner's IT with violence but is distinguished from the IT gen- eral pattern of attempting to control the partner. But VR is solely theoretical as there is no measure of motivation for violence to test this category. *Mutual violent control* (MVC) refers to a partner who reacts with severe violence and controlling behaviors. Thus, both partners in this dynamic would be considered intimate terrorists who are battling for control in a relationship.[48]

The research of Hines and Douglas (2010a) examined men who sustained intimate terrorism by women and found that the IPV they experienced was severe and was both mentally and physically damaging. Their most frequent response to their partner's IPV was to escape from her, and their efforts to leave were routinely blocked physically. But most often their strong psychological and emotional connections to their partners and especially children prevented them from leaving. Most men in the study did not strike back, but those that did use violence against their female partners engaged in violent resistance. Follow-up research from Hines and Douglas (2010b) on IT by women towards men found that a male help seekers sample (i.e., men who contacted a national domestic abuse helpline) consisted of victims of IT and violence by the male victims was consistent with violent resistance compared to men in a community sample who were involved in IPV that was indicative of SCV. Hines and Douglas (2018) discovered that men who were victims of IT had signifi- cantly worse mental health than men who experienced SCV. Further, male victims of IT experienced significant severe and frequent partner violence (PV) that included physical (e.g., minor/severe physical aggression), sexual (e.g., minor/severe sexual aggression), and nonphysical (e.g., minor/severe psychological aggression, controlling behaviors, threatened legal/administrative aggression, actual legal/administrative aggression) forms of IPV and sustained significantly more types of both minor and severe injuries. Moreover, male victims of IT experienced worse mental and physical health than men who experienced MVC. Male victims of IT had significantly greater levels of PTSD symptom severity in comparison to male victims of SCV. In addition, significant differences were discovered between IT and SCV male victims in depression symptom severity and physical health indicators.

The highest rates of violence, including domestic violence in the industrialized world, can be found in the U.S. Intimate partner violence (IPV/domestic violence) is a pattern of behaviors that includes physical assault, psychological and emotional abuse, and sexual assault and coercion. IPV is a human problem rather than a sex/gender problem. Over 40 years of research indicates that men and women both experience IPV by their opposite sex partners. Verbal abuse, sexual aggression, threats, and controlling behaviors are not solely perpetuated by men. Men are approximately 50 percent of all victims of IPV each year. The long-held assumption that women's motive for IPV against their male partners is self-defense or retaliation in response to presumably violent male partners has been refuted by research studies that demonstrate that most women do not report self-defense or retaliation as a motive for IPV. Women use IPV against their male partners at rates and frequencies that are often reciprocal and symmetrical (bidirectional) to that of their male partners. The Centers for Disease Control and Prevention (CDC) National Intimate Partner and Sexual Violence Survey (NISVS/2014) revealed that approximately 37 percent (4,595,000) of Black males suffer physical violence (e.g., ranging from being slapped to having a knife or gun used against them) by an intimate partner during their lifetime, while Black women reported a lifetime prevalence of 41 percent (5,955,000). Native American men reported a lifetime prevalence of 45 percent (365,000), Latino men 26 percent (4,277,000), and white men 28 percent (21,524,000). Native American women reported a lifetime prevalence of approximately 46 percent (399,000), Latina women 35 percent (5,317,000), and white women approximately 32 percent (25,746,000). The lifetime prevalence of physical violence by an intimate partner for lesbian identified victims was 40 percent (659,000), while gay male victims reported 25 percent (685,000). Sexual minorities report higher rates of IPV than those who identify as heterosexual. Lesbians report greater numbers of IPV than heterosexual women, while heterosexual men report higher rates of IPV than gay men. Bidirectional violence was the most frequently reported IPV among lesbians, bisexuals, and gay men.[49]

Khurana et al. (2021) reviewed the National Electronic Injury Surveillance System-All Injury Program data from 2005 to 2015 for all IPV-related injuries in both male and female patients and discovered that IPV accounts for approximately 1 percent of emergency department visits, while 17 percent account for males, and approximately 83 percent account for females. Male IPV patients were more likely to be Black males (approximately 41 percent compared to approximately 29 percent), the most likely causes of injury were being struck, and the head/neck was the most common anatomical location, but compared to female IPV patients they sustained more injuries due to cutting (28 percent compared to approximately 4 percent), more lacerations (approximately 47 percent compared to 13 percent), more injuries to the upper extremity (approximately 26 percent compared to 14 percent), fewer contusions/abrasions (30 percent compared to 49 percent), and were more likely to be hospitalized (approximately 8 percent compared to approximately 4 percent) due to more severe injuries. They were also significantly more likely to have injuries due to being bitten, pedestrian (e.g., being struck by a vehicle), fire/burn (e.g., being exposed to flames, heat, or chemicals), and firearm/GSW (gunshot wound/e.g., injury caused by bullet or projectile). They suggest that Black men may be more at risk for IPV victimization, but additional stereotypes (caricatures) and barriers may prevent them from being recognized as victims of IPV. Rates of IPV are significantly higher in Black American than in European American communities. But West (2016) has asserted that national studies have had limitations due to the data of ethnic differences in rates of violence among Blacks (e.g., Black Americans compared to Black immigrant populations and second-generation Caribbeans/Africans) not being further disaggregated, which results in an "ethnic lumping" that obscures the data.

Black Americans (individuals or couples) consistently report higher rates of overall IPV that includes severe, bidirectional, and recurrent past and lifetime victimization and perpetration compared to their white and Latino/a, and Asian American counterparts in general population, community, and university samples. The rates of physical and psychological aggression among Black men and women are comparable. Bidirectional violence is the most frequently reported pattern of relationship violence in the Black community. Moreover, the bidirectional violence has been described as severe by one-third of Black couples. Unidirectional aggression (IT) is likely to be female perpetrated among Black Americans. Caetano et al. (2005) found high rates of female-to-male partner violence (violence rates of 30 percent) perpetrated by Black wives against their Black husbands. The correlation between race and domestic violence is substantially reduced or disappears altogether when comparing European Americans to Black Americans in similar ecological contexts. Black Americans are placed at greater risk for domestic violence due to SES, contextual variables, and forms of racial oppression. The chronic unemployment and underemployment of Black males are stressors that are significantly associated with domestic violence.[50]

From 1976 to 1985, Black males were significantly more likely than Black females to be victims of intimate partner homicide (IPH). But by 2005, Black women were two times more likely than Black men to be victims of IPH. IPH among Black Americans had significantly declined over the past 30 years from a high of 1,529 victims in 1976 to 475 victims in 2005 representing a 69 percent decline. IPH among Black males declined by 83 percent compared to a 55 percent decline among Black females. Velopulos et al. (2019) examined male and female victims of IPH and bidirectionality through the National Violent Death Reporting System (NVDRS/2003–2015) and found a total of 6,131 persons in opposite-sex relationships and 181 in same-sex relationships were murdered due to IPV. Women and Black men were disproportionately victimized, and alcohol and preceding arguments were a significant factor of male victims. Female perpetrators of IPH were more likely than males to use a stabbing instrument (e.g., knife or blade), but firearms were the most common weapon among both female and male perpetrators. Bidirectionality was highest among male victims (5 percent vs. approximately 1 percent) of female perpetrators and among same-sex pairings regardless of the sex of the victims. IPV is a risk factor for IPH and IPH caused by IPV is a public health crisis for both women and Black men. Men under-report their injuries, are less likely to be forthcoming about the cause of their injuries, and are less likely to report IPV than women. This is partly due to not recognizing it as criminal, and fear of being ridiculed or being falsely accused as the primary aggressor. In addition, societal biases that IPV is primarily perpetrated by men against women prevents men from getting the help they need. Further, the overrepresentation of Black male victims of IPV and female-perpetrated homicides has not prompted more research on Black male victims as research continues to be sparse and almost nonexistent.[51]

CLINICAL IMPLICATIONS

The marginalization of Black males is understudied, and their vulnerability remains invisible. The marginalization and vulnerability of Black males is traumatizing. The areas that are within the scope of clinical practice are suicide, sexual victimization, and IPV. But these areas as well as the other significant structural determinants of BMN highlighted in Chapters 7 and 8 need to be immediately addressed through urgent and responsive public policy to change societal conditions. Otherwise, simply recommending clinical intervention without advocating that the structural determinants addressed in Chapters 7 and 8 be removed inadvertently endorses genocidal logics and what Wilderson (2018) states Black psychologists and Black psychoanalysts do, which is *help Black people make it through the day*.

It is important to integrate a structural and systemic lens when working with Black males to comprehensively approach clinical work with Black males. This includes how they are socially located (i.e., the socially engineered conditions they are made to live and die through) along with barriers and challenges they are navigating or might have to navigate. The ideas about Black males are predominantly based on deficit models (i.e., deviance and pathology orientations) and not empirical data. Clinicians need to evaluate their own anti-Black misandric beliefs and how they potentially are perpetuating anti-Black misandric micro/aggressions. Further, it is important to understand Black manhood as apatriarchal and center conceptualizations of Black manhood that are strengths-based and independent of feminist or intersectionality ideology and are free of notions of privilege, hypermasculinity, hypersexuality, criminality, or any other constructed caricature of Black male deviance that obscures the vulnerability of Black men. The mental health field faces a challenge in this regard as feminist theory and intersectionality are deeply embedded in graduate programs, organizations, and publications. Black maleness is situated as a category of condemnation and is positioned as an antagonism to women and LGBTQ+ populations. Any attempts to discuss Black male oppression often dissolves into a zero-sum game in opposition to other groups' oppression including Black women. The zero-sum logic can cause people to become dysregulated and take a defensive stance with attempts to discredit the experiences of Black men and engage in the oppression Olympics while demonizing Black men (anti-Black misandric micro/aggressions). This is a form of double victimization with attempts at silencing Black men. A public health perspective recommends that it is important to focus on those most at risk to adequately address a problem. Therefore, a space to talk about the impossibility of Black male life is extremely significant and a revolutionary act.

Suicide

Raced-based everyday discrimination (i.e., anti-Black misandric micro/aggressions) is associated with higher rates of death/suicide ideation among Black men and has an indirect effect through depressive symptoms. In addition, being unfairly fired, police violence, racial-residential segregation (i.e., being prevented from moving into a neighborhood), financial insecurity, job instability, trauma, residing in areas of concentrated poverty, and alcohol abuse/dependency all heighten suicide risk among Black men, while strong social networks protect against suicidal behaviors. Being unfairly fired, police violence, and being prevented from pursuing an education are associated with a suicide plan while police violence and being prevented from pursuing an education are associated with suicide attempts. Among Black male youth, racial discrimination, online exposure to race-related traumatic events, extreme levels of socioeconomic disadvantage (i.e., poverty and racial-residential segregation), insecure attachment with caregivers, abuse and neglect (also referred to as adverse childhood experiences/ACES), lack of social support, depression, anxiety, and community violence are associated with suicide ideation and suicide. Anti-Black misandric micro/aggressions often leave Black men feeling frustrated, defeated, and hopeless. Stewart (1980) asserts that Black male suicides are due to racial discrimination that is reflected in the structural violence of the political economy through income and employment differentials that produces economic frustration. Thus, Black males are removed from the civilian population through institutional decimation (e.g., death by suicide). According to Durkheim (1951), all types of suicide are associated with social conditions. Therefore, the social environment (i.e., external factors) is the primary cause of suicide and not individual temperament (i.e., internal factors). Durkheim's concept of fatalistic suicide has been posited as an explanation of Black male suicide due to Black men "being trapped" where their existence is heavily regulated, and their passions and futures are violently obstructed in an oppressive white patriarchal America. Thus, their options are to exist (i.e., a slow painful death) with incessant regulation and abuse/terrorism/death, fight back through active resistance (i.e., meaning-making and the maintenance of one's dignity, and what Newton (1973) has referred to as *revolutionary suicide*, which includes his philosophy of extending the moment by giving all to the present), or simply exit through death. According to Newton (1973), young Black males who have been deprived of human dignity, crushed by oppressive forces, and denied their right to live as proud and free human beings die by suicide (what he refers to as reactionary suicide) in response to social conditions that overwhelm them and condemn them to helplessness. Part of this process involves a spiritual death (i.e., condemned to a living death) that is even more painful and degrading than death of the flesh as one lapses into a life of quiet desperation. Collapsing into resignation in the fight against the various forms of anti-Black oppression is indicative of a spiritual death. Therefore, social structures in the U.S. produce structural violence (i.e., institutional decimation) directed towards Black males that contributes to their suicide.

Suicide is a multifaceted phenomenon that requires a multidimensional approach for prevention and treatment, which includes a sociological/ecological (i.e., the relationship between society and the environment; the stratification of Black males and anti-Black misandry) and psychological (i.e., internal drives; low self-esteem and a negative locus of control) lens. Clinicians should examine environmental factors and life stressors that may activate an individual's predisposition to suicidal behaviors. This should be followed by assessing if an individual feels defeated or humiliated, which prompts feelings of entrapment that lead to suicide ideation. Racial discrimination (i.e., anti-Black misandry) may emerge as a factor that is connected to the suicide ideation. Clinicians will need to help Black males process depression as well as navigate racial discrimination in a way that helps them feel empowered.[52]

Sexual Victimization

Black men are at a greater risk of rape due to their inferior status (i.e., racial undercaste) in the U.S. as racialized out-group men. Male victims of sexual abuse are often identified due to the threat they pose to others (e.g., a sexual offense) where they are often recognized as a perpetrator and not a victim. The repressive social conditions of anti-Black racism and poverty contributes to broken families which places Black males at greater risk of sexual victimization. In addition, Black boys are at greater risk for sexual coercion and assaults due to incarceration, foster care, and social unwantedness. Black boys are at greater risk of actual or attempted intercourse and extrafamilial abuse. Male victims who are sexually violated are more likely to be physically abused and experience violent sexual abuse than their female counterparts. Child sexual abuse of males increases the probability of suffering multiple traumas, future violence, self-harm, suicide attempts, substance abuse/dependency, guilt, shame, emasculation, anxiety, depression, personality disorders, compulsive masturbation, sexual dysfunction, sexual risk-taking, sexual aggression, IPV (victim and perpetrator), homophobia (if sexually victimized by a male perpetrator), endorsing hypersexuality stereotypes of women in their racial group (if sexually victimized by a female perpetrator from the same racial group), and marriage problems. The sexual victimization of Black males can be socially and psychologically debilitating due to a fear that a disclosure would not be believed as well as self-blame and guilt particularly among men who became physically aroused during the abuse. Heterosexual sexual coercion (sexual abuse) is often reinterpreted by young males as consensual with the belief that they were knowledgeable and partly in control. There is an embedded belief in the U.S. that sex with an older woman is not traumatic but a pleasurable experience. This belief is reinforced within gender and race theory scholarship on masculinity where the recognition of female sexual offenders and male victims is nearly obsolete. This includes feminist theory scholarship that asserts that women are oppressed by patriarchy and are never perpetrators of sexual violence but only victims. Research indicates that women exert violence against others independent of male influence or presence. But women and girls are afforded an innocence that affords an invisibility as perpetrators due to the politics of sex/gender and female victimhood (e.g., reinforcing regressive notions of female vulnerability that include ideas that women are noble, pure, passive, and ignorant), which ultimately makes it difficult for the public, law enforcement, and professionals to recognize this violence clearly and fully. Moreover, beliefs that women are less physically able to commit harmful acts due to the female body's form reinforce sex/gender stereotypes and scripts about sexual behavior. Sexual violence (e.g., sexual assault or rape) by female perpetrators against male victims does not have to include being physically overpowered or physically dominated. Black males who are sexually victimized by females may be unable and unwilling to trust women in relationships. Female-perpetrated sexual abuse of Black males is believed to provide the greatest risk of future violence by Black male victims directed towards others. They might become more aggressive and dominant particularly in heterosexual intimate relationships with women, which might result in sex offending as well as higher levels of physical violence. The sexual victimization of Black males by police officers is often obscured by heteronormative assumptions about sex and sexuality. They include beliefs that an erotic element does not exist in the police brutality of Black men, the sexual assault of men is rare, heteronormative men (i.e., men who claim a heterosexual identity or appear to be heterosexual) don't have homosexual desire/arousal/attractions (i.e., homoeroticism), and sexuality is confined to what takes place in bed. These assumptions allow stop-and-frisk policies to continue unabated where Black males are sexually harassed/violated/victimized by police officers who might specialize in these tactics because they find them exciting (i.e., sexually arousing), thus the connection between sadism/predation and anti-Black racism remains invisible.[53]

It is imperative that an ecosystemic approach (individual, familial, cultural, and societal factors) that incorporates the effects of anti-Black racism and systemic oppression be used in working with Black boys who are victims of child sexual abuse. The marking of Black male bodies with the myth of hypersexuality makes it difficult for researchers and clinicians to recognize the statutory rape and sexual coercion of Black men and boys. Black males are thought to be invulnerable to sexual coercion, sexual abuse, and statutory rape. In addition, the lack of language and a cultural script that identifies older women and girls forcing them to perform cunnilingus or penetrate their vaginas against their will creates a significant barrier in identifying and defining acts of rape or sexual violence perpetrated against them. Other forms of sexual violence against Black males includes coercively being fellated or orally penetrated, forcibly being manually stimulated or made to manually stimulate, and being made to penetrate anally or being penetrated anally. Black male sexual vulnerability to Black women and girls leaves many Black men and boys without the language to articulate their sexual trauma and the ability to think of themselves as victims of sexual violence. But a prevailing racial script in the Black community is that the sexual victimization of Black boys is rare, and a white problem that does not affect Black children, specifically Black male children. Therefore, the sexual violation of Black boys is believed to be inconsequential to their socialization and psychological development throughout their development into adulthood. Anti-Black misandry manifests in beliefs that Black males are not victims of societal sexual violence but perpetrators, which denies them of the ability to be victims of sexually predatory acts. It is not unlikely that untreated Black male victims of sexual violence are living with trauma. Therefore, it is imperative that clinicians provide compassionate and responsive care in order to afford them the opportunity to heal and not be consumed by the wound of trauma.[54]

IPV

IPV is indicative of a relationship-system collapse. Men under-report their injuries, are less likely to be forthcoming about the cause of their injuries, and are less likely to report IPV than women. This is partly due to not recognizing it as criminal, and fear of being ridiculed, not being believed, or being falsely accused as the primary aggressor. Many men do not hit back due to moral objections to hitting a woman and fear that they could be arrested and lose custody of their children (i.e., societal sanctions for hitting a woman). This includes a restraining order filed against them under false pretenses or false accusations that they physically or sexually abused the children. Male victims of IPV suffer from higher rates of PTSD, depression, stress, psychosomatic symptoms, and alcohol abuse. In addition, they are at risk for emotional hurt, fear, helplessness, anger, revenge seeking, sadness, self-blame, shame and humiliation, weight loss, and psychological distress. Men often find it difficult to leave a violent relationship due to the strong emotional attachment to their partners (traumatic bonding in cases of IT) as well as the fear of leaving their children with a violent parent believing that if they remain in the household, they can at least protect the children. Therefore, their psychological investment in their families is a significant barrier to leaving. Other barriers include having no place to go and a lack of financial resources to support leaving. Societal tolerance for female violence is greater than male violence. In addition, societal biases that IPV is primarily perpetrated by men against women prevents men from getting the help they need from domestic violence hotlines, domestic violence agencies, hospital employees, social workers, district attorneys, and police officers. District attorneys tend to prefer that law enforcement officers do not arrest both the man and woman in cases of mutual abuse (SCV) as it complicates the case. Men are often turned away, ridiculed, accused of being a batterer, and arrested. According to Al'Uqdah et al. (2016), solely blaming Black men for the high rates of IPV in the Black community contributes to the maintenance of negative environments that perpetuate IPV due to the diminished willingness of service providers to counteract the larger societal factors that contribute to IPV in the Black community as a result of framing Black men as the sole perpetrators of IPV.[55]

According to Fontes (2007), the feminist movement has become politically enmeshed in the domestic violence movement where they are now synonymous, and any discussion of male victims is viewed as a threat to their paradigm and movement. This includes funding being provided primarily for female victims, which ultimately creates obstacles for male victims in accessing needed services. Based on their research, Hines and Douglas (2018) recommends no longer considering feminist patriarchal theory as the principal theory/explanations for IPV (SCV & IT) or in guiding policy and practice. Currently, men arrested for IPV are required to complete the Duluth Model (Paymar & Pence, 1993), which is a men-only group that addresses patriarchal beliefs and power and control. The Duluth Model continues to be required even though there is no empirical evidence to support its theoretical supposition and as an effective treatment in reducing recidivism of family violence.

Anti-Black racism, poverty, residing in disadvantaged neighborhoods, unemployment and underemployment, low SES, childhood abuse (experiencing child abuse or witnessing domestic violence in family of origin), attachment insecurity, exposure to community violence, and alcohol abuse/dependency are predictors of IPV for Black Americans, which places the entire family system at risk. An ecological model that examines interpersonal violence as the outcome of a complex interaction among multiple factors at four levels (e.g., *individual, relationship, community*, and *ecological*) is recommended. The *individual level* includes a person's sociodemographic characteristics, formative history (e.g., exposure to child abuse), and substance use that increase their risk of interpersonal violence. The *relationship level* includes interactions between the person and their partner, family members, and peers. The *community level* includes the environment in which the person lives (e.g., exposure to neighborhood crime). The *ecological model* incorporates larger societal factors (e.g., norms, policies, and inequalities) that create an environment where violence is sustained. Clinicians need to be aware of anti-Black misandric biases they may hold that may be demonstrated through devaluing, blaming, or treating Black men harshly. Anti-Black misandry may be demonstrated by Black clinicians as feelings of distrust, anger, and disappointment towards Black men followed by harsh treatment in clinical settings. Parenting support and techniques to prevent or lessen the psychological impact of IPV on children (e.g., poor self-esteem, anxiety and trauma symptoms, depression, aggression, disrupted peer relationships, and poor academic performance) should be provided as well as protection and safety planning.[56]

The clinician needs to differentiate whether it is SCV or IT that is taking place in a relationship by assessing the pattern of physical assaults, significance of controlling and emotionally abusive behavior, motivation for violence, impact of the violence, and partner's subjective experience. Part of delineating SCV from IT is assessing the partner's subjective experience, meaning do they fear their partner or fear being assaulted or injured by their partner? This can be problematic in evaluating among some males as men are acculturated to not feel afraid of their female partners when they may be in real danger of physical harm. Further, a male might be reluctant to admit fear out of the fear of appearing vulnerable. Thus, this part of the evaluation should not rely solely on the subjective experience whether the male feels afraid of his female partner but rather if the abuse warrants additional help from further victimization. Addressing the client's desire to either remain or leave the relationship is imperative. SCV can be initially assessed by using the Situational Violence Screening Tool (SVST; Friend et al., 2011) or the Revised Conflict Tactics Scale (CTS2; Straus et al., 1996) and can be appropriately treated within couples therapy when the risk of continued violence is low. This includes Domestic Violence-Focused Couples Therapy (DVFCT), the Creating Healthy Relationships Program (CHRP), or an attachment-focused couple therapy where there is a continuous assessment of safety (it is important to note that many state guidelines mandate against couple therapy in cases of court-ordered IPV treatment even though there have been promising results in treating SCV with couple therapy). Behavioral Couples Therapy (BCT) is recommended if one partner is struggling with alcohol or drug abuse. BCT was developed to address substance abuse and has been found to be effective in reducing IPV. BCT addresses the substance abuse first before focusing on relationship functioning.[57]

The context of the IPV should be assessed separately and privately during individual sessions. Couple therapy would not be appropriate if either partner does not feel safe. The accounts of IPV within the relationship should be similar and congruent among both partners as significant discrepancies may be indicative of an inability to assume accountability which is contraindicated for treatment. Utilizing polarizing language such as *perpetrator* and *victim* when working with couples of SCV who have chosen to remain in the relationship can leave them feeling less supported by the therapist especially when they do not view their conflict in these terms. Using these terms also confuses instead of elucidates their conflicts. Part of this process entails taking accountability for violence without blaming one's partner and the maladaptive responses to situations. Moreover, a joint commitment to safety that is demonstrated by a "no-violence" contract where both partners agree to discontinue violence in the relationship during treatment is a precondition to couples therapy. The contract provides clear expectations and boundaries and the refusal to sign the contract would indicate a lack of motivation and commitment by one or both partners in ending IPV in their relationship. But a contract can also create a barrier during treatment where clients are reluctant to disclose any conflicts that escalated into violence between appointments. Therefore, it is important that the contract is not used as a pass/fail test. Enlisting support from family members, local religious leaders, and trusted community elders and advocates can be instrumental in working with Black Americans. It is essential that clinicians understand that many in the Black community might be cautious of service agencies due to the differential treatment by the child welfare system and the disproportionate rate of child removal and out-of-home placement of Black children and arrest rates of Black males for domestic violence.[58]

NOTES

1 Curry, 2017; Flaherty, 2017.
2 Stein, 2015; Fredrickson, 1971; Fanon, 1952; Curry, 2014, 2017, 2020, 2021; Curry & Curry, 2020; Hipple et al., 2020; Edwards et al., 2019; Anderson & Curry, 2021; James, 1999; Oluwayomi, 2020; Wolfers et al., 2015; Ogungbure, 2019a, 2019b; Mbembé, 2003; Rogers, 2014; Durr, 2015; Uhuru, 2021; Finkelhor et al., 2005; Jones-Eversley et al., 2020; Levine et al., 2001; Miller, 1996; Marable, 2007; Brunkard et al., 2008; Daniels, 2021; Sykes et al., 2021; Gramlich, 2022; Arseniev-Koehler et al., 2021; DeAngelis, 2021.
3 Stein, 2015; Fredrickson, 1971; Fanon, 1952; Curry, 2014, 2017, 2020, 2021; Curry & Curry, 2020; Hipple et al., 2020; Edwards et al., 2019; Anderson & Curry, 2021; James, 1999; Oluwayomi, 2020; Wolfers et al., 2015; Ogungbure, 2019a, 2019b; Mbembé, 2003; Rogers, 2014; Durr, 2015; Uhuru, 2021; Finkelhor et al., 2005; Jones-Eversley et al., 2020; Levine et al., 2001; Miller, 1996; Marable, 2007; Brunkard et al., 2008; Daniels, 2021; Sykes et al., 2021; Gramlich, 2022; Arseniev-Koehler et al., 2021; DeAngelis, 2021.
4 Stein, 2015; Fredrickson, 1971; Fanon, 1952; Curry, 2014, 2017, 2020, 2021; Curry & Curry, 2020; Hipple et al., 2020; Edwards et al., 2019; Anderson & Curry, 2021; James, 1999; Oluwayomi, 2020; Wolfers et al., 2015; Ogungbure, 2019a, 2019b; Mbembé, 2003; Rogers, 2014; Durr, 2015; Uhuru, 2021; Finkelhor et al., 2005; Jones-Eversley et al., 2020; Levine et al., 2001; Miller, 1996; Marable, 2007; Brunkard et al., 2008; Daniels, 2021; Sykes et al., 2021; Gramlich, 2022; Arseniev-Koehler et al., 2021; DeAngelis, 2021.
5 Stein, 2015; Fredrickson, 1971; Fanon, 1952; Curry, 2014, 2017, 2020, 2021; Curry & Curry, 2020; Hipple et al., 2020; Edwards et al., 2019; Anderson & Curry, 2021; James, 1999; Oluwayomi, 2020; Wolfers et al., 2015; Ogungbure, 2019a, 2019b; Mbembé, 2003; Rogers, 2014; Durr, 2015; Uhuru, 2021; Finkelhor et al., 2005; Jones-Eversley et al., 2020; Levine et al., 2001; Miller, 1996; Marable, 2007; Brunkard et al., 2008; Daniels, 2021; Sykes et al., 2021; Gramlich, 2022; Arseniev-Koehler et al., 2021; DeAngelis, 2021.

6 Stein, 2015; Fredrickson, 1971; Fanon, 1952; Curry, 2014, 2017, 2020, 2021; Curry & Curry, 2020; Hipple et al., 2020; Edwards et al., 2019; Anderson & Curry, 2021; James, 1999; Oluwayomi, 2020; Wolfers et al., 2015; Ogungbure, 2019a, 2019b; Mbembé, 2003; Rogers, 2014; Durr, 2015; Uhuru, 2021; Finkelhor et al., 2005; Jones-Eversley et al., 2020; Levine et al., 2001; Miller, 1996; Marable, 2007; Brunkard et al., 2008; Daniels, 2021; Sykes et al., 2021; Gramlich, 2022; Arseniev-Koehler et al., 2021; DeAngelis, 2021.

7 Stein, 2015; Fredrickson, 1971; Fanon, 1952; Curry, 2014, 2017, 2020, 2021; Curry & Curry, 2020; Hipple et al., 2020; Edwards et al., 2019; Anderson & Curry, 2021; James, 1999; Oluwayomi, 2020; Wolfers et al., 2015; Ogungbure, 2019a, 2019b; Mbembé, 2003; Rogers, 2014; Durr, 2015; Uhuru, 2021; Finkelhor et al., 2005; Jones-Eversley et al., 2020; Levine et al., 2001; Miller, 1996; Marable, 2007; Brunkard et al., 2008; Daniels, 2021; Sykes et al., 2021; Gramlich, 2022; Arseniev-Koehler et al., 2021; DeAngelis, 2021.

8 Stein, 2015; Fredrickson, 1971; Fanon, 1952; Curry, 2014, 2017, 2020, 2021; Curry & Curry, 2020; Hipple et al., 2020; Edwards et al., 2019; Anderson & Curry, 2021; James, 1999; Oluwayomi, 2020; Wolfers et al., 2015; Ogungbure, 2019a, 2019b; Mbembé, 2003; Rogers, 2014; Durr, 2015; Uhuru, 2021; Finkelhor et al., 2005; Jones-Eversley et al., 2020; Levine et al., 2001; Miller, 1996; Marable, 2007; Brunkard et al., 2008; Daniels, 2021; Sykes et al., 2021; Gramlich, 2022; Arseniev-Koehler et al., 2021; DeAngelis, 2021.

9 Stein, 2015; Fredrickson, 1971; Fanon, 1952; Curry, 2014, 2017, 2020, 2021; Curry & Curry, 2020; Hipple et al., 2020; Edwards et al., 2019; Anderson & Curry, 2021; James, 1999; Oluwayomi, 2020; Wolfers et al., 2015; Ogungbure, 2019a, 2019b; Mbembé, 2003; Rogers, 2014; Durr, 2015; Uhuru, 2021; Finkelhor et al., 2005; Jones-Eversley et al., 2020; Levine et al., 2001; Miller, 1996; Marable, 2007; Brunkard et al., 2008; Daniels, 2021; Sykes et al., 2021; Gramlich, 2022; Arseniev-Koehler et al., 2021; DeAngelis, 2021.

10 Stein, 2015; Fredrickson, 1971; Fanon, 1952; Curry, 2014, 2017, 2020, 2021; Curry & Curry, 2020; Hipple et al., 2020; Edwards et al., 2019; Anderson & Curry, 2021; James, 1999; Oluwayomi, 2020; Wolfers et al., 2015; Ogungbure, 2019a, 2019b; Mbembé, 2003; Rogers, 2014; Durr, 2015; Uhuru, 2021; Finkelhor et al., 2005; Jones-Eversley et al., 2020; Levine et al., 2001; Miller, 1996; Marable, 2007; Brunkard et al., 2008; Daniels, 2021; Sykes et al., 2021; Gramlich, 2022; Arseniev-Koehler et al., 2021; DeAngelis, 2021.

11 Stein, 2015; Fredrickson, 1971; Fanon, 1952; Curry, 2014, 2017, 2020, 2021; Curry & Curry, 2020; Hipple et al., 2020; Edwards et al., 2019; Anderson & Curry, 2021; James, 1999; Oluwayomi, 2020; Wolfers et al., 2015; Ogungbure, 2019a, 2019b; Mbembé, 2003; Rogers, 2014; Durr, 2015; Uhuru, 2021; Finkelhor et al., 2005; Jones-Eversley et al., 2020; Levine et al., 2001; Miller, 1996; Marable, 2007; Brunkard et al., 2008; Daniels, 2021; Sykes et al., 2021; Gramlich, 2022; Arseniev-Koehler et al., 2021; DeAngelis, 2021.

12 Stein, 2015; Fredrickson, 1971; Fanon, 1952; Curry, 2014, 2017, 2020, 2021; Curry & Curry, 2020; Hipple et al., 2020; Edwards et al., 2019; Anderson & Curry, 2021; James, 1999; Oluwayomi, 2020; Wolfers et al., 2015; Ogungbure, 2019a, 2019b; Mbembé, 2003; Rogers, 2014; Durr, 2015; Uhuru, 2021; Finkelhor et al., 2005; Jones-Eversley et al., 2020; Levine et al., 2001; Miller, 1996; Marable, 2007; Brunkard et al., 2008; Daniels, 2021; Sykes et al., 2021; Gramlich, 2022; Arseniev-Koehler et al., 2021; DeAngelis, 2021.

13 Stein, 2015; Fredrickson, 1971; Fanon, 1952; Curry, 2014, 2017, 2020, 2021; Curry & Curry, 2020; Hipple et al., 2020; Edwards et al., 2019; Anderson & Curry, 2021; James,

1999; Oluwayomi, 2020; Wolfers et al., 2015; Ogungbure, 2019a, 2019b; Mbembé, 2003; Rogers, 2014; Durr, 2015; Uhuru, 2021; Finkelhor et al., 2005; Jones-Eversley et al., 2020; Levine et al., 2001; Miller, 1996; Marable, 2007; Brunkard et al., 2008; Daniels, 2021; Sykes et al., 2021; Gramlich, 2022; Arseniev-Koehler et al., 2021; DeAngelis, 2021.

14 Stein, 2015; Fredrickson, 1971; Fanon, 1952; Curry, 2014, 2017, 2020, 2021; Curry & Curry, 2020; Hipple et al., 2020; Edwards et al., 2019; Anderson & Curry, 2021; James, 1999; Oluwayomi, 2020; Wolfers et al., 2015; Ogungbure, 2019a, 2019b; Mbembé, 2003; Rogers, 2014; Durr, 2015; Uhuru, 2021; Finkelhor et al., 2005; Jones-Eversley et al., 2020; Levine et al., 2001; Miller, 1996; Marable, 2007; Brunkard et al., 2008; Daniels, 2021; Sykes et al., 2021; Gramlich, 2022; Arseniev-Koehler et al., 2021; DeAngelis, 2021.

15 Stein, 2015; Fredrickson, 1971; Fanon, 1952; Curry, 2014, 2017, 2020, 2021; Curry & Curry, 2020; Hipple et al., 2020; Edwards et al., 2019; Anderson & Curry, 2021; James, 1999; Oluwayomi, 2020; Wolfers et al., 2015; Ogungbure, 2019a, 2019b; Mbembé, 2003; Rogers, 2014; Durr, 2015; Uhuru, 2021; Finkelhor et al., 2005; Jones-Eversley et al., 2020; Levine et al., 2001; Miller, 1996; Marable, 2007; Brunkard et al., 2008; Daniels, 2021; Sykes et al., 2021; Gramlich, 2022; Arseniev-Koehler et al., 2021; DeAngelis, 2021.

16 Stein, 2015; Fredrickson, 1971; Fanon, 1952; Curry, 2014, 2017, 2020, 2021; Curry & Curry, 2020; Hipple et al., 2020; Edwards et al., 2019; Anderson & Curry, 2021; James, 1999; Oluwayomi, 2020; Wolfers et al., 2015; Ogungbure, 2019a, 2019b; Mbembé, 2003; Rogers, 2014; Durr, 2015; Uhuru, 2021; Finkelhor et al., 2005; Jones-Eversley et al., 2020; Levine et al., 2001; Miller, 1996; Marable, 2007; Brunkard et al., 2008; Daniels, 2021; Sykes et al., 2021; Gramlich, 2022; Arseniev-Koehler et al., 2021; DeAngelis, 2021.

17 Gibbs, 1988; Bridge et al., 2015, 2018; CDC, 1998, 2019, 2020; Joe et al., 2018; Graves et al., 2010; Bell & Clark, 1998; Davis & Short, 1978; Jiang et al., 2015; Ialongo et al., 2002; Crosby & Molock, 2006; Barnes, 2010; Xiao et al., 2021; Lindsey et al., 2019; Joe & Kaplan, 2001.

18 Gibbs, 1988; Bridge et al., 2015, 2018; CDC, 1998, 2019, 2020; Joe et al., 2018; Graves et al., 2010; Bell & Clark, 1998; Davis & Short, 1978; Jiang et al., 2015; Ialongo et al., 2002; Crosby & Molock, 2006; Barnes, 2010; Xiao et al., 2021; Lindsey et al., 2019; Joe & Kaplan, 2001.

19 Wynter, 2001, 2003; Scott, 2000; Fein, 1979; Goff et al., 2008; Newton, 1967; Wilderson, 2018; Fredrickson, 1971; Bar-Tal & Teichman, 2005; Newton, 1967; Wilkinson, 1977; Delgado & Stefancic, 1991; Uhuru, 2021; Smiley & Fakunle, 2016; Livingstone Smith & Panaitiu, 2015.

20 Wynter, 2001, 2003; Scott, 2000; Fein, 1979; Goff et al., 2008; Newton, 1967; Wilderson, 2018; Fredrickson, 1971; Bar-Tal & Teichman, 2005; Newton, 1967; Wilkinson, 1977; Delgado & Stefancic, 1991; Uhuru, 2021; Smiley & Fakunle, 2016; Livingstone Smith & Panaitiu, 2015.

21 Wynter, 2001, 2003; Scott, 2000; Fein, 1979; Goff et al., 2008; Newton, 1967; Wilderson, 2018; Fredrickson, 1971; Bar-Tal & Teichman, 2005; Newton, 1967; Wilkinson, 1977; Delgado & Stefancic, 1991; Uhuru, 2021; Smiley & Fakunle, 2016; Livingstone Smith & Panaitiu, 2015.

22 Wynter, 2001, 2003; Scott, 2000; Fein, 1979; Goff et al., 2008; Newton, 1967; Wilderson, 2018; Fredrickson, 1971; Bar-Tal & Teichman, 2005; Newton, 1967; Wilkinson, 1977; Delgado & Stefancic, 1991; Uhuru, 2021; Smiley & Fakunle, 2016; Livingstone Smith & Panaitiu, 2015.

23 Wynter, 2001, 2003; Scott, 2000; Fein, 1979; Goff et al., 2008; Newton, 1967; Wilderson, 2018; Fredrickson, 1971; Bar-Tal & Teichman, 2005; Newton, 1967; Wilkinson, 1977;

Delgado & Stefancic, 1991; Uhuru, 2021; Smiley & Fakunle, 2016; Livingstone Smith & Panaitiu, 2015.

24 Wynter, 2001, 2003; Scott, 2000; Fein, 1979; Goff et al., 2008; Newton, 1967; Wilderson, 2018; Fredrickson, 1971; Bar-Tal & Teichman, 2005; Newton, 1967; Wilkinson, 1977; Delgado & Stefancic, 1991; Uhuru, 2021; Smiley & Fakunle, 2016; Livingstone Smith & Panaitiu, 2015.

25 Wynter, 2001, 2003; Scott, 2000; Fein, 1979; Goff et al., 2008; Newton, 1967; Wilderson, 2018; Fredrickson, 1971; Bar-Tal & Teichman, 2005; Newton, 1967; Wilkinson, 1977; Delgado & Stefancic, 1991; Uhuru, 2021; Smiley & Fakunle, 2016; Livingstone Smith & Panaitiu, 2015.

26 Wynter, 2001, 2003; Scott, 2000; Fein, 1979; Goff et al., 2008; Newton, 1967; Wilderson, 2018; Fredrickson, 1971; Bar-Tal & Teichman, 2005; Newton, 1967; Wilkinson, 1977; Delgado & Stefancic, 1991; Uhuru, 2021; Smiley & Fakunle, 2016; Livingstone Smith & Panaitiu, 2015.

27 Wynter, 2001, 2003; Scott, 2000; Fein, 1979; Goff et al., 2008; Newton, 1967; Wilderson, 2018; Fredrickson, 1971; Bar-Tal & Teichman, 2005; Newton, 1967; Wilkinson, 1977; Delgado & Stefancic, 1991; Uhuru, 2021; Smiley & Fakunle, 2016; Livingstone Smith & Panaitiu, 2015.

28 Wynter, 2001, 2003; Scott, 2000; Fein, 1979; Goff et al., 2008; Newton, 1967; Wilderson, 2018; Fredrickson, 1971; Bar-Tal & Teichman, 2005; Newton, 1967; Wilkinson, 1977; Delgado & Stefancic, 1991; Uhuru, 2021; Smiley & Fakunle, 2016; Livingstone Smith & Panaitiu, 2015.

29 Jones, 2006; Johnson & Leighton, 1995; Randall, 2015; Miller, 1991, 2004; Moses, 2002; Curry, 2021; Storr, 2011; Du Bois, 1903; Norgaard, 1995; Boyd & Allen, 1995; Stewart & Scott, 1978; Bell, 1993; Staples, 1987a; Farrell et al., 1983; Patterson, 1952; Willhelm, 1986; Fatal Force: Police Shootings Database, n.d.; Fatal Encounters, n.d.; Wolfers et al., 2015; Ogungbure, 2019a, 2019b; Curry, 2017; Rodríguez, 2011; EJI, 2017; Tolnay & Beck, 1995.

30 Jones, 2006; Johnson & Leighton, 1995; Randall, 2015; Miller, 1991, 2004; Moses, 2002; Curry, 2021; Storr, 2011; Du Bois, 1903; Norgaard, 1995; Boyd & Allen, 1995; Stewart & Scott, 1978; Bell, 1993; Staples, 1987a; Farrell et al., 1983; Patterson, 1952; Willhelm, 1986; Fatal Force: Police Shootings Database, n.d.; Fatal Encounters, n.d.; Wolfers et al., 2015; Ogungbure, 2019a, 2019b; Curry, 2017; Rodríguez, 2011; EJI, 2017; Tolnay & Beck, 1995.

31 Jones, 2006; Johnson & Leighton, 1995; Randall, 2015; Miller, 1991, 2004; Moses, 2002; Curry, 2021; Storr, 2011; Du Bois, 1903; Norgaard, 1995; Boyd & Allen, 1995; Stewart & Scott, 1978; Bell, 1993; Staples, 1987a; Farrell et al., 1983; Patterson, 1952; Willhelm, 1986; Fatal Force: Police Shootings Database, n.d.; Fatal Encounters, n.d.; Wolfers et al., 2015; Ogungbure, 2019a, 2019b; Curry, 2017; Rodríguez, 2011; EJI, 2017; Tolnay & Beck, 1995.

32 Jones, 2006; Johnson & Leighton, 1995; Randall, 2015; Miller, 1991, 2004; Moses, 2002; Curry, 2021; Storr, 2011; Du Bois, 1903; Norgaard, 1995; Boyd & Allen, 1995; Stewart & Scott, 1978; Bell, 1993; Staples, 1987a; Farrell et al., 1983; Patterson, 1952; Willhelm, 1986; Fatal Force: Police Shootings Database, n.d.; Fatal Encounters, n.d.; Wolfers et al., 2015; Ogungbure, 2019a, 2019b; Curry, 2017; Rodríguez, 2011; EJI, 2017; Tolnay & Beck, 1995.

33 Jones, 2006; Johnson & Leighton, 1995; Randall, 2015; Miller, 1991, 2004; Moses, 2002; Curry, 2021; Storr, 2011; Du Bois, 1903; Norgaard, 1995; Boyd & Allen, 1995; Stewart & Scott, 1978; Bell, 1993; Staples, 1987a; Farrell et al., 1983; Patterson, 1952; Willhelm, 1986; Fatal Force: Police Shootings Database, n.d.; Fatal Encounters, n.d.; Wolfers et al., 2015; Ogungbure, 2019a, 2019b; Curry, 2017; Rodríguez, 2011; EJI, 2017; Tolnay & Beck, 1995.

34 Jones, 2006; Johnson & Leighton, 1995; Randall, 2015; Miller, 1991, 2004; Moses, 2002; Curry, 2021; Storr, 2011; Du Bois, 1903; Norgaard, 1995; Boyd & Allen, 1995; Stewart &

Scott, 1978; Bell, 1993; Staples, 1987a; Farrell et al., 1983; Patterson, 1952; Willhelm, 1986; Fatal Force: Police Shootings Database, n.d.; Fatal Encounters, n.d.; Wolfers et al., 2015; Ogungbure, 2019a, 2019b; Curry, 2017; Rodríguez, 2011; EJI, 2017; Tolnay & Beck, 1995.

35 Jones, 2006; Johnson & Leighton, 1995; Randall, 2015; Miller, 1991, 2004; Moses, 2002; Curry, 2021; Storr, 2011; Du Bois, 1903; Norgaard, 1995; Boyd & Allen, 1995; Stewart & Scott, 1978; Bell, 1993; Staples, 1987a; Farrell et al., 1983; Patterson, 1952; Willhelm, 1986; Fatal Force: Police Shootings Database, n.d.; Fatal Encounters, n.d.; Wolfers et al., 2015; Ogungbure, 2019a, 2019b; Curry, 2017; Rodríguez, 2011; EJI, 2017; Tolnay & Beck, 1995.

36 Jones, 2006; Johnson & Leighton, 1995; Randall, 2015; Miller, 1991, 2004; Moses, 2002; Curry, 2021; Storr, 2011; Du Bois, 1903; Norgaard, 1995; Boyd & Allen, 1995; Stewart & Scott, 1978; Bell, 1993; Staples, 1987a; Farrell et al., 1983; Patterson, 1952; Willhelm, 1986; Fatal Force: Police Shootings Database, n.d.; Fatal Encounters, n.d.; Wolfers et al., 2015; Ogungbure, 2019a, 2019b; Curry, 2017; Rodríguez, 2011; EJI, 2017; Tolnay & Beck, 1995.

37 Jones, 2006; Johnson & Leighton, 1995; Randall, 2015; Miller, 1991, 2004; Moses, 2002; Curry, 2021; Storr, 2011; Du Bois, 1903; Norgaard, 1995; Boyd & Allen, 1995; Stewart & Scott, 1978; Bell, 1993; Staples, 1987a; Farrell et al., 1983; Patterson, 1952; Willhelm, 1986; Fatal Force: Police Shootings Database, n.d.; Fatal Encounters, n.d.; Wolfers et al., 2015; Ogungbure, 2019a, 2019b; Curry, 2017; Rodríguez, 2011; EJI, 2017; Tolnay & Beck, 1995.

38 Smith et al., 2017.

39 Smith et al., 2017; Curry, 2017, 2019; Chapleau et al., 2008; Holmes & Slap, 1998; Struckman-Johnson, 1988; Rosin, 2014; Foston, 2003; Goldstein, 1997; Binion, 2021; Stern, 2019; Satterfield, 2022; Morgan-Smith, 2019; Samson, 2020; Barton, 2019; Ebony, 2019; Fruen & Smith, 2020; Woodard, 2014; Greene, 2020; Mumford, 2017; Rothman, 2013; Bandes et al., 2019; Blackmon, 2008; Woodyatt, 2022; Geller et al., 2014.

40 French et al., 2015.

41 Smith et al., 2017; Curry, 2017, 2019; Chapleau et al., 2008; Holmes & Slap, 1998; Struckman-Johnson, 1988; Rosin, 2014; Foston, 2003; Goldstein, 1997; Binion, 2021; Stern, 2019; Satterfield, 2022; Morgan-Smith, 2019; Samson, 2020; Barton, 2019; Ebony, 2019; Fruen & Smith, 2020; Woodard, 2014; Greene, 2020; Mumford, 2017; Rothman, 2013; Bandes et al., 2019; Blackmon, 2008; Woodyatt, 2022; Geller et al., 2014.

42 Smith et al., 2017; Curry, 2017, 2019; Chapleau et al., 2008; Holmes & Slap, 1998; Struckman-Johnson, 1988; Rosin, 2014; Foston, 2003; Goldstein, 1997; Binion, 2021; Stern, 2019; Satterfield, 2022; Morgan-Smith, 2019; Samson, 2020; Barton, 2019; Ebony, 2019; Fruen & Smith, 2020; Woodard, 2014; Greene, 2020; Mumford, 2017; Rothman, 2013; Bandes et al., 2019; Blackmon, 2008; Woodyatt, 2022; Geller et al., 2014.

43 Ogungbure, 2018; Hernton, 1965; Stein, 2015; Lemelle, 1995; Hickey, 2006; Blake, 2020; Morris, 2016; Saint-Aubin, 1994; Marriott, 2000; Williams-Myers, 1995; Samson, 2020; Klein, 2016; Dines, 2003; Kitossa, 2020; Fredrickson, 1971; Woodyatt, 2022.

44 Ogungbure, 2018; Hernton, 1965; Stein, 2015; Lemelle, 1995; Hickey, 2006; Blake, 2020; Morris, 2016; Saint-Aubin, 1994; Marriott, 2000; Williams-Myers, 1995; Samson, 2020; Klein, 2016; Dines, 2003; Kitossa, 2020; Fredrickson, 1971; Woodyatt, 2022.

45 Ogungbure, 2018; Hernton, 1965; Stein, 2015; Lemelle, 1995; Hickey, 2006; Blake, 2020; Morris, 2016; Saint-Aubin, 1994; Marriott, 2000; Williams-Myers, 1995; Samson, 2020; Klein, 2016; Dines, 2003; Kitossa, 2020; Fredrickson, 1971; Woodyatt, 2022.

46 Ogungbure, 2018; Hernton, 1965; Stein, 2015; Lemelle, 1995; Hickey, 2006; Blake, 2020; Morris, 2016; Saint-Aubin, 1994; Marriott, 2000; Williams-Myers, 1995; Samson, 2020; Klein, 2016; Dines, 2003; Kitossa, 2020; Fredrickson, 1971; Woodyatt, 2022.

47 Ogungbure, 2018; Hernton, 1965; Stein, 2015; Lemelle, 1995; Hickey, 2006; Blake, 2020; Morris, 2016; Saint-Aubin, 1994; Marriott, 2000; Williams-Myers, 1995; Samson, 2020; Klein, 2016; Dines, 2003; Kitossa, 2020; Fredrickson, 1971; Woodyatt, 2022.

48 Malley-Morrison & Hines, 2004, 2007; McNeely et al., 2001; Hamel, 2007; Archer, 2000; Breiding et al., 2014; Johnson & Ferraro, 2000; Hines & Malley-Morrison, 2001; Medeiros & Straus, 2006; Cook, 2009; Mann, 1988; McCleod, 1984; Shupe et al., 1987; Steinmetz & Lucca, 1988; Fox & Zawitz, 2006; Malley-Morrison et al., 2007; Light-Allende, 2004; West, 2012; Fontes, 2007; Hughes et al., 2010; Palmetto et al., 2013; Langhinrichsen-Rohling et al., 2012; McNeely & Torres, 2009; McNeely & Robinson-Simpson, 1987; Caetano et al., 2005; Hampton et al., 2005; Benson et al., 2004; Hall, 2012; DeMaris, 1992; Johnson, 2008; Mihalic & Elliott, 1997; Moffitt et al., 2001; Douglas & Hines, 2011; Goldenberg et al., 2016; Cho & Wilke, 2010; Brown, 2004; Kernsmith & Craun, 2008; Melton & Belknap, 2003; Drijber et al., 2013; Fiebert, 2014; Whitaker et al., 2007.

49 Malley-Morrison & Hines, 2004, 2007; McNeely et al., 2001; Hamel, 2007; Archer, 2000; Breiding et al., 2014; Johnson & Ferraro, 2000; Hines & Malley-Morrison, 2001; Medeiros & Straus, 2006; Cook, 2009; Mann, 1988; McCleod, 1984; Shupe et al., 1987; Steinmetz & Lucca, 1988; Fox & Zawitz, 2006; Malley-Morrison et al., 2007; Light-Allende, 2004; West, 2012; Fontes, 2007; Hughes et al., 2010; Palmetto et al., 2013; Langhinrichsen-Rohling et al., 2012; McNeely & Torres, 2009; McNeely & Robinson-Simpson, 1987; Caetano et al., 2005; Hampton et al., 2005; Benson et al., 2004; Hall, 2012; DeMaris, 1992; Johnson, 2008; Mihalic & Elliott, 1997; Moffitt et al., 2001; Douglas & Hines, 2011; Goldenberg et al., 2016; Cho & Wilke, 2010; Brown, 2004; Kernsmith & Craun, 2008; Melton & Belknap, 2003; Drijber et al., 2013; Fiebert, 2014; Whitaker et al., 2007.

50 Malley-Morrison & Hines, 2004, 2007; McNeely et al., 2001; Hamel, 2007; Archer, 2000; Breiding et al., 2014; Johnson & Ferraro, 2000; Hines & Malley-Morrison, 2001; Medeiros & Straus, 2006; Cook, 2009; Mann, 1988; McCleod, 1984; Shupe et al., 1987; Steinmetz & Lucca, 1988; Fox & Zawitz, 2006; Malley-Morrison et al., 2007; Light-Allende, 2004; West, 2012; Fontes, 2007; Hughes et al., 2010; Palmetto et al., 2013; Langhinrichsen-Rohling et al., 2012; McNeely & Torres, 2009; McNeely & Robinson-Simpson, 1987; Caetano et al., 2005; Hampton et al., 2005; Benson et al., 2004; Hall, 2012; DeMaris, 1992; Johnson, 2008; Mihalic & Elliott, 1997; Moffitt et al., 2001; Douglas & Hines, 2011; Goldenberg et al., 2016; Cho & Wilke, 2010; Brown, 2004; Kernsmith & Craun, 2008; Melton & Belknap, 2003; Drijber et al., 2013; Fiebert, 2014; Whitaker et al., 2007.

51 Malley-Morrison & Hines, 2004, 2007; McNeely et al., 2001; Hamel, 2007; Archer, 2000; Breiding et al., 2014; Johnson & Ferraro, 2000; Hines & Malley-Morrison, 2001; Medeiros & Straus, 2006; Cook, 2009; Mann, 1988; McCleod, 1984; Shupe et al., 1987; Steinmetz & Lucca, 1988; Fox & Zawitz, 2006; Malley-Morrison et al., 2007; Light-Allende, 2004; West, 2012; Fontes, 2007; Hughes et al., 2010; Palmetto et al., 2013; Langhinrichsen-Rohling et al., 2012; McNeely & Torres, 2009; McNeely & Robinson-Simpson, 1987; Caetano et al., 2005; Hampton et al., 2005; Benson et al., 2004; Hall, 2012; DeMaris, 1992; Johnson, 2008; Mihalic & Elliott, 1997; Moffitt et al., 2001; Douglas & Hines, 2011; Goldenberg et al., 2016; Cho & Wilke, 2010; Brown, 2004; Kernsmith & Craun, 2008; Melton & Belknap, 2003; Drijber et al., 2013; Fiebert, 2014; Whitaker et al., 2007.

52 Goodwill et al., 2021; O'Connor, 2011a, 2011b; Graves et al., 2010; Bell & Clark, 1998; McLoyd & Lozoff, 2001; Barnes, 2010; Jacobs et al., 1999; Xiao et al., 2021; Lindsey et al., 2019.

53 Mendel, 1995; Hlavka, 2016; Hines & Finkelhor, 2007; Coxell & King, 2010; Rush, 1980; Curry & Utley, 2018; Duncan & Williams, 1998; Crowder, 2014; Hernandez et al., 1993; Curry, 2019, 2023b; Goldstein, 1997; Stemple & Meyer, 2014; Stemple et al.,

2017; Struckman-Johnson, 1988; Turner et al., 2017; Foston, 2003; McGuffey, 2008; Fontes et al., 2001.

54 Mendel, 1995; Hlavka, 2016; Hines & Finkelhor, 2007; Coxell & King, 2010; Rush, 1980; Curry & Utley, 2018; Duncan & Williams, 1998; Crowder, 2014; Hernandez et al., 1993; Curry, 2019, 2023b; Goldstein, 1997; Stemple & Meyer, 2014; Stemple et al., 2017; Struckman-Johnson, 1988; Turner et al., 2017; Foston, 2003; McGuffey, 2008; Fontes et al., 2001.

55 Hines & Douglas, 2010a; Cook, 2009; Migliaccio, 2001; Greene & Bogo, 2002; Hamel, 2007; Malley-Morrison & Hines, 2007; West, 2012, 2016; Fox & Benson, 2006; Hines & Malley-Morrison, 2001; Slootmaekers & Migerode, 2018, 2020; McNeely et al., 2001; Babcock et al., 2017.

56 Hines & Douglas, 2010a; Cook, 2009; Migliaccio, 2001; Greene & Bogo, 2002; Hamel, 2007; Malley-Morrisson et al., 2007; West, 2012, 2016; Fox & Benson, 2006; Hines & Malley-Morrison, 2001; Slootmaekers & Migerode, 2018, 2020; McNeely et al., 2001; Babcock et al., 2017; Keilholtz & Spencer, 2022.

57 Hines & Douglas, 2010a; Cook, 2009; Migliaccio, 2001; Greene & Bogo, 2002; Hamel, 2007; Malley-Morrisson et al., 2007; West, 2012, 2016; Fox & Benson, 2006; Hines & Malley-Morrison, 2001; Slootmaekers & Migerode, 2018, 2020; McNeely et al., 2001; Babcock et al., 2017; Keilholtz & Spencer, 2022.

58 Hines & Douglas, 2010a; Cook, 2009; Migliaccio, 2001; Greene & Bogo, 2002; Hamel, 2007; Malley-Morrisson et al., 2007; West, 2012, 2016; Fox & Benson, 2006; Hines & Malley-Morrison, 2001; Slootmaekers & Migerode, 2018, 2020; McNeely et al., 2001; Babcock et al., 2017; Keilholtz & Spencer, 2022.

CHAPTER 9

COPING MECHANISMS AND INTERVENTIONS

COPING MECHANISMS

John Henryism

The Black American folktale of John Henry refers to the railroad worker/steel-driving man who was known among the 19th century railroad and tunnel workers for his remarkable physical strength and endurance demonstrated in his work. Legend has it that with powerful blows, he beat a mechanical steam drill with a nine-pound hammer in a steel-driving contest that pit man against machine and won the contest but dropped dead moments later from complete physical and mental exhaustion. James et al. (1983) developed the John Henryism framework which refers to prolonged high-effort active coping with chronic psychosocial stressors that are associated with an elevated risk for adverse health outcomes (e.g., elevated blood pressure). John Henryism can manifest in Black men working extremely hard under pressure to disprove stereotypes of laziness and inability. It includes an individual's perception that he can meet the demands of his environment through hard work and determination with an emphasis on environmental mastery (i.e., attempting to control environmental stressors; also referred to as personal efficacy and locus of control). Said differently, John Henryism includes the belief that one can control psychosocial environmental stressors (i.e., social and economic oppression; e.g., chronic financial strain, job insecurity, anti-Black racial micro/aggressions) through a combination of hard work and determination. The John Henryism framework is characterized by the three main components of efficacious mental and physical vigor, a strong commitment to hard work, and a single-minded determination to succeed. Black men who score higher on John Henryism (after being assessed) tend to suffer from hypertension (high blood pressure). Black male workers attempt to neutralize anti-Black misandric micro/aggressions through hard work with the belief they will be able to transcend their experiences and achieve security and upward mobility in their jobs.[1]

James et al. (1984) found that high John Henryism men felt that being Black had hindered their chances for job success, were more psychologically involved with their jobs (e.g., job success), experienced low job security, and lack of support from supervisors. The noxious environments in which Black Americans live and work expose them to unrelieved psychosocial stress that make them susceptible to John Henryism. These conditions generate psychological stress that requires an exorbitant amount of daily energy to manage. Racial discrimination erodes their economic security and psychological well-being and operates as a pernicious psychosocial stressor. Research from Angner et al. (2011) revealed that John Henryism was negatively associated with happiness. Hudson et al. (2016b) discovered that greater levels of John Henryism were associated with an increase in depression among Black men. A couple of *ProPublica* (2020) articles titled "Black Men Have the Shortest Lifespans of Any Americans: This Theory Helps to Explain Why" and "How COVID-19 Hollowed Out a Generation of Young Black Men" use the John Henryism framework to explain Black male death and dying. The authors of the second article investigated the deaths of Black men from COVID-19 by gathering stories, reviewing news articles, obituaries, medical examiners' reports, and interviewing family and friends along with researchers and

DOI: 10.4324/9781003430551-10

attributed their deaths to John Henryism. A composite was formulated from the interviews about the young Black men who died from COVID-19. The Black men were described as hard-working, ambitious, and optimistic and persistent who attempted to lift others along with themselves. They were described as significant community members that communities would turn to for assistance to recover from the pandemic (e.g., entrepreneurs who were also employers; confidants like coaches, pastors and barbers; family men who were forced to take care of their parents who got sick earlier while they were taking care and raising their own children). The authors assert that the weathering of their bodies began when they were boys attempting to navigate white spaces or push through adverse anti-Black experiences (i.e., Racial Battle Fatigue/RBF). The weathering continues into adulthood while navigating the publics' projections of danger (i.e., white delusions and caricatures) with unyielding vigilance. The article speaks to the epidemiological frameworks of John Henryism, weathering, RBF, and how they overlap in the lives of young Black males through a cycle of striving and succumbing that ultimately end in their deaths.[2]

Double-Consciousness

Du Bois (1903) refers to double-consciousness (i.e., two-ness: an American and a Negro) as two thoughts, two unreconciled strivings, two warring ideals – the sense of always looking at one's self through the eyes of others. It serves as a second sight that provides Black men with insight into how they are being viewed by white America and other groups. Therefore, Black males are constantly navigating through and struggling with how they constitute themselves (i.e., their authentic human selves) versus the objectified dehumanizing caricatures created by white delusions that are projected onto Black male bodies where they are permanently positioned as a problem.

The multiple self-states of double-consciousness is an emotional and cognitive depleting process of survival. Double-consciousness can manifest as an internal struggle with a consciousness of white Western neo-colonialism that is invested in the hypervaluation of whiteness with the rejection of the latter in order to be an integrated whole. The Cool Pose thesis (Majors & Billson, 1993) is a prominent framework that is used to explain the disposition of working-class Black males. This framework is rooted in culture of poverty and even criminology theories. The fundamental proposition of the Cool Pose thesis is that Black males display stoicism and conceal emotions in order to not be perceived as weak or vulnerable and in control (i.e., cool presence). This framework includes a superficial structural or systemic analysis and is described as "descriptive" and "speculative and exploratory." Unnever and Chouhy (2021) found that Black males including poor Black males in urban areas were equally as likely as white males to feel pressure to conceal their feelings when they felt sad or anxious. Their research challenges the legitimacy of the Cool Pose thesis. Jackson (2018) advocated for a move beyond this framework to have a deeper understanding of emotion management strategies among Black men. He uses Erving Goffman's (1959) concept of the frontstage and backstage to describe how Black men navigate individuals within various settings. These emotional strategies help them to navigate targeted (anti-Black misandric) systemic oppression and discrimination. The frontstage is where they conceal specific emotions in order to provide a specific presentation of themselves to an audience of peers, coworkers, etc. The backstage is where they are able to let their guard down (i.e., step out of character) and rely on their close friends as a primary source of social and emotional support. Jackson's description of the frontstage and backstage is what this author would refer to as double-consciousness where Black men are navigating white spaces along with white projections and delusions including Black spaces that are more affirming, safe, and where they are able to be their authentic selves. Double-consciousness is different from code-switching in that code-switching refers to the act (i.e., behavior) of navigating white and Black spaces, while double-consciousness describes the psychological processes of navigating white and Black spaces.[3]

According to Corrigan (2020), emotions are racialized and politicized in the U.S. There are significant ethnic differences in emotion judgments, display rules, and emotional expressions among Black, white, Asian, and Latino/a Americans. Dawel et al. (2023) found no difference between men's and women's self-display rules. Emotional expression is complex and includes structural components that often influence emotion expression. Black male emotional expression tends to be surveilled with an expectation of a specific emotional expression script that routinely is superficial where an analysis of the structural component of emotion expression is absent. When Black males do express vulnerable emotions, they tend to be negated and invalidated. It is important to note that theories about Black male dispositions are inherently pathologizing. These characterizations are not only simplistic but reinforce caricatures and obscure the nuance and complexity of Black males. Anyone who is not feeling safe will not be emotionally vulnerable, and this is not unique to Black males. The idea that individuals would show up in an unsafe environment in an emotionally vulnerable manner is incongruent with decades worth of research. Therefore, theories of Black males demonstrating a unique emotional disposition (e.g., Cool Pose) while feeling unsafe are problematic and reinforce dehumanization (i.e., speciation). Double-consciousness provides a more viable framework that incorporates a structural analysis that is dynamic and non-essentialist in understanding Black male emotional expression.[4]

Racial Identity

Racial identity refers to the significance and meaning that Black Americans place on race in defining themselves. The ability to identify racism is dependent upon a person's racial identity status. Racial identity can serve as a protective factor (e.g., lower psychological distress in response to perceived racial discrimination) against racial discrimination. The process of racial identity development is characterized by the rejection of white culture in one's definition of self and includes the internal development of a positive racial identity. Racial identity can range from external (i.e., dominant racial group identification; conformity) to internal (i.e., own-racial-group identification; internalization) ego statuses that are dynamic and conform to a developmental or progressive stage process. An externally focused racial identity status is characterized by color-blind ideology, conformity, or beliefs that race is not a significant factor in a person's everyday life or the life of others. Therefore, the ability to recognize race-based encounters (i.e., racism; race-based trauma) is contingent on a person's internally defined racial identity status. Research from Ellison (1992) revealed that Black males with military backgrounds expressed lower levels of racial identification and separatist sentiment than nonveteran Black males. This may indicate that military culture promotes a race distancing orientation that is a part of patriotism. Carter et al. (2017a) found an association between externally defined or less developed racial identity status attitudes and higher racial trauma symptoms. Decreased psychological distress and racial trauma symptoms were correlated with internally defined or more differentiated racial identity statuses. Therefore, an internally defined Black racial identity serves as a protective factor (e.g., a positive resource of cultural pride) against racial trauma for Black men.[5]

Hope and Resilience

Liberalism traffics tropes of hope, change, progress, and equality as containment strategies in lieu of transformational policy (e.g., reparations). Warren's (2015) analysis of the politics of hope reveals the relationship between the utilization (i.e., capitalization/exploitation) of the spiritual concept of hope and political hope that acts as a deceptive political instrument that only serves to perpetuate anti-Blackness. Black existence is organized by political institutions, mandates, logics, and language as an apparatus to govern and discipline Black Americans. This serves as an articulation and socializing belief that hope and politics are synonymous (i.e., one has to engage in politics in order to have hope). The historical record of voting for Black Americans proves to be an ineffective practice in obtaining redress, equality, and political subjectivity (i.e., concrete transformations of anti-Blackness), but Black Americans are positioned as a faithful voting block as an act of historical commemoration and obligation (i.e., a sense of duty and indebtedness due to the Black Americans who marched and died for the opportunity to vote). Therefore, this mechanism becomes a vicious and abusive continual feedback loop where Black Americans are thrust into a perpetual struggle that is not time-bound and thus shielded from critique. Black despair and expectation are reconfigured through Black political action in pursuit of the elusive and impossible in an anti-Black political structure. The research of Gilens and Page (2014) revealed that economic elites and organized groups who represent business interests wield significant power over U.S. government policy while average citizens and large interest-based groups have very little or no independent government policy influence. The politics of hope reconfigures despair as possibility, struggle as triumph, and lack as proximity. The politics of hope have no historical or sociological grounding as evidence and is an object of political fantasy that serves as a containment strategy and calls for the Black downtrodden to embrace optimism, which is a form of violence. The fundamental strategies that undergird and maintain the politics of hope include positioning it as the only alternative to the problem of anti-Blackness, shielding it from rigorous historical, sociological, and philosophical analysis, framing the political sphere as the only source of legitimate and recognizable agency, and the demonization of critiques leveled at the politics of hope. The politics of hope under the auspices of optimism, positivity (i.e., being positive), and happiness provides an elixir for Black suffering. The politics of hope as a solution to anti-Blackness doesn't exist in politics and only serves as an illusion that actually repeats anti-Blackness while simultaneously disavowing that anti-Blackness is a problem. A binary sequence between action/inaction is provided as an explanation for permissible action that serves to silence and discredit critical engagement, critique, and protest of political hope ideology. According to Warren (2015), the distribution of fraudulent hope is a form of necropolitics that leaves Black Americans endangered.

Smith et al. (2012) examined hope, RBF, and race-related stress among Black men and found that Black men with high to moderate levels of hope experienced more stress associated with racial microaggressions and societal problems than Black men who had low hope. Possessing a more realistic assessment of the racial discrimination that Black men might encounter provided additional coping mechanisms for the low hope group. The high hope group of Black men were slightly more formally educated, older, held full-time jobs, higher incomes, and were married in greater numbers but were at greater risk for race-related stress. Moreover, the research of Assari et al. (2018) found that Black males of a higher socioeconomic status (SES) were at an increased risk of having a major depressive episode (MDE). It is not uncommon for high-SES Black Americans to report more experiences of racial discrimination due to increased contact with whites, but the research on hope from Smith et al. (2012) might be able to illuminate this dynamic where the endorsement of hope might be a mediating factor of depression among high-SES Black males.

Resilience is often emphasized based on a strengths-based approach or perspective in clinical work. It is conceptualized as highlighting an individual's adaptive resources/capacities in navigating structural inequality. Resilience is defined by the ability to be able to recover after experiencing trauma, assault, injury, or any other adverse experience and is a preferred approach than prevailing pathological models for understanding Black people. But resilience is often framed from a Western perspective that emphasizes individualism. Resilience does not provide a structural or systemic analysis. Consequently, structural violence (i.e., institutional decimation) in the form of anti-Black misandric aggression directed towards Black men is not examined, but instead how well they are able to adjust and cope is the focus. In addition, the health effects (e.g., weathering, John Henryism, RBF) of coping with these conditions are completely absent from thought. Resilience is a product of neoliberalism and is ideologically invested in the maintenance of status quo. Oppression is positioned as a permanence that does not warrant critique, engagement, or protest. Therefore, resilience solely is an ideologically and ethically inadequate framework for application in working with Black males.[6]

Black Rage, Anger, Shame, and Pain

Emotion refers to a collection of processes that contribute to how one relates to the social and physical world. Emotion is characterized by a complex reaction pattern that involves physiological, experiential, and behavioral elements that helps people appraise the significance of situations for their well-being. People's lay conceptions (distinct from scientific conceptualizations of primary and secondary emotions) of emotions includes a continuum that ranges from uniquely human secondary emotions (e.g., shame, resentment, love, hope, disappointment) to nonuniquely human primary emotions (e.g., anger, pain, pleasure, surprise, fear, excitement). Secondary emotions include a longer duration, less intensity, reveal more morality and sensitivity, are more cognitively complex, less visible, and appear later in life. Vaes et al. (2003) found in-group members discriminate against out-group members based on the expression of human emotions. The in-group tended to attribute secondary emotions (i.e., uniquely human emotions) to their group than to the out-group which was a form of dehumanization (i.e., denial of human essence). In-group members who expressed secondary emotions were met with conformity, prosocial reactions, and kind responses, while out-group members who expressed secondary emotions prompted opposite reactions (e.g., distanced themselves from the out-group member). In addition, secondary emotions facilitated an approach response to in-group members but activated an avoidance response towards out-group members. The in-group demonstrated a shared common humanity that was denied to the out-group. An in-group member who expresses themselves using secondary emotions potentially are perceived as more human where the human category is reserved for the in-group. Their research provides evidence of a specific form of dehumanization that the in-group moderates through emotion expression. Therefore, it is plausible that Black men are discriminated against, avoided, and dehumanized in their emotion expression regardless of the expression of uniquely or nonuniquely human emotions.[7]

Black rage serves an existential function through the affirmation of Black humanity and dignity amidst a hostile sociopolitical landscape. Rage is a protective reaction to hurt and the disorganizing effects of underlying fear or shame (i.e., secondary anger). Rage can be a manifestation of secondary anger or primary adaptive anger that has deteriorated (e.g., excessive arousal and loss of meaning in the initial focus of the embodied anger) into secondary anger. Almost all Black people are subjected to anti-Black oppression, making the experience of rage almost inevitable. Rage is a normal and even expected response to the painful degradation of racial oppression. Anger that is not expressed can fester and be transformed into rage. The primary distinction between anger and rage is intensity and can be conceptualized as anger that has not been expressed and festers, thus transforming into rage. The protective function of rage serves as a mechanism of resistance or a buffer against racial trauma. An individual can feel empowered while expressing rage in response to a painful and humiliating experience that is associated with subjugation. When rage is suppressed and internalized, it can present as despair or arrested anger that leads to depression. Internalized rage can contribute to weathering (early health deterioration), substance abuse/dependency, and death/suicidal ideation or suicide plan. Suppressed rage can be externalized into explosive volatility. Black Americans are routinely forced to suffer their pain and humiliation in silence, which creates an optimal context for the cultivation of rage. Anger is a powerful emotion that is characterized by a biological tendency to defend oneself from attack, self-protection from intrusion, or to help transcend barriers. Anger can be elicited as a reaction to a perceived wrongdoing, violations, or abandonment while ranging from regenerative to destructive. Greenberg and Paivio (1997) describe three types of anger, but this section will focus on the two types that are relevant. *Primary anger* describes an immediate and direct response to a perceived environmental threat that is characterized by an affective cognitive response. Further, it can be differentiated into *primary adaptive anger* when activated to protect the individual from immediate danger or can become *primary maladaptive anger* when it no longer serves an adaptive function in response to a present situation. *Secondary anger* (i.e., *reactive* or *defensive anger*) describes a reaction to another primary emotion where the *secondary anger* is actually a secondary emotion, and the concealed emotion is the primary emotion. The expression of anger is employed to conceal more intense and intolerable emotions such as fear, sadness, and shame. Anger provides a sense of agency, while fear, sadness, and shame leave a person feeling vulnerable. The research of Mabry and Kiecolt (2005) revealed that Black Americans neither feel nor express more anger than whites. Consequently, a sense of control for Black Americans reduces feelings of anger and anger expression. Carter and Forsyth (2010) found feeling disrespected and angry were the most frequent reactions to racial discrimination followed by feeling insulted, disappointed, frustrated, outraged, hurt, and shocked. Pittman's (2011) research indicated that the use of anger to cope with racial discrimination by Black Americans negatively affected their general well-being and caused psychological distress. Black men expressed anger (referred to as active anger) to cope with acute racism at a higher rate than Black women. This author would describe the expressed anger described in this research study as potentially primary maladaptive anger, where the participants were thrust into a state of hypervigilance due to incessant racial trauma even in moments they were not actively exposed to a racist incident (i.e., anti-Black racial micro/aggression), or it could have been secondary anger that would have likely concealed their feelings of fear, sadness, or shame. Christ et al. (2020) found that rumination (i.e., repetitive focus on the experience of distress including the causes and consequences of the distress) mediated overall PTSD symptoms and anger reactions (i.e., negative alterations in cognitions/mood and physiological arousal). Therefore, it is plausible that rumination can be instrumental in the maintenance of primary maladaptive anger or secondary anger in situations where Black men have experienced racial trauma that leaves them feeling vulnerable and ruminating about the incident(s).[8]

Herman (2011) has described PTSD as a shame disorder in relation to interpersonal traumas that are repeated and chronic and involves a relationship of dominance and subordination where the victim experiences humiliation, degradation, and shame. An extreme manifestation of shame is the reaction to degradation or stigmatization that produces a sense of inferiority and powerlessness. La Bash and Papa (2014) found that shame in addition to fear contributes to the development of PTSD symptoms in survivors of interpersonal traumas. Shame appears to be a more dominant emotion than fear in survivors of interpersonal traumas due to an ongoing sense of threat. Shame reactions of inferiority or continuous self-criticism (i.e., condemnation of the self) can contribute to an ongoing sense of threat. Both shame and fear evoke withdrawal and avoidance behaviors that would need to be assessed in order to distinguish between shame and fear in PTSD assessment.

Fear is characterized by the motivational or experiential response to physical threat that is vital to survival. Both shame and guilt are considered social or moral emotions that delineate the boundaries of socially acceptable behavior but are two distinct emotions. Shame describes the global self, which includes a stable, trait-like, morally unacceptable aspect of the core self that one is powerless to moderate; whereas guilt describes a specific action that an individual has committed that motivates prosocial responses such as atonement/reparations for a specific time-bound transgression. Research from Øktedalen et al. (2015) revealed that patients with higher levels of shame and guilt displayed a higher level of PTSD symptoms and that within-person change in shame and guilt predicted a change in PTSD symptoms. In addition, Orth et al. (2006) found that shame elicits rumination, which leads to depression. Moreover, shame is thought to be instrumental in depression, social anxiety, and death/suicidal ideation. Shame is an emotion that is characterized by a felt sense of defectiveness (e.g., vulnerable, worthless, unlovable, inadequate, and weak) and devaluation (e.g., inferiority), where a part of the self is believed to be corrupted (which corrupts the whole self) by an irredeemable act or by a contaminating event that prompts perceived judgement from others and leaves one feeling powerless. Inferiority is often a felt experience as a marker of an individual's supposed defect, but Black males are societally consigned to an inferior status as racialized out-group men that is routinely reinforced though devaluation [i.e., Black male negation (BMN)]. Shame is felt as an inner turmoil and torment (i.e., an inner wound or self-disintegration) that is evoked by a sense of failure (e.g., deficiency) or by being the object of condemnation or contempt (e.g., ridicule, rejection, or rebuke). The external component of shame includes the preoccupation and perception of contempt from others (i.e., expectation of social devaluation) directed at the self and the internal component includes the internalization of those external perceptions that inform one's view of self (i.e., preoccupation with self-devaluation) that confirms their inferiority or defect (i.e., negative evaluations of the entire self). The painfully diminished sense of self (e.g., feeling small) feels exposed, which destabilizes an individual's internal security. An individual experiencing shame will often isolate (i.e., withdraw) to escape, hide, or express self-protective anger (i.e., secondary anger) in order to conceal the supposed defect or failure and protect themselves (avoidance behaviors) out of fear of condemnation and rejection, which impedes connection and exacerbates shame through loneliness and despair, and confirmation of the defect and failure based on reactions to the self-protective anger. They are not only disconnected from others but disconnected from themselves (i.e., fragmented) due to a lack of internal security that produces a sense of embodiment and coherence. Empathy for the self is lost, and a lack of empathy is experienced from others. The lack of empathy for oneself might be exemplified by continuous self-criticism that exacerbates the shame. Shame like fear is a biologically hardwired experience. The intense physiological response of shame can overwhelm higher cortical functions where speech and thought are inhibited. Further, shame increases proinflammatory cytokine activity and cortisol, which can lead to adverse health outcomes (i.e., weathering). It can be indicated through facial and postural indicators such as gaze aversion (e.g., lowered eyes), bowed head and body, and hiding behaviors (i.e., shrinking and disappearing). The paralyzing effect of shame can occur as a reinforcing feedback loop where consistent devaluation reinforces a sense of ontological failure.[9]

Shame is a universal system that is part of human cooperative biology that regulates social hierarchy and peer relationships. Disgust and contempt are indicative of emotions of status demarcation in hierarchical societies that is directed toward those who are consigned to a lower status. The relational dominance and subordination are inherently shaming. This is exemplified by U.S. chattel slavery that was the most extreme form of social subordination, where enslaved Black Americans existed in a permanently dishonored status that represented a social death (it has been argued and demonstrated throughout this text that the primary mechanisms of U.S. chattel slavery are still operating as well as the racial undercaste status of Black Americans).[10]

Lynchings as a technology of murder also exemplified an extreme form of social subordination. The emotion of shame defends against social devaluation and is part of a neurocognitive system. This system is activated to cues of potential or actual devaluation. Cognitive mechanisms are employed that deters an individual from taking action that would incur more social devaluation, the ability for others to learn about and spread potentially damaging information is limited, the degree and costs of subsequent social devaluation is limited, and an individual is mobilized to adaptively respond to a new social landscape if devaluation occurs. An individual will feel pain with the prospect of or actually being devalued. They avoid action that would cause or exacerbate devaluation and conceal damaging information. An individual withdraws, appeases, or produces a nonverbal display that communicates subordination when others discover reputation-damaging information. Discrediting information becoming common knowledge prompts people to behave in a more cooperative manner, which is thought to restore one's reputation as a good cooperative partner. If cooperation fails or is not cost-effective, a remaining negotiating tool might be aggression, which provides a sense of being empowered than the shame of feeling weak. Individuals with multiple socially valued characteristics can pose more cost on others before being devalued themselves and could limit the cost of devaluation when it occurs and as a result are less prone to shame. When an individual is deemed to be less valuable or less able to enforce their interests, they are devalued by the people whom they interact. Thus, the person is harmed more and helped less incurring fitness costs (i.e., the ability to reproduce and survive). The social ecology of shame presents a significant adaptive problem in the prevention of social devaluation along with minimizing its costs. Direct experiences with racial discrimination are associated with higher levels of shame.[11]

Shame contributes to the weathering of Black males through proinflammatory cytokine activity and cortisol. Moreover, shame is a part of the social dominance and racial hierarchy apparatus in the U.S. The dominance and subordination of Black males is part and parcel of the patriarchal caste system. Black males are reminded daily of their undercaste status by the disgust and contempt that is directed towards them, which demarcates their status. Black men are routinely exposed to degradation, where their attempts to navigate the degradation can result in internalized feelings of inferiority (i.e., shame) and powerlessness. This author posits that shame contributes to the development and maintenance of racial trauma, where the routine societal devaluation (i.e., BMN) of Black males can leave them feeling defective and without agency. Black men can experience shame due to not being able to transcend anti-Black racism (i.e., anti-Black misandric micro/aggressions). Not being able to finan-cially provide for their families can also produce shame. In addition, the inability to protect oneself from police violence and vigilantism can produce a sense of shame (e.g., feeling weak and helpless) while encountering the ongoing threat to one's bodily integrity leading to with-drawal for self-protection. The shame can elicit rumination and lead to depression, which can leave them simultaneously grappling with racial trauma and depression. Black men are often objects of condemnation that include incessant messages that they are failures, and not only by an action but their being (i.e., ontology) is a failure, which can evoke shame. This might be expressed through self-protective anger that might further isolate them or self-criticism.[12]

The essence of emotional pain is an embodied feeling of being broken or shattered that is often precipitated by a trauma or crisis. The pain (brokenness) is typically a visceral experience that has been described as a feeling of being ripped apart. Pain is distinguished from sadness, fear, and anger as it is preceded by some damage that has occurred. But pain is adaptive as it mobilizes self-protective action along with the learned avoidance of potential damaging experiences. It indicates damage to the self and is a higher-level emotional expe-rience compared to a single emotion. Racial trauma can leave Black men feeling broken due to the continuous assaults they experience.[13]

CLINICAL IMPLICATIONS

A humanistic-experiential psychotherapy approach can be optimal in working with Black men. However, the problems with humanistic philosophy/humanism (see Chapter 8: "No Humans Involved (N.H.I.)/Dehumanization" for details) must be considered, and the heavy reliance on self-determination within humanistic approaches can be a limitation as the options for the self-determination of Black men in the U.S. are severely restricted. There-fore, a contextualized humanistic-experiential approach is recommended in working with Black men, where the realities (i.e., anti-Black misandric micro/aggressions) of Black male experience are integrated in the therapy. Clinicians working with Black men who are dis-playing John Henryism (e.g., overworking or exerting high effort to cope in order to control/manage their environment) will need to help them feel empowered in their lives and engage in healthier coping mechanisms while discovering other fulfilling aspects of their lives that are independent of their employment. A double-consciousness framework is significant in helping clinicians and Black males describe their nimble ability to navigate white spaces and dehumanizing objectification while operating as a fully integrated human being. More-over, it is essential that therapists address the emotional and cognitive depletion that causes exhaustion due to the double-consciousness of Black males.[14]

The Cross (1971, 1991) model of Nigrescence (to become Black) is the most widely used model of Black American racial identity. The Nigrescence model includes five stages (also referred to as attitudes or statuses: preencounter, encounter, immersion/emersion, internal-ization, internalization-commitment) of racial identity development that Black Americans experience that are a part of developing a psychologically healthy Black identity. The first stage of *preencounter* entails a belief that race is not an important component of identity. This may include the idealization of whiteness (dominant white society) or emphasizing another identity component such as sex/gender, class, or religion. The second stage of *encounter* includes a profound racialized experience or a collection of racialized experiences. Therefore, individuals are prompted to reexamine their identity or develop a Black identity. The third stage of *immersion/emersion* is described as an idealization of Black culture and rejection of white culture. Black culture is obsessively identified with, but there is an internal lack of commitment to endorse all Black cultural values and traditions. The fourth stage of *internalization* encompasses a feeling state of inner security and satisfaction with being Black. This includes a less idealized perspective of the meaning of race where a less dichotomous view of being Black and white are integrated. The fifth stage of *internalization/commitment* is characterized by individuals translating their internalized identities into action. These stages are not static but a dynamic process that is situational/contextual as well as stable and has been described as a gradual emergence of stage characteristics with the ability to return to a previous stage while experiencing that stage in a different manner. It is not uncommon that a person is primarily operating in one stage while simultaneously engaged with characteristics from other stages. It is important to note that the Nigresence model has evolved from a developmental stage model to an attitudinal model. Pierre and Mahalik (2005) found that Black men whose attitudes reflected preencounter and immersion racial identity attitudes and who did not demonstrate resistance against anti-Blackness reported greater psychological distress and lower self-esteem.[15]

The multidimensional model of racial identity (MMRI) integrates a number of existing theories on group identity and cultural experiences that inform the unique racial/group identity of Black Americans. A phenomenological approach is used in studying racial identity with a focus on a person's self-perceptions of what it means to be Black. The MMRI defines Black American racial identity as the significance and qualitative meaning that individuals attribute to their membership within the Black racial group within their self-concepts.[16]

The following two questions encompass this definition: *How important is race in the individual's perception of self? What does it mean to be a member of this racial group?* The assumptions that undergird the MMRI are that identities are situationally and contextually influenced as well as being stable properties of the person, individuals have a number of different hierarchically ordered identities (e.g., race in the context of other identities is able to be investigated), individuals' perception of their racial identity is the most significant indicator of their identity, and the status of an individual's racial identity instead of its development is a fundamental focus of the MMRI. The MMRI includes four dimensions (*salience, centrality, regard,* and *ideology*) of racial identity with an emphasis on the significance and the qualitative meaning of race in the self-concepts of Black Americans. Racial *salience* refers to the extent to which an individual's race is a relevant aspect of one's self-concept situationally and contextually. Racial *centrality* refers to the significance individuals ascribe to race. Racial *regard* refers to a person's judgments about their race and includes *private regard* (perceptions of being Black American and assessments of other Black Americans) and *public regard* (an individual's assessment of how Black Americans are viewed by society). *Ideology* consists of an individual's beliefs, opinions, and attitudes regarding how Black Americans should act and includes *assimilationist, humanist, oppressed minority,* and *nationalist perspectives. Assimilationist* ideology emphasizes the similarities between Black Americans and American society. *Humanist* ideology is characterized by an emphasis on the similarities among all humans. *Oppressed minority* ideology focuses on the similarities between Black Americans and other oppressed populations. *Nationalist* ideology emphasizes the uniqueness of the being Black experience (i.e., the Black American experience). Sellers et al. (2006) found that greater racial centrality and private regard were related to greater psychological well-being. While the Nigrescence model of racial identity development has utility, the MMRI provides a more nuanced and comprehensive understanding of racial identity. The *multidimensional inventory of black identity (MIBI)* can be useful in assessing a client's racial identity status.[17]

Clinicians should abstain from engaging in the politics of hope (i.e., promoting fraudulent hope). It is imperative that the barriers that Black men are likely to navigate are made explicit and honestly addressed (i.e., racial realism) while avoiding baseless platitudes. Divesting from various forms of naïve political vulnerability is important for one's health. A more realistic assessment of the anti-Black misandric aggression that Black men might encounter can serve as a protective factor and provide a sense of agency. In addition, a strengths-based approach will need to move beyond a sole focus on resilience and incorporate a structural and systemic analysis as well as integrate a biopsychosocial approach.[18]

It is important that clinicians are aware of their responses when working with Black men who are emotionally expressing themselves. Not recognizing and responding to their emotional expression can perpetuate dehumanization. Biases that Black males don't emotionally express themselves or engage in non-normative emotional responses constitute a form of dehumanization. Black men need to feel seen, heard, understood, and accepted in order to facilitate a therapeutic alliance.

It is often unsafe for Black men to express anger let alone rage. Therefore, clinicians will need to explicitly acknowledge their client's rage and create space for its expression with an open invitation. Validating the rage and creating a space for its expression along with the exploration of constructive mechanisms for continued expression are fundamental in forging a therapeutic relationship. The lives of Black males have been shaped by oppression (i.e., anti-Black misandric micro/aggression), and rage is a natural reaction to oppression. Working effectively with rage in therapy includes the identification of rage and its connection to the presenting problem, validating rage, identification of other related emotions, and exploring constructive ways of channeling rage. The "angry Blacks" trope/caricature is a form of dehumanization that prevents Black Americans from being able to fully emotionally express themselves (i.e., articulate their pain) without condemnation. Thus, a pervasive fear among many Black Americans persists of being misunderstood or reinforcing racial tropes/caricatures if one embraces anger or rage. Further, the very mechanisms of racial oppression (i.e., anti-Black racism) socialize many Black Americans to remain silent about their racial oppression and the anger and rage that accompanies it. Therefore, an invitation to speak openly in therapy about their racial oppression, anger, and rage can initially be met with denial from the client. Clinicians will need to maintain a curious approach in their attempts to identify rage along with patience, persistence, and respect. Some clients might feel safer discussing rage indirectly through various mediums such as art, music, literature, or storytelling, where they feel most comfortable accessing intense and even threatening emotions. The identification and expression of rage should be followed by the validation of its existence and continued expression. Therapists who find it difficult to validate their clients' rage run the risk of replicating the same social processes (i.e., anti-Black racism) that led to the suppression of rage. Clinicians who are uncomfortable (e.g., avoidant) and have adverse reactions to strong negative affect will need to engage in personal work to expand their ability to be with rage/anger. Otherwise, therapists will not be able to guide their clients through dysfunctional dimensions of rage, which is important in transitioning toward managing and constructively channeling rage. The identification and expression of other emotions associated with rage should be addressed in therapy as well, where clients access other related emotions such as pain and grief (e.g., sadness and loss) that frequently accompanies rage in order to facilitate resolution. Processing grief often involves expressing angry protest at a loss before sadness can be accessed. Therapists will need to help clients feel empowered by developing healthier long-term coping strategies that incorporates existing strengths and resources that facilitate the constructive expression of rage in a racially oppressive society.[19]

Anger indicates that a person's boundaries are being invaded, they are being hurt, their rights are being violated, their wants or needs are not being sufficiently met, or that progress toward a goal is being obstructed. Anger helps people set boundaries and points to their unmet needs of interpersonal security (e.g., safety). The therapist cultivates safety and is to provide a supportive relationship that includes acknowledging and validating the client's experience of anger. This is followed by empathetic reflections along with empathetic affirmations that helps to deepen emotional experiencing by exploring associated feelings, thoughts, and needs. The therapist empathetically guides the client into deeper exploration of their vulnerability. The primary adaptive anger (i.e., assertive anger) with the underlying needs of safety or support can deteriorate into secondary anger that has an undifferentiated emotional quality. The deterioration into secondary anger includes excessive arousal and loss of meaning in the initial focus of the embodied anger. The therapist helps the client to regain their focus by resymbolizing the violation that occurred and restoring their productive assertion (i.e., assertive anger) or at the very least assist the client to develop some meta-awareness regarding their loss of focus. In addition, it is important that therapists help clients differentiate their emotions and process them separately. Differentiating and processing each emotion should address the effects of rumination (e.g., negative alterations in cognitions/mood and physiological arousal) in secondary anger. Moreover, secondary anger frequently conceals sadness that is due to deprivation.[20]

The power imbalance between client and therapist along with client disclosure of their most intimate thoughts and feelings that leaves them feeling exposed in a nonreciprocal exchange partly positions the therapeutic relationship as inherently shaming. Therefore, various levels of shame are a constant in therapeutic work with clients as they are frequently selecting what part of their inner experience they can reveal safely and what part must remain hidden. Directly addressing shame in the psychotherapy relationship normalizes shame reactions. Further, therapist self-disclosure can be effective in reducing shame within the therapeutic relationship, and it is important in developing rapport with Black male clients. This is not a gratuitous process but one that is intentional and contextually relevant. The therapist self-discloses at a deep and personal level within their comfort, which can facilitate credibility and promote rapport with Black men in therapy. Identifying racial-trauma-related shame early during treatment and helping clients reduce the level of shame is essential in increasing the effectiveness of treatment of racial trauma. Trauma-related shame can be initially assessed by using the *Trauma Related Shame Inventory* (*TRSI*; Øktedalen et al., 2014). Shame is associated with low self-compassion, high self-criticism, and low self-esteem. The emotional processing of racial trauma can be impeded by shame (e.g., treatment stagnation, prolonged treatment, and reduced treatment outcome). Clinicians working with shame will need to demonstrate empathy, accessibility, attunement, and unconditional positive regard (e.g., non-judgmental understanding) in order to facilitate corrective experiences.[21]

The therapeutic relationship along with exposing the source of shame has the capability to facilitate resolution from race-based shame (RBS/this can change a person's relationship with their conditions, i.e., not internalizing degradation or condemnation, but does not change their conditions) where the therapist serves as a secure attachment figure. Stabilization and safety are essential prerequisites where the therapist assists the client to facilitate stability and safety in their daily life (e.g., work, school, and home) that includes a support system (e.g., friends, family, church, etc.). Further, adequate emotion regulation and distress tolerance skills are a fundamental prerequisite as the focus on the experience of shame can be distressing. Clients will need to engage in a racial trauma narrative where the client recalls (i.e., expresses traumatic emotional episodic memories) the incident(s) which facilitates the integration of the memory into the client's self-narrative (meaning-making). Helping clients put language to their internal experience is essential in therapeutic work where they focus on an internal bodily felt experience. Clients need to be able to differentiate their internal emotional states with specificity (referred to as emotional granularity), which helps them process their experiences and has an emotional regulating effect by organizing internal chaos.[22]

Greenberg's (2021) theory of changing emotion with emotion is described as a process of transformation that includes the synthesis of opposing emotions. The dreaded and painful underlying maladaptive emotions are accessed and transformed with new adaptive emotions. The underlying maladaptive emotion is not extinguished but transformed with new experience (e.g., new narrative and meaning). The therapist is to process this experience with the client. Moreover, helping clients recognize and overcome avoidance while acknowledging painful feelings of shame are instrumental in the therapeutic work. An imaginal encounter between the experiencing part of the self or the part that is more resourced and resilient (i.e., stronger, wiser, and more compassionate part), and the shame-based part (i.e., critical part) or those who have abused or devalued the client can be evoked in this process after an alliance and relationship has been established with the client along with the creation of safety. This entails changing emotion with emotion by changing the shame (e.g., withdrawal and avoidance responses of feeling defeated and demoralized) by evoking approach responses such as empowered anger (primary adaptive anger), comfort-seeking sadness, or expansive pride (e.g., racial pride), or other positive emotions (e.g., self-compassion) that unravel the paralyzing effects of shame.

Shame is frequently transformed by the adaptive emotions of empowered anger where one asserts oneself and stands up to the abusers in imaginal confrontations in order to empower oneself and challenge self-condemnation and contempt (e.g., anger transforms shame into confidence) or comfort-seeking sadness where one reaches out to others for support and connection (e.g., sadness transforms shame into calm or relief). Racial pride is another option in transforming shame where one positively identifies with their racial group, which is affirming and cultivates a sense of pride (i.e., a positive self-image) due to belonging to that racial group and forms a secure identity (e.g., pride transforms shame into a stable and positive identity).[23]

Devaluation that may be internalized as racial inferiority will need to be confronted, neutralized, and assimilated for a person to experience a coherent sense of self. Shame causes emotional pain where the need to be acknowledged as valuable (e.g., value and agency/autonomy – the space for one's own pursuits) is violated. In addition, emotional pain is caused when the need to be safe (e.g., a sense of being protected) is violated because of the terror or fear evoked from racial trauma. Part of this process entails helping the client to identify their needs that are underneath the shame. Furthermore, spontaneous, and genuine shared laughter (i.e., playfulness) relieves shame and restores a sense of social connection.[24]

Resolving emotional pain involves a stage process. The previously avoided (e.g., fear of annihilation and fear of seeing self) and feared painful feelings are approached which transitions to allowing brokenness (i.e., allowing the pain) where the client views and accepts the self as broken, which helps the client begin to tolerate and eventually process the aversive pain. This is followed by staying with the brokenness where the client begins to examine what is broken and engage and organize the pieces of the shattered self. The client acknowledges and owns their sense of brokenness (i.e., re-owning of previously avoided painful experience) and expresses and processes associated feelings where primary maladaptive emotions are changed by adaptive emotions. These processes lead to the transformation of self (i.e., resolution), where the client can access the underlying need or affective goal (e.g., to feel safe). The need that was accessed is a healthy internal resource that can be used to challenge maladaptive cognitions (i.e., dysfunctional beliefs) that contributed to the painful state. A sense of release and relief along with the integration of a more self-nurturing and affirming stance are markers of the transformation of self and coherence. This process facilitates the tolerance of pain and internal reorganization that produces change where the sense of brokenness is acknowledged along with allowing, accepting, experiencing, and expressing formerly avoided overregulated feelings. Like shame, this process can be facilitated with the incorporation of an imaginal encounter.[25]

Group psychotherapy can be a valuable psychotherapeutic modality where group members are among peers (e.g., no power imbalances) with similar struggles whom they can provide compassionate support to as well as receive it. Thus, providing them with a sense of value to the group as well as deserving of the support they receive. Moreover, the group can cultivate a sense of acceptance and belonging that can serve as a potent antidote to feelings of shame and devaluation.[26]

The word *shame* may not resonate with clients initially so words like *worthless, uncomfortable,* and *embarrassed* might initially be more effective. In addition, clients will frequently reject or disown descriptions of their whole being; therefore, it is often helpful for the therapist to talk about parts of the client feeling worthless, uncomfortable, or embarrassed. Clients more readily accept disowned aspects of themselves and their experiences if engaged as parts of oneself. Clients struggling with shame will often be highly defended as a form of self-protection, which can create a barrier between the therapist and client. The therapist can cultivate empathy by holding in their mind the client's experience, which includes their internal emotional state and vulnerability.[27]

INTERVENTIONS

Macrointerventions

Reparations

A program of reparations is owed to Black Americans who descend from U.S. enslavement and as a promising intervention can be transformative in scope to address structural and systemic inequities. A reparations program is part of a human rights framework that emphasizes retributive or restorative justice compared to a civil rights framework that emphasizes equalizing access.[28]

According to Darity (2008), a program of reparations includes three objectives: **acknowledgment** with public recognition of a grievous injustice perpetrated by the responsible institution or group and includes a formal apology; **redress** for the injustice includes compensatory actions that attempt to mitigate the enduring consequences (e.g., lasting intergenerational effects) of the grievous injustice (e.g., the design and implementation of a U.S. reparations program for Black Americans that would eliminate historically created racial disparities caused by slavery, legal segregation, and ongoing discrimination); and **closure** of the grievances brought forth by the group subjected to the injustice and includes the settling of accounts that facilitates a healing process (e.g., an effective reparations program would settle any future claims on behalf of Black Americans for the wrongs of slavery, Jim/Jane Crow, and past discrimination).

The injustices of slavery, the Jim/Jane Crow regime after Reconstruction that lasted nearly a century, and ongoing anti-Black discrimination are three types of injustices that motivate a program of reparations for Black Americans. The federal government through legislative action would be responsible for the inauguration of a reparations program on behalf of Black Americans. Native Americans who were forcibly exiled from their lands received land and billions of dollars through various benefits and programs. Japanese

Americans who had been incarcerated in internment camps during World War II were paid reparations ($1.5 billion) that was facilitated by federal legislative action through the Civil Liberties Act of 1988 and recently Guam residents were paid reparations from the U.S. government. In addition, the U.S. assisted in the facilitation of reparations for Jews who were victims of the Nazi Holocaust as well as various investments through the Marshall Plan. The magnitude of reparations owed to Black Americans can be calculated by beginning with the present-day value of 40 acres and a mule. Forty acres and a mule refer to General Sherman issued Special Field Orders No. 15 on January 16, 1865, that established the provision that newly freed Black Americans would be provided no more than 40 acres of confiscated Confederate land (coastal land in S. Carolina and Georgia) to be provided to Black families. Forty acres would be allocated to a family of four, and ten acres would be provided to each formerly enslaved Black American which would have equated to 40–45 million acres total. The *mule* referred to actual mules left over from the war given to some families, and it also metaphorically referred to the farm implements, and supplies provided as a grant to each family of the formerly enslaved as startup equipment. Moreover, the Freedman's Bureau Act of March 3, 1865, was more expansive and included an explicit racial land redistribution provision that was pursuant to the Southern land confiscation acts of 1861, 1862, 1863, and 1864. It mirrored General Sherman's order in that no more than 40 acres were to be provided to freedmen but also included the provision that the land would be leased out to the freedman for three years and that the rent was not to exceed 6 percent of the assessed value of the land based on state tax appraisals (conducted by state tax authorities) in 1860. The occupants had the option of purchasing the land and receiving the title at the end of the three years. This and the Southern Homestead Act of 1866 faced fierce opposition from President Andrew Johnson who by the end of 1865 ordered the removal of the formerly enslaved Black Americans from the coastal lands and restored the lands to the former white enslavers. Their wealth was handed back to them after being traitors to their country. Moreover, white enslavers in Washington, DC, were paid reparations for their lost property (i.e., the formerly enslaved Black Americans).[29]

The primary goal of a reparations program for Black Americans will be to close the racial/lineage wealth gap which will have the effect of moving Black Americans out of a racial undercaste status. The distribution of reparations can be issued as a down payment as well as a portfolio. In addition to the down payment, a trust fund could be established for eligible Black Americans who could apply for grants for multiple asset-building projects (e.g., homeownership, education, business start-up funds, or vouchers to purchase financial assets) and businesses would be incentivized to participate. Further, a robust affirmative action program that is specifically for Black Americans who descend from U.S. enslavement and is comprehensive in scope beyond simply the prevention of anti-Black discrimination would need to be a part of a reparations program. There will need to be protections in place to protect the newly acquired capital of Black Americans from predatory capitalists through mechanisms such as consumerism. A program of reparations will need to be a robust, long-term multigenerational program that will more than likely need to be flexible and responsive to the objectives of the program with a primary emphasis on closing the racial/lineage wealth gap. Resources will need to be devoted to achieving this goal until it is met. For individuals to be eligible for reparations, they would need to establish that they are descendants of formerly enslaved Black Americans in the U.S. and provide proof that they have self-identified as *Black*, *African American*, *Negro*, or *Colored* at least ten years prior to the adoption of a reparations program. Individuals living as white thus benefitting from white privilege but precipitously claiming a Black identity in order to access reparations would not qualify for a reparations program.[30]

Craemer et al. (2020) compared the 2018 Black-white wealth gap that was approximately $352,250 (this is the bare minimum amount proposed for Black American reparations per person in 2018 dollars and should close the Black-white wealth gap if properly structured) along with portions of the estimated cost of slavery and discrimination of Black American descendants of U.S. slavery. The estimated costs of slavery were between approximately $12 to $13 trillion in 2018 dollars (this estimate was established using Darity's land-based and Marketti's price-based estimation methods). When Craemer's wage-based method was used, the estimate was higher and ranged from approximately $19 trillion at 3 percent interest to $6.2 quadrillion at 6 percent interest. The value of lost freedom (LF – the inability to make decisions regarding one's own life) was $35 trillion (this was calculated based on Japanese American World War II internment reparations that included a 3 percent interest rate) and with the addition of a 6 percent interest rate totaled $16 quadrillion. They asserted that further research would have to be conducted to estimate the cost of lost opportunities (LC) and pain and suffering (PS). Additional research would be required to estimate the costs of colonial slavery and racial discrimination to Black American descendants of slavery following the abolition of slavery in the U.S. The wealth gap is a comprehensive marker of the cumulative disadvantages that afflicts the present generation. The wealth gap embodies the cumulative effects of past atrocities (i.e., white supremacy/terrorism), which includes colonial slavery, U.S. slavery, post–Civil War massacres, Jim/Jane Crow discrimination, New Deal discrimination, segregation during World War II, postwar discrimination, and post–civil rights discrimination. Himmelstein et al. (2022) found a reduction in life expectancy gaps by 65 percent to approximately 103 percent between Black and white individuals when reparations were used to close the mean racial wealth gap in simulations. Differences in wealth are associated with the life expectancy gap that exists between Black and white Americans that potentially can be narrowed or ameliorated by reparations payments that eliminate the racial wealth gap and the subsequent racial inequities in mortality. Moreover, the research of Richardson et al. (2021) revealed that a reparations program targeted toward Black Americans would have decreased COVID-19 risk and included mitigating effects across racial groups, thus benefitting the general population. They found that reparations payments made before the pandemic could have reduced the coronavirus transmission rate in the state of Louisiana between 31 to 68 percent. A recent poll indicated that 62 percent of Americans opposed (38 percent supported) reparations in the form of financial payments to Black Americans as compensation for slavery. This opposition remained even amid awareness of contemporary racial inequality. Seventy-two percent of whites opposed cash payments as a form of reparations and 28 percent supported while 86 percent of Black Americans supported while 14 percent opposed. White Americans cite the difficulty in determining monetary value of the impact of slavery along with the fact that there is no one still living who was directly involved in slavery. White Americans also deny the ongoing legacy of slavery and express concerns regarding the undeserving nature of Black Americans as prospective recipients of reparations. Reichelmann and Hunt (2021) state that white Americans received the largest gains from slavery and its compounded effects (i.e., unjust enrichment) and propose that their widespread opposition to reparations is motivated by their desire to maintain this advantage (racial hierarchy).[31]

Transitional Justice

In addition to reparations that operates within a retributive (e.g., punishment of perpetrators of wrongdoing) or restorative justice (e.g., the repair of ruptured relationships is prioritized among victim, offender, and community caused by wrongdoing, which includes an apology and reparations followed by forgiveness) framework, this author recommends a transitional justice framework for addressing the wrongs that have been perpetuated against Black males. Transitional justice is comprised of both legal and philosophical theory and is a global practice that pursues redress for past and present wrongdoing with the intention of vindicating victims while holding perpetrators accountable and transforming relationships [e.g., among citizens (horizontal interactions) and between citizens and public officials (vertical interactions)]. Transitional justice has been instituted in dozens of countries (e.g., S. Africa to Columbia) that emerged from periods of war, genocide, dictatorship, and repression. Part of the transitional justice framework includes identifying what is damaged along with acknowledgment of the damage followed by addressing the damage before a repair can be attempted. In addition, a boundary is drawn between what was accepted in the past and what will be acceptable in the future to prevent the recurrence of atrocity. Truth commissions, criminal investigations and prosecutions, reparations, lustration (the vetting of government officials for ties to repressive regimes or activity), and other legal and institutional changes are all measures used to achieve the aims of transitional justice.[32]

Restorative justice offers valuable guidance for a specific wrong, but transitional justice provides the capacity to address systemic problems. Forgiveness or letting go of anger does not change the sources of racial oppression (i.e., anti-Black racism) and can encourage the victimized to capitulate their own degradation. Retributive justice assumes state legitimacy where the intentional infliction of punishment is compatible with the state's recognition of equality among all citizens, while transitional justice analyzes how to establish the legitimacy of the state with an initial baseline equality among all citizens.[33]

Transitional justice not only satisfies the moral claims of victims and holds perpetrators accountable but transforms society so that systemic wrongdoing does not occur again. Obtaining an accurate understanding of the core problems with relationships among members of society is a fundamental aspect of transitional justice where relationships can only be transformed if there is a thorough understanding of the conditions that enabled the injustice to persist and the relationship between past wrongs and present interaction. Transitional justice is a robust generational project that requires ongoing political will and multiple processes. Transitional justice would need to confront Black male negation (BMN, e.g., extermination and genocide/gendercide) and the interconnected structures/institutions (i.e., institutional decimation, e.g., legal and judicial system, education, employment, housing, health care system, and other economic institutions) along with the individuals who are decision-makers within these structures and institutions. Whether deliberate or indeliberate, politicians, academics, law enforcement, and various other professionals will need to be made accountable for contributing to BMN whether through anti-Black misandric ideology or through action (anti-Black misandric aggression).[34]

Microinterventions

Racial Realism

According to Bell (1992), the aim for integration in racist America is unobtainable for Black Americans and creates persistent frustration and despair that is self-defeating. Therefore, he advocates for *racial realism*, which is the acknowledgment of racism as a permanent fixture in the U.S., where Black people will remain in a subordinate status (i.e., racial undercaste) and never gain full equality (i.e., racial equality ideology). Any political victories hailed as successful are temporary and short-lived that become irrelevant as adaptive racial patterns maintain white dominance. This can be verified by honestly reviewing Black history within the U.S. Bell cites examples of legal precedents that were thought to be permanent and were overturned as well as the 400+ years of Black freedom struggle as evidence of the permanence of racism. In addition, Bell (1980) introduced the concept of *interest convergence*, where the interests of Blacks in obtaining racial equality will only be accommodated when it converges with the interests of whites. Racial realism and interest convergence are both foundational theories of critical race theory (CRT). Historian Mary Dudziak (2000/*Cold War Civil Rights*) elucidated the dynamic of interest convergence during the Cold War and how it prompted desegregation in an attempt to revamp the international image of the U.S. with its treatment of Black Americans. The primary interests of white America was the presentation of democracy as the best option in its geopolitical struggle for global influence as U.S. allies were concerned about American anti-Black racism, which was a propaganda theme utilized by the Soviet Union, and created an obstacle for U.S. Cold War goals of promoting democracy in Africa, Asia, and Latin America. Therefore, a civil rights agenda was able to gain traction because it aligned with white interests of global domination (imperialism). The commitment to racial equality (i.e., racial equality syndrome) perpetuates the disempowerment of Black Americans, while racial realism can empower Black Americans where that energy could be invested in ensuring that Black Americans attain a more meaningful status as a permanent subordinate group. Therefore, racial realism cultivates the opportunity to be responsive to the recurring aspects of Black subordinate status. Forgoing the illusion of idealism with a focus on realism provides freedom of thought and the ability to plan accordingly. Further, issues of Black poverty, joblessness, and lack of health care can be directly addressed without falling into the delusional trap of equality. Removing the distortion of racial equality ideology provides a protective factor for Black Americans where they are better equipped to cope (e.g., self-care and self-affirmation) with their racial subordination (i.e., anti-Black racism). Racial realism can lead to policy positions and campaigns that provide a sense of agency (i.e., engagement and commitment) through resistance/struggle (an antidote to despair and defeat) and meaning through Black humanity.[35]

Legal reform of qualified immunity, *Graham v. O'Connor* and *Terry v. Ohio*, could potentially take place under the auspice of racial realism. The legal protection of qualified immunity [created 50 years ago by the Supreme Court with *Pierson v. Ray* (1967)] that is afforded to police officers should be removed as it serves as an impenetrable legal shield for police violence. Qualified immunity is a judicially created doctrine (i.e., a form of sovereign immunity) that protects government officials (including police officers) from being held personally liable (i.e., civil suits) for violating constitutional rights. Therefore, it is almost impossible to win a civil suit against a police officer for the violation of a person's civil rights (e.g., the right to be free from excessive force) even if they committed unlawful acts. Further, the burden of proof for the use of excessive force should be shifted from victims of police violence to police officers. This potentially can be accomplished by overturning *Graham v. O'Connor* (1989). Moreover, the unreasonable search and seizures of stop-and-frisk that are non-consensual encounters and associated with the PTSD and the sexual victimization of Black males should be discontinued. The overturning of *Terry v. Ohio* (1968) would likely be necessary in this process.[36]

Coping Strategies and Groups

Research from Hudson et al. (2016a) examined racial discrimination and coping among Black men in St. Louis (MO) and found that participants described experiences of anti-Black misandric aggression in multiple settings that included the workplace, school, residential, and within the criminal justice system. Their coping strategies included drinking, smoking, religiosity, and familial support. The men indicated that they found relief in group settings where they could discuss their stressors. Black men are routinely challenged with navigating when, where, and how to resist oppression (i.e., anti-Black misandric micro/aggression) versus when, where, how to accommodate it. Utsey (1997) recommends that Black men confront the perpetrators of racist behavior (this is contingent upon their safety). Therefore, the racism (i.e., anti-Black misandric micro/aggression) is not ingested but placed with the perpetrator.[37]

Individual therapy is a significant viable option for Black men experiencing psychological and emotional distress due to frequent encounters with racial discrimination (i.e., racial trauma). The maintenance of health and wellness requires a holistic approach that promotes psychological, emotional, and spiritual well-being (i.e., physical health, diet, family, recreational activities, spirituality, etc.).[38]

Participation in support groups for Black men experiencing racism-related stress related to societal racism can provide a sense of community (e.g., belonging) where group members feel seen, heard, understood, and accepted. Elligan and Utsey (1999) recommend an African-centered group approach such as Ntu psychotherapy, which includes the five phases of harmony, awareness, alignment, actualization, and synthesis, and the five principles of harmony, balance, interconnectedness, cultural awareness, and authenticity. Thus, helping Black men develop effective coping skills and ameliorate the impact of societal racism and oppression. The group Elligan and Utsey (1999) designed had seven group members, was intergenerational (ages ranged from late twenties to mid-seventies), and met for 12 regular group sessions (three months) with one social outing to a jazz club. The various Ntu stages were a focus throughout the 12 weeks. Emotional themes of anger, fear, joy, and happiness emerged during the group that were a part of the group discussions. Common themes that emerged as discussion points included the use of spirituality/religion as a coping mechanism, being "pulled over at gunpoint" by the police for false charges, humiliating experiences in front of white coworkers or classmates that respectively took place in workplace and school settings, stress due to substance abuse fatalities within one's family, John Henryism (e.g., the belief that Black men have to work "ten times" as hard as white men in order to achieve similar goals), raising healthy and proud Black children, getting married, getting divorced, intragroup white supremacy within the Black American/African diaspora, discussions of the slave trade, and coping strategies utilized by other non-African/Black American cultures. Further, the group dispelled the myth of the Cool Pose caricature (i.e., macho, cool, and emotionally distant). Outcomes from the group included reported decreases in frequency of interpersonal conflicts with significant others (e.g., girlfriend or spouse), a decrease in anger and frustration, an increase in appreciation and love for other Black men, and a sense of community/social support with other group members. In addition, the Black barbershop can also be a site of mental health collaboration, whereas the importance of Black men's hair grooming process is centered around negotiating health, community connections, family dynamics, and emotions.[39]

According to Baker-Fletcher (1993), somebodiness was the most comprehensive component of Martin Luther King's (1967) philosophy on human dignity. Johnson (2016) examined somebodiness, which was defined by the Black men in his study as sense of worth, purpose, and community. The Black men in the study believed that they were a person of worth because they were created by God (i.e., personal worth and value). They desired and were on a quest to discover their purpose while manifesting a positive outcome with one's life (i.e., existential purpose and meaning), and they yearned to help others particularly Black youth in the community. Investing in the community was particularly redemptive for those who had denigrated themselves and their communities. Thus, somebodiness was a central psychological theme in the lives of Black men. The participants were motivated by a greater sense of worth, purpose, and community. They asserted that their worth came from God and could not be taken away and expected to be treated with dignity and respect. Their self-constitution of somebodiness assisted them in resisting dehumanization while feeling, seeing, and imagining themselves as persons of infinite worth regardless of societal ascription.

Family, friends, teachers, and the community influenced their notions of a successful and productive life as well as what would be required to cultivate that life. Dignity and integrity were foundational in their conceptualizations of success, where being successful was not as important than how one achieved success. The communal orientation of somebodiness manifested in their individual identification with Black Americans as a group and the obligations they felt to the Black community (i.e., collective uplift). The multidimensional and culturally relevant concept of somebodiness can assist therapists in effectively serving Black men. Clinicians should assume that every Black man desires to experience himself as a person of infinite worth and is capable of a meaningful contribution regardless of his presentation, situation, or circumstance.[40]

It is important to note that there are limitations to clinical interventions as the issues highlighted throughout this volume require long-term robust and transformative public policy that examines the structural and intentional processes generating racial hierarchy and caste. A move toward interventions (reparations, redistribution of wealth, etc.) on a national level is imperative. This can reorganize U.S. society to address systemic (structural and institutional) issues that are socially engineered to create the conditions (institutional decimation) that Black men are made to live through and that is largely responsible for their demise (death and dying). The macrointerventions of reparations and transitional justice proposed in this chapter provide the opportunity for a course correct through transformative systemic interventions. The microinterventions provide clinicians with the tools to be able to provide responsive care and clinical interventions that inform treatment approaches. Moreover, this volume is an essential resource for therapists to recognize and articulate the racial trauma of Black men and respond appropriately by utilizing the frameworks of the unified theory of racism (UTR), integrated model of racial trauma (IMRT), transgenerational trauma points (TTP), plantation politics, Black male negation (BMN), and race-based shame (RBS).

NOTES

1 James, 1994; Bennett et al., 2004; Singer et al., 2020; Johnson & Martin, 2020; Link & Phelan, 2001; James et al., 1983.
2 James, 1994; Bennett et al., 2004; Singer et al., 2020; Johnson & Martin, 2020; Link & Phelan, 2001; James et al., 1983.
3 Du Bois, 1903; Wynter, 2006; Matsumoto, 1993.
4 Du Bois, 1903; Wynter, 2006; Matsumoto, 1993.
5 Sellers et al., 1998; Thompson & Carter, 1997.
6 Williams, 2016.
7 Frijda, 1986, 2016; Greenberg, 2021.
8 Greenberg, 2015, 2021; Hardy & Laszloffy, 1995; Paivio & Carriere, 2007; Tarba, 2015; Paivio, 1999; Nolen-Hoeksema et al., 2008; Pascual-Leone et al., 2012; Hussen, 2013.
9 Carter & Forsyth, 2010; Sznycer et al., 2018; Kaufman, 1996; DeYoung, 2015; Miller, 1998; Patterson, 1982; Tangney & Dearing, 2002; Dickerson et al., 2004.
10 Carter & Forsyth, 2010; Sznycer et al., 2018; Kaufman, 1996; DeYoung, 2015; Miller, 1998; Patterson, 1982; Tangney & Dearing, 2002; Dickerson et al., 2004.

11 Carter & Forsyth, 2010; Sznycer et al., 2018; Kaufman, 1996; DeYoung, 2015; Miller, 1998; Patterson, 1982; Tangney & Dearing, 2002; Dickerson et al., 2004.

12 Carter & Forsyth, 2010; Sznycer et al., 2018; Kaufman, 1996; DeYoung, 2015; Miller, 1998; Patterson, 1982; Tangney & Dearing, 2002; Dickerson et al., 2004.

13 Bolger, 1999; Greenberg & Bolger, 2001.

14 Johnson, 2006; Tate, 1973; White, 1970; Rice & Greenberg, 1992; Rogers, 1961, 1980; Gendlin, 1981, 1996.

15 Cross & Vandiver, 2001; Helms, 1990, 1995; Parham, 1989; Thompson & Carter, 1997.

16 Sellers et al., 1998.

17 Sellers et al., 1998.

18 Jaima, 2021.

19 Hardy & Laszloffy, 1995; Greenberg, 2015; Pascual-Leone et al., 2012; Tarba, 2015; Christ et al., 2020.

20 Hardy & Laszloffy, 1995; Greenberg, 2015; Pascual-Leone et al., 2012; Tarba, 2015; Christ et al., 2020.

21 Øktedalen et al., 2015; Gilbert & Procter, 2006; Greenberg & Iwakabe, 2011; Herman, 2011; Kaufman, 1996; DeYoung, 2015; Nathanson, 1992; Timulak, 2015; Mlotek & Paivio, 2017; Kashdan et al., 2015; Lee, 1999.

22 Øktedalen et al., 2015; Gilbert & Procter, 2006; Greenberg & Iwakabe, 2011; Herman, 2011; Kaufman, 1996; DeYoung, 2015; Nathanson, 1992; Timulak, 2015; Mlotek & Paivio, 2017; Kashdan et al., 2015.

23 Øktedalen et al., 2015; Gilbert & Procter, 2006; Greenberg & Iwakabe, 2011; Greenberg, 2015; Herman, 2011; Kaufman, 1996; DeYoung, 2015; Timulak, 2015; Mlotek & Paivio, 2017; Kashdan et al., 2015; Nathanson, 1992.

24 Øktedalen et al., 2015; Gilbert & Procter, 2006; Greenberg & Iwakabe, 2011; Greenberg, 2015; Herman, 2011; Kaufman, 1996; DeYoung, 2015; Timulak, 2015; Mlotek & Paivio, 2017; Kashdan et al., 2015.

25 Bolger, 1999; Greenberg & Bolger, 2001.

26 Bolger, 1999; Greenberg & Bolger, 2001.

27 Øktedalen et al., 2015; Gilbert & Procter, 2006; Greenberg & Iwakabe, 2011; Greenberg, 2015; Herman, 2011; Kaufman, 1996; DeYoung, 2015; Timulak, 2015; Mlotek & Paivio, 2017; Kashdan et al., 2015.

28 Darity, 2008.

29 Darity, 2008.

30 Darity, 2008, 2021; Hofschneider, 2020; Darity & Mullen, 2020a, 2020b; Williams & Collins, 2004; Williams, 2017; Ray & Perry, 2020; Harriot, 2020; Graham, 2021; Feagin, 2004, 2014; Carnell, 2021.

31 Darity, 2008, 2021; Hofschneider, 2020; Darity & Mullen, 2020a, 2020b; Williams & Collins, 2004; Williams, 2017; Ray & Perry, 2020; Harriott, 2020; Graham, 2021; Feagin, 2004, 2014; Carnell, 2021.

32 Murphy, 2021.

33 Murphy, 2021.

34 Murphy, 2021.

35 Bell, 1976, 1991, 1993.

36 Chung et al., 2020; Sobel, 2020; Sullivan, 2021; Curry, 2021; Alexander, 2010; Cooper, 2015.

37 Bell, 1994, 1996.

38 Bell, 1994, 1996; Utsey et al., 2001.

39 Elligan & Utsey, 1999; Mbilishaka et al., 2021.

40 Johnson, 2016.

REFERENCES

Abbas, C. C., Schmid, J. P., Guler, E., Wiedemar, L., Begré, S., Saner, H., Schnyder, U., & Von Känel, R. (2009). Trajectory of posttraumatic stress disorder caused by myocardial infarction: A two-year follow-up study. *The International Journal of Psychiatry in Medicine, 39*(4), 359–376.

Acebo, A. (2012). Life, liberty, and the pursuit of whiteness: A revolution of identity politics in America. *Columbia Journal of Race and Law, 2*, 149–166.

Adair, M., & Howell, S. (1988). *The subjective side of politics.* Tools for Change.

Addo, F. R., & Darity, W. A., Jr. (2021). Disparate recoveries: Wealth, race, and the working class after the great recession. *The Annals of the American Academy of Political and Social Science, 695*(1), 173–192.

Agency for Healthcare Research and Quality. (2018). *National healthcare quality and disparities report* (AHRQ Publication No. 19-0070-EF). Department of Health and Human Services. www.ahrq.gov/sites/default/files/wysiwyg/research/findings/nhqrdr/2018qdr-final-es.pdf

Aja, A. A., Zaw, K., Beesing, G., Price, A. E., Bustillo, D., Darity, W. A., Jr., Clealand, D., Paul, M., & Hamilton, D. (2019). *The color of wealth in Miami.* A joint publication of The Kirwan Institute for the Study of Race and Ethnicity at the Ohio State University, the Samuel DuBois Cook Center on Social Equity at Duke University, and the Insight Center for Community Economic Development.

Ajilore, O., & Thames, A. D. (2020). The fire this time: The stress of racism, inflammation and COVID-19. *Brain, Behavior, and Immunity, 88*, 66–67.

Alang, S., McAlpine, D., McCreedy, E., & Hardeman, R. (2017). Police brutality and Black health: Setting the agenda for public health scholars. *American Journal of Public Health, 107*(5), 662–665.

Alexander, H. (2022, January 28). BLM will not confirm who controls its $60m after founder stepped down. *Mail Online.* www.dailymail.co.uk/news/article-10449911/Black-Lives-Matter-not-con firm-controls-60m-funds-founder-stepped-down.html

Alexander, M. (2010). *The new Jim Crow: Mass incarceration in the age of colorblindness.* New Press.

Alexis, M. (1998). The economics of racism. *The Review of Black Political Economy, 26*(3), 51–75.

Allen, A. T. (2014). Feminism and fatherhood in Western Europe, 1900–1950s. *Journal of Women's History, 26*(2), 39–62.

Allen, R. L. (1969). *Black awakening in capitalist America.* Doubleday.

Allen, R. L. (2005). Reassessing the internal (neo) colonialism theory. *The Black Scholar, 35*(1), 2–11.

Allen, R. L. (2010). Forty years later: Reflections on the writing of Black awakening in capitalist America. *The Black Scholar, 40*(2), 2–10.

Allen, T. (1994). *The invention of the White race.* Verso.

Allport, G. W. (1954). *The nature of prejudice.* Addison-Wesley.

Al'Uqdah, S. N., Maxwell, C., & Hill, N. (2016). Intimate partner violence in the African American community: Risk, theory, and interventions. *Journal of Family Violence, 31*(7), 877–884.

Amato, P. R. (2005). The impact of family formation change on the cognitive, social, and emotional well-being of the next generation. *The Future of Children*, 75–96.

American Psychiatric Association. (1968). *Diagnostic and statistical manual of mental disorders* (2nd ed.). American Psychiatric Association.

American Psychiatric Association. (1980). *Diagnostic and statistical manual of mental disorders* (3rd ed.). American Psychiatric Association.

American Psychiatric Association. (2013). *Diagnostic and statistical manual of mental disorders* (5th ed.). American Psychiatric Association.

Amir, M. (1971). *Patterns in forcible rape.* University of Chicago Press.

Anderson, P. D. (2021, September 8). *The theory of intersectionality emerges out of racist, colonialist ideology, not radical politics – rethinking the CRT debate part 3.* Black Agenda Report. www.blackagendare port.com/theory-intersectionality-emerges-out-racist-colonialist-ideology-not-radical-politics-rethinking

Anderson, R., & Curry, T. J. (2021). Black radical nationalist theory and Afrofuturism 2.0. In P. Butler (Ed.), *Critical Black futures: Speculative theories and explorations* (pp. 119–138). Palgrave Macmillan.

Andrasfay, T., & Goldman, N. (2021). Reductions in 2020 US life expectancy due to COVID-19 and the disproportionate impact on the Black and Latino populations. *Proceedings of the National Academy of Sciences, 118*(5).

Angner, E., Hullett, S., & Allison, J. J. (2011). "I'll die with the hammer in my hand": John Henryism as a predictor of happiness. *Journal of Economic Psychology, 32*(3), 357–366.

Ani, M. (1994). *Yurugu: An African-centered critique of European cultural thought and behavior.* African World Press.

Ansley, F. L. (1997). White supremacy (and what we should do about it). *Critical White Studies: Looking Behind the Mirror,* 592–595.

Archer, J. (2000). Sex differences in aggression between heterosexual partners: A meta-analytic review. *Psychological Bulletin, 126*(5), 651–680.

Arseniev-Koehler, A., Foster, J. G., Mays, V. M., Chang, K. W., & Cochran, S. D. (2021). Aggression, escalation, and other latent themes in legal intervention deaths of non-Hispanic Black and White men: Results from the 2003–2017 national violent death reporting system. *American Journal of Public Health, 111*(S2), S107–S115.

Asante-Muhammad, D., & Devine, J. (2021, April 21). *Rebuilding Black-owned businesses after Covid-19.* Institute for Policy Studies. https://ips-dc.org/rebuilding-black-owned-businesses-after-covid-19

Assari, S. (2018). Health disparities due to diminished return among Black Americans: Public policy solutions. *Social Issues and Policy Review, 12*(1), 112–145.

Assari, S., Cochran, S. D., & Mays, V. M. (2021). Money protects White but Not African American men against discrimination: Comparison of African American and White Men in the same geographic areas. *International Journal of Environmental Research and Public Health, 18*(5), 2706.

Assari, S., Lankarani, M. M., & Caldwell, C. H. (2018). Does discrimination explain high risk of depression among high-income African American men? *Behavioral Sciences, 8*(4), 40.

Austin, A. (2012, January 19). *A good credit score did not protect Latino and Black borrowers.* Economic Policy Institute. www.epi.org/publication/latino-black-borrowers-high-rate-subprime-mortgages

Austin, A. (2021). *The jobs crisis for Black men is a lot worse than you think.* Center for Economic and Policy Research.

Aviv, A., Valdes, A. M., & Spector, T. D. (2006). Human telomere biology: Pitfalls of moving from the laboratory to epidemiology. *International Journal of Epidemiology, 35,* 1424–1429.

Azar, K. M., Shen, Z., Romanelli, R. J., Lockhart, S. H., Smits, K., Robinson, S., Brown, S., & Pressman, A. R. (2020). Disparities In outcomes among COVID-19 patients in a large health care system in California: Study estimates the COVID-19 infection fatality rate at the US county level. *Health Affairs, 39*(7), 1253–1262.

Babcock, J. C., Armenti, N. A., & Warford, P. (2017). The trials and tribulations of testing couples-based interventions for intimate partner violence. *Partner Abuse, 8*(1), 110–124.

Bailey, Z. D., Feldman, J. M., & Bassett, M. T. (2021). How structural racism works – racist policies as a root cause of US racial health inequities. *New England Journal of Medicine, 384*(8), 768–773.

Bailey, Z. D., Krieger, N., Agénor, M., Graves, J., Linos, N., & Bassett, M. T. (2017). Structural racism and health inequities in the USA: Evidence and interventions. *The Lancet, 389*(10077), 1453–1463.

Baker, F. M., & Bell, C. C. (1999). Issues in the psychiatric treatment of African Americans. *Psychiatric Services, 50*(3), 362–368.

Baker-Fletcher, G. K. (1993). *Somebodyness: Martin Luther King, Jr., and the theory of dignity.* Fortress Press.

Baldus, D. C., Pulaski, C., & Woodworth, G. (1983). Comparative review of death sentences: An empirical study of the Georgia experience. *The Journal of Criminal Law and Criminology (1973–), 74*(3), 661–753.

Baldwin, J. (1963). *The fire next time.* Dial Press.

Bandes, S. A. (1999). Patterns of injustice: Police brutality in the courts. *Buffalo Law Review, 47,* 1275–1341.

Bandes, S. A., Pryor, M., Kerrison, E. M., & Goff, P. A. (2019). The mismeasure of Terry stops: Assessing the psychological and emotional harms of stop and frisk to individuals and communities. *Behavioral Sciences & the Law, 37*(2), 176–194.

Banks, K. H., Kohn-Wood, L. P., & Spencer, M. (2006). An examination of the African American experience of everyday discrimination and symptoms of psychological distress. *Community Mental Health Journal*, *42*(6), 555–570.

Baptiste, N. (2014, October 13). Staggering loss of Black wealth due to subprime scandal continues unabated. *The American Prospect*. https://prospect.org/api/content/c5278216-cb68-540e-b41f-522696be117c

Baradaran, M. (2018). *The color of money*. Harvard University Press.

Barbash, E. (2017). Different types of trauma: Small "t" versus large "T". *Psychology Today*, p. 13.

Barclay, A. G., & Cusumano, D. R. (1967). Testing masculinity in boys without fathers. *Transaction*, *5*(2), 33–35.

Barclay, D. (2001, December 2). Torn from the land: The lynching trail. *The Sunday Herald-Sun* (Durham, NC), pp. Al, A3.

Bargh, J. A., & Chartrand, T. L. (1999). The unbearable automaticity of being. *American Psychologist*, *54*(7), 462–479.

Barker, D., Nalder, K., & Newham, J. (2021). Clarifying the ideological asymmetry in public attitudes toward political protest. *American Politics Research*, *49*(2), 157–170.

Barlow, M. H. (1998). Race and the problem of crime in "Time" and "Newsweek" cover stories, 1946 to 1995. *Social Justice*, *25*(2(72)), 149–183.

Barnes, D. L. (2010). Suicide. In R. L. Hampton, T. P. Gullotta, & R. L. Crowel (Eds.), *Handbook of African American health* (pp. 444–460). The Guilford Press.

Barnes, L. L., De Leon, C. F. M., Wilson, R. S., Bienias, J. L., Bennett, D. A., & Evans, D. A. (2004). Racial differences in perceived discrimination in a community population of older blacks and whites. *Journal of Aging and Health*, *16*(3), 315–337.

Baron, A. S., & Banaji, M. R. (2006). The development of implicit attitudes: Evidence of race evaluations from ages 6 and 10 and adulthood. *Psychological Science*, *17*(1), 53–58.

Bar-Tal, D., & Teichman, Y. (2005). *Stereotypes and prejudice in conflict: Representations of Arabs in Israeli Jewish society*. Cambridge University Press.

Barton, L. (2019, February 6). *The minimising of the sexual assault of Black boys*. Media Diversified. https://mediadiversified.org/2019/02/06/the-minimising-of-the-sexual-assault-of-black-boys

Baum, D. (2016, April). Legalize it all: How to win the war on drugs. *Harper's Magazine*. https://harpers.org/archive/2016/04/legalize-it-all

Bauman, J. F. (1987). *Public housing, race, and renewal: Urban planning in Philadelphia, 1920–1974*. Temple University Press.

Baumgartel, S., Guilmette, C., Kalb, J., Li, D., Nuni, J., Porter, D., & Resnik, J. (2015). *Time-in-cell: The ASCA-Liman 2014 national survey of administrative segregation in prison* (Public Law Research Paper 552). Yale Law School.

Bayer, P., & Charles, K. K. (2018). Divergent paths: A new perspective on earnings differences between Black and White men since 1940. *The Quarterly Journal of Economics*, *133*(3), 1459–1501.

Beattie, G. (2013). *Our racist heart? An exploration of unconscious prejudice in everyday life*. Routledge.

Bechteler, S., Kane-Willis, K., Butler, K., & Espinosa-Ravi, I. (2020). *An epidemic of inequities: Structural racism and COVID-19 in the Black community*. Chicago Urban League. https://chiul.org/wp-content/uploads/2020/05/ChicagoUrbanLeague_An-Epidemic-of-Inequities_5-12-20.pdf

Beck, A. J. (2015). *Use of restrictive housing in U.S. prisons and jails, 2011–12*. U.S. Bureau of Justice Statistics. www.ojp.gov/ncjrs/virtual-library/abstracts/use-restrictive-housing-us-prisons-and-jails-2011-12

Beck, A. J. (2021). *Race and ethnicity of violent crime offenders and arrestees, 2018*. U.S. Bureau of Justice Statistics. https://bjs.ojp.gov/library/publications/race-and-ethnicity-violent-crime-offenders-and-arrestees-2018

Becker, G. S. (1967). *Human capital and the personal distribution of income: An analytical approach* (No. 1). Institute of Public Administration.

Beckett, K. (1997). *Making crime pay: The politics of law and order in the contemporary United States*. Oxford University Press.

Belgrave, F. Z., & Allison, K. W. (2018). *African American psychology: From Africa to America*. Sage Publications.

Bell, C. C. (1994). Finding a way through the maze of racism. *Emerge*, *5*(11), 80.

Bell, C. C. (1996). Treatment issues for African-American men. *Psychiatric Annals, 26*(1), 33–36.

Bell, C. C., & Clark, D. C. (1998). Adolescent suicide. *Pediatric Clinics of North America, 45*(2), 365–380.

Bell, D. A. (1976). Racial remediation: An historical perspective on current conditions. *Notre Dame Law, 52*, 5–29.

Bell, D. A. (1980). Brown v. board of education and the interest-convergence dilemma. *Harvard Law Review*, 518–533.

Bell, D. A. (1988). White superiority in America: Its legal legacy, its economic costs. *Villanova Law Review, 33*, 767–779.

Bell, D. A. (1991). Racism is here to stay: Now what. *Howard Law Journal, 35*, 79–93.

Bell, D. A. (1992). Racial realism. *Connecticut Law Review, 24*(2), 363–379.

Bell, D. A. (1993). The racism is permanent thesis: Courageous revelation or unconscious denial of racial genocide. *Capital University Law Review, 22*, 571–587.

Bendick, M., Jr., Jackson, C. W., & Reinoso, V. A. (1994). Measuring employment discrimination through controlled experiments. *The Review of Black Political Economy, 23*(1), 25–48.

Bennett, G. G., Merritt, M. M., Edwards, C. L., & Sollers, J. J., III (2004). Perceived racism and affective responses to ambiguous interpersonal interactions among African American men. *American Behavioral Scientist, 47*(7), 963–976.

Bennett, G. G., Merritt, M. M., Sollers, J. J., III, Edwards, C. L., Whitfield, K. E., Brandon, D. T., & Tucker, R. D. (2004). Stress, coping, and health outcomes among African-Americans: A review of the John Henryism hypothesis. *Psychology & Health, 19*(3), 369–383.

Benson, M. L., Wooldredge, J., Thistlethwaite, A. B., & Fox, G. L. (2004). The correlation between race and domestic violence is confounded with community context. *Social Problems, 51*(3), 326–342.

Berman, M., Horwitz, S., & Lowery, W. (2016, February 11). Justice department sues the city of Ferguson to force policing reform. *Washington Post*. www.washingtonpost.com/news/post-nation/wp/2016/02/10/ferguson-demands-changes-to-agreement-reforming-police-tactics-justice-dept-criticizes-unnecessary-delay

Bertrand, M., & Mullainathan, S. (2004). Are Emily and Greg more employable than Lakisha and Jamal? A field experiment on labor market discrimination. *American Economic Review, 94*(4), 991–1013.

Bhattacharyya, G. (2009). *Dangerous Brown men: Exploiting sex, violence and feminism in the "war on terror".* Bloomsbury Publishing.

Bialik, C. (2017, January 21). How unconscious sexism could help explain Trump's win. *FiveThirtyEight*. https://fivethirtyeight.com/features/how-unconscious-sexism-could-help-explain-trumps-win

Biddle, S. (2020, July 9). Police surveilled George Floyd protests with help from twitter-affiliated startup Dataminr. *The Intercept*. https://theintercept.com/2020/07/09/twitter-dataminr-police-spy-surveillance-black-lives-matter-protests

Biddle, S. (2021, April 22). U. S. Marshals used drones to spy on Black lives matter protests in Washington, DC. *The Intercept*. https://theintercept.com/2021/04/22/drones-black-lives-matter-protests-marshals

Binion, B. (2021, May 25). Baton Rouge cops strip-searched a minor during a traffic stop and entered a family's home without a warrant: The city just settled for $35,000. *Reason.Com*. https://reason.com/2021/05/25/baton-rouge-cops-strip-searched-minor-traffic-stop-ken-camallo-clarence-green

Binswanger, I. A., Stern, M. F., Deyo, R. A., Heagerty, P. J., Cheadle, A., Elmore, J. G., & Koepsell, T. D. (2007). Release from prison – a high risk of death for former inmates. *New England Journal of Medicine, 356*(2), 157–165.

Bird, C. (1968). *Born female: The high cost of keeping women down*. Pocket Book.

Bishop, J. H. (1980). Jobs, cash transfers and marital instability: A review and synthesis of the evidence. *Journal of Human Resources*, 301–334.

Blackburn, E. H., Epel, E. S., & Lin, J. (2015). Human telomere biology: A contributory and interactive factor in aging, disease risks, and protection. *Science, 350*, 1193–1198.

Blackmon, D. A. (2008). *Slavery by another name: The re-enslavement of Black Americans from the civil war to world war II*. Anchor.

Blair, I. V. (2002). The malleability of automatic stereotypes and prejudice. *Personality and Social Psychology Review, 6*(3), 242–261.

Blake, J. (2020, May 27). There's one epidemic we may never find a vaccine for: Fear of Black men in public spaces. *CNN*. www.cnn.com/2020/05/26/us/fear-black-men-blake/index.html

Blau, F. D., & Graham, J. W. (1990). Black-White differences in wealth and asset composition. *The Quarterly Journal of Economics, 105*(2), 321–339.

Blau, P. M., & Duncan, O. D. (1967). *The American occupational structure*. John Wiley & Sons.

Blaut, J. M. (1992). The theory of cultural racism. *Antipode, 24*(4), 289–299.

Blee, K. M. (2008). *Women of the Klan: Racism and gender in the 1920s*. University of California Press.

Blee, K. M., & Tickamyer, A. R. (1995). Racial differences in men's attitudes about women's gender roles. *Journal of Marriage and the Family*, 21–30.

Blumenbach, J. F., & Bendyshe, T. (1865). *The anthropological treatises of Johann Friedrich Blumenbach*. Anthropological Society.

Blumstein, A. (1982). On the racial disproportionality of United States' prison populations. *Journal of Criminal Law & Criminology, 73*, 1259–1281.

Blumstein, A. (1993). Making rationality relevant: The American society of criminology 1992 presidential address. *Criminology, 31*(1), 1–16.

Blumstein, A., & Beck, A. J. (1999). Population growth in US prisons, 1980–1996. *Crime and Justice, 26*, 17–61.

Blustein, D. L. (2008). The role of work in psychological health and well-being: A conceptual, historical, and public policy perspective. *American Psychologist, 63*(4), 228–240.

Bobo, L., & Thompson, V. (2010). Racialized mass incarceration: Poverty, prejudice and punishment. In H. R. Markus & P. M. Moya (Eds.), *Doing race: 21 essays for the 21st century* (pp. 322–355). W. W. Norton & Company.

Bolger, E. (1999). Grounded theory analysis of emotional pain. *Psychotherapy Research, 9*(3), 342–362.

Bonastia, C. (2015, June). Low-hanging fruit: The impoverished history of housing and school desegregation. *Sociological Forum, 30*, 549–570.

Bond, M. J., & Herman, A. A. (2016). Lagging life expectancy for Black men: A public health imperative. *American Journal of Public Health, 106*(7), 1167–1169.

Bonilla-Silva, E. (2001). *White supremacy and racism in the post-civil rights era*. Lynne Rienner Publishers.

Bonilla-Silva, E. (2006). *Racism without racists: Color-blind racism and the persistence of racial inequality in the United States*. Rowman & Littlefield Publishers.

Bonilla-Silva, E., Goar, C., & Embrick, D. G. (2006). When Whites flock together: The social psychology of White habitus. *Critical Sociology, 32*(2–3), 229–253.

Boone, M. L., Neumeister, D. W., & Charney, C. L. (2003). Neurobiological mechanisms of psychological trauma. In R. J. Usano & A. E. Norwood (Eds.), *Trauma and disaster: Responses and management* (pp. 1–30). American Psychiatric Publishing.

Bor, J., Venkataramani, A. S., Williams, D. R., & Tsai, A. C. (2018). Police killings and their spillover effects on the mental health of Black Americans: A population-based, quasi-experimental study. *The Lancet, 392*(10144), 302–310.

Borgman, A. (2019). *Commodity racism, cultural appropriation, and the perpetuation of oppressive food discourse: A thesis* [Doctoral dissertation, Oregon Health & Science University].

Borjas, G. J., Freeman, R. B., & Katz, L. F. (1991). *On the labor market effects of immigration and trade*.

Borrell, L. N., Kiefe, C. I., Williams, D. R., Diez-Roux, A. V., & Gordon-Larsen, P. (2006). Self-reported health perceived racial discrimination, and skin color in African Americans in the CARDIA study. *Social Science & Medicine, 63*(6), 1415–1427.

Bound, J., & Holzer, H. J. (1991). *Industrial shifts, skills levels, and the labor market for White and Black males*. National Bureau of Economic Research.

Bovell-Ammon, B. J., Xuan, Z., Paasche-Orlow, M. K., & LaRochelle, M. R. (2021). Association of incarceration with mortality by race from a national longitudinal cohort study. *JAMA Network Open, 4*(12), e2133083.

Bowser, B. P. (1991). *Black male adolescents: Parenting and education in community context*. University Press of America.

Bowser, B. P. (2017). Racism: Origin and theory. *Journal of Black Studies*, *48*(6), 572–590.

Boyd, H., & Allen, R. L. (1995). *Brotherman: The odyssey of Black men in America – an anthology*. One World/ Ballantine.

Bracic, A., Israel-Trummel, M., & Shortle, A. F. (2019). Is sexism for White people? Gender stereotypes, race, and the 2016 presidential election. *Political Behavior*, *41*(2), 281–307.

Brame, R., Bushway, S. D., Paternoster, R., & Turner, M. G. (2014). Demographic patterns of cumulative arrest prevalence by ages 18 and 23. *Crime & Delinquency*, *60*(3), 471–486.

Brandt, A. M. (1978). Racism and research: The case of the Tuskegee syphilis study. *Hastings Center Report*, 21–29.

Brayne, S. (2020). *Predict and surveil: Data, discretion, and the future of policing*. Oxford University Press.

Brehm, J. W. (1966). *A theory of psychological reactance*. Academic Press.

Breiding, M. J., Chen, J., & Black, M. C. (2014). *Intimate partner violence in the United States – 2010*. National Center for Injury Prevention and Control, Centers for Disease Control and Prevention.

Breslau, N. (2001). The epidemiology of posttraumatic stress disorder: What is the extent of the problem? *Journal of Clinical Psychiatry*, *62*, 16–22.

Brewin, C. R. (2020). Complex post-traumatic stress disorder: A new diagnosis in ICD-11. *BJPsych Advances*, *26*(3), 145–152.

Bridge, J. A., Asti, L., Horowitz, L. M., Greenhouse, J. B., Fontanella, C. A., Sheftall, A. H., Kelleher, K. J., & Campo, J. V. (2015). Suicide trends among elementary school – aged children in the United States from 1993 to 2012. *JAMA Pediatrics*, *169*(7), 673–677.

Bridge, J. A., Horowitz, L. M., Fontanella, C. A., Sheftall, A. H., Greenhouse, J., Kelleher, K. J., & Campo, J. V. (2018). Age-related racial disparity in suicide rates among US youths from 2001 through 2015. *JAMA Pediatrics*, *172*(7), 697–699.

Briere, J. N., & Scott, C. (2014). *Principles of trauma therapy: A guide to symptoms, evaluation, and treatment (DSM-5 update)*. Sage Publications.

Bright, S. B. (1995). The death penalty as the answer to crime: Costly, counterproductive and corrupting. *Santa Clara Law Review*, *36*, 1069–1096.

Britton, T. (2019). *Does locked up mean locked out? The effects of the anti-drug act of 1986 on Black male students' college enrollment*. University of California.

Britt-Spells, A. M., Slebodnik, M., Sands, L. P., & Rollock, D. (2018). Effects of perceived discrimination on depressive symptoms among Black men residing in the United States: A meta-analysis. *American Journal of Men's Health*, *12*(1), 52–63.

Brody, E. B. (1961). Social conflict and schizophrenic behavior in young adult Negro males. *Psychiatry*, *24*(4), 337–346.

Broeck, S. (2011). Re-reading de Beauvoir after race: Woman-as-slave revisited. *International Journal of Francophone Studies*, *14*(1–2), 167–184.

Broman, C. L. (1996). The health consequences of racial discrimination: A study of African Americans. *Ethnicity & Disease*, *6*(1–2), 148–153.

Broman, C. L., Mavaddat, R., & Hsu, S. Y. (2000). The experience and consequences of perceived racial discrimination: A study of African Americans. *Journal of Black Psychology*, *26*(2), 165–180.

Bromberg, W., & Simon, F. (1968). The protest psychosis: A special type of reactive psychosis. *Archives of General Psychiatry*, *19*(2), 155–160.

Brondolo, E., Libby, D. J., Denton, E.-G., Thompson, S., Beatty, D. L., Schwartz, J., & Gerin, W. (2008). Racism and ambulatory blood pressure in a community sample. *Psychosomatic Medicine*, *70*(1), 49–56.

Brooks, S. K., & Greenberg, N. (2021). Psychological impact of being wrongfully accused of criminal offences: A systematic literature review. *Medicine, Science and the Law*, *61*(1), 44–54.

Brophy, A. (2002). *Reconstructing the dreamland: The Tulsa Riot in 1921*. Oxford University Press.

Brown, E. M. (2003). *The condemnation of Little B: New age racism in America*. Beacon Press.

Brown, E. M. (2016, June 23). *Why Black homeowners are more likely to be Caribbean-American than African-American in New York: A theory of how early West Indian migrants broke racial cartels in housing* (GWU Legal Studies Research Paper No. 2016-23). GWU.

Brown, G. A. (2004). Gender as a factor in the response of the law-enforcement system to violence against partners. *Sexuality and Culture*, *8*(3), 3–139.

Brown, T. N. (2001). Measuring self-perceived racial and ethnic discrimination in social surveys. *Sociological Spectrum, 21*(3), 377–392.

Browne, S. (2015). *Dark matters*. Duke University Press.

Brownmiller, S. (1975). *Against our will: Men, women and rape*. Simon & Schuster.

Brunkard, J., Namulanda, G., & Ratard, R. (2008). Hurricane Katrina deaths, Louisiana, 2005. *Disaster Medicine and Public Health Preparedness, 2*(4), 215–223.

Bryant-Davis, T. (2007). Healing requires recognition: The case for race-based traumatic stress. *The Counseling Psychologist, 35*(1), 135–143.

Bryant-Davis, T., & Ocampo, C. (2005). Racist incident – based trauma. *The Counseling Psychologist, 33*(4), 479–500.

Buck, P. D. (2001). *Worked to the bone: Race, class, power, and privilege in Kentucky*. Monthly Review Press.

Bulhan, H. A. (1985). *Frantz Fanon and the psychology of oppression*. Plenum Press.

Bumiller, K. (2008). *In an abusive state*. Duke University Press.

Buolamwini, J., & Gebru, T. (2018, January). Gender shades: Intersectional accuracy disparities in commercial gender classification. In *Conference on fairness, accountability and transparency* (pp. 77–91). PMLR.

Burd-Sharps, S., Lewis, K., & Martins, E. B. (2008). *The measure of America: American human development report, 2008–2009*. Social Science Research Council.

Butler, P. (2013). Black male exceptionalism? The problems and potential of Black male-focused interventions. *Du Bois Review: Social Science Research on Race, 10*(2), 485–511.

Buxton, J. L., Suderman, M., Pappas, J. J., Borghol, N., McArdle, W., Blakemore, A. I., Hertzman, C., Power, C., Szyf, M., & Pembrey, M. (2014). Human leukocyte telomere length is associated with DNA methylation levels in multiple subtelomeric and imprinted loci. *Scientific Reports, 4*(1), 1–8.

Byars-Winston, A., Fouad, N., & Wen, Y. (2015). Race/ethnicity and sex in US occupations, 1970–2010: Implications for research, practice, and policy. *Journal of Vocational Behavior, 87*, 54–70.

Bynum, B. (2000). Discarded diagnoses. *The Lancet, 356*(9241), 1615.

Byrne, K. (2016). The tautology of blackface and the objectification of racism: A "how-to" guide. *The European Legacy, 21*(7), 664–674.

Caetano, R., Ramisetty-Mikler, S., & Field, C. A. (2005). Unidirectional and bidirectional intimate partner violence among White, Black, and Hispanic couples in the United States. *Violence and Victims, 20*(4), 393–406.

Callimachi, R. (2020, July 6). Breonna Taylor's family claims she was alive after shooting but given no aid. *The New York Times*. www.nytimes.com/2020/07/06/us/breonna-taylor-lawsuit-claims.html

Camp, N. P., Voigt, R., Jurafsky, D., & Eberhardt, J. L. (2021). The thin blue waveform: Racial disparities in officer prosody undermine institutional trust in the police. *Journal of Personality and Social Psychology, 121*(6), 1157–1171.

Camp, S. M. (1998). *Viragos: Enslaved women's everyday politics in the Old South*. University of Pennsylvania.

Campbell, S. (2022, April 4). Black lives matter secretly bought a $6 million house. *Intelligencer*. https://nymag.com/intelligencer/2022/04/black-lives-matter-6-million-dollar-house.html

Capps, K., & Cannon, C. (2021, March 15). *Redlined, now flooding: Maps of historic housing discrimination show how neighborhoods that suffered redlining in the 1930s face a far higher risk of flooding today*. www.bloomberg.com/tosv2.html?vid=&uuid=eb07f4a4-a8d9-11ec-8c35-4370715a6871&url=L2dyYXBoaWNzLzIwMjEtZmxvb2Qtcmlzay1yZWRsaW5pbmctP3NybmQ9Y2l0eWxhYiZTY-19jaWQ9YjMxMWNlNDY0MCZtY2tZ19laWQ9NjFiNzc5ZGQzZQ==

Carbado, D. W., Crenshaw, K. W., Mays, V. M., & Tomlinson, B. (2013). Intersectionality: Mapping the movements of a theory. *Du Bois Review: Social Science Research on Race, 10*(2), 303–312.

Card, D., & DiNardo, J. E. (2002). Skill-biased technological change and rising wage inequality: Some problems and puzzles. *Journal of Labor Economics, 20*(4), 733–783.

Carlson, E. B. (1997). *Trauma assessments: A clinician's guide*. Guilford Press.

Carnell, Y. (2021, February 1). *Reparations: A transformative Black agenda*. www.youtube.com/watch?v=W0Em0lLq9FY

Carson, E. A. (2018). *Prisoners in 2016*. U.S. Bureau of Justice Statistics. https://bjs.ojp.gov/library/publications/prisoners-2016

Carter, R. T. (2007). Racism and psychological and emotional injury: Recognizing and assessing race-based traumatic stress. *The Counseling Psychologist, 35*(1), 13–105.

Carter, R. T., & Forsyth, J. M. (2009). A guide to the forensic assessment of race-based traumatic stress reactions. *Journal of the American Academy of Psychiatry and the Law, 37*(1), 28–40.

Carter, R. T., & Forsyth, J. M. (2010). Reactions to racial discrimination: Emotional stress and help-seeking behaviors. *Psychological Trauma: Theory, Research, Practice, and Policy, 2*(3), 183–191.

Carter, R. T., Forsyth, J. M., Mazzula, S., & Williams, B. (2005). Racial discrimination and race-based traumatic stress. In R. T. Carter (Ed.), *Handbook of racial – cultural psychology and counseling: Training and practice* (Vol. 2, pp. 447–476). Wiley.

Carter, R. T., & Helms, J. E. (2002, September). *Racial discrimination and harassment: A race based traumatic stress disorder.* Paper presented at the American College of Forensic Examiners Conference, Orlando, FL.

Carter, R. T., Johnson, V. E., Roberson, K., Mazzula, S. L., Kirkinis, K., & Sant-Barket, S. (2017a). Race-based traumatic stress, racial identity statuses, and psychological functioning: An exploratory investigation. *Professional Psychology: Research and Practice, 48*(1), 30–37.

Carter, R. T., Lau, M. Y., Johnson, V., & Kirkinis, K. (2017b). Racial discrimination and health outcomes among racial/ethnic minorities: A meta-analytic review. *Journal of Multicultural Counseling and Development, 45*(4), 232–259.

Carter, R. T., Mazzula, S., Victoria, R., Vazquez, R., Hall, S., Smith, S., Sant-Barket, S., Forsyth, J., Bazelais, K., & Williams, B. (2013). Initial development of the race-based traumatic stress symptom scale: Assessing the emotional impact of racism. *Psychological Trauma: Theory, Research, Practice, and Policy, 5*(1), 1–9.

Carter, R. T., & Pieterse, A. L. (2005). Race: A social and psychological analysis of the term and its meaning. In R. T. Carter (Ed.), *Handbook of racial – cultural psychology and counseling: Theory and research* (Vol. 1, pp. 41–63). Wiley.

Carter, R. T., & Pieterse, A. L. (2020). *Measuring the effects of racism.* Columbia University Press.

Carter, R. T., & Sant-Barket, S. M. (2015). Assessment of the impact of racial discrimination and racism: How to use the race-based traumatic stress symptom scale in practice. *Traumatology, 21*(1), 32–39.

Casas, J. M. (2005). Race and racism: The efforts of counseling psychology to understand and address the issues associated with these terms. *The Counseling Psychologist, 33*(4), 501–512.

Castelli, L., Zogmaister, C., & Tomelleri, S. (2009). The transmission of racial attitudes within the family. *Developmental Psychology, 45*(2), 586–591.

Castillo, L. G. D. (2018). Unconscious racial prejudice as psychological resistance: A limitation of the implicit bias model. *Critical Philosophy of Race, 6*(2), 262–279.

Cavalli-Sforza, L. L., Cavalli-Sforza, L., Menozzi, P., & Piazza, A. (1994). *The history and geography of human genes.* Princeton University Press.

Cazenave, N. A. (1979). Middle-income Black fathers: An analysis of the provider role. *Family Coordinator*, 583–593.

Cazenave, N. A. (1983). Black male-Black female relationships: The perceptions of 155 middle-class Black men. *Family Relations*, 341–350.

CDC. (1998). Suicide among Black youths – United States, 1980–1995. *MMWR: Morbidity and Mortality Weekly Report, 47*(10), 193–196.

CDC. (2019). *Cases of Coronavirus disease (COVID-19) in the U.S.* www.cdc.gov/coronavirus/2019-ncov/casesupdates/cases-in-us.html

CDC. (2020). https://www.cdc.gov/nchs/data/nvsr/nvsr72/nvsr72-10.pdf

CDC. (2021, November 24). *Racism and health.* Centers for Disease Control and Prevention. www.cdc.gov/healthequity/racism-disparities/index.html

Cebul, B. (2020, July 22). Tearing down Black America. *Boston Review.* https://bostonreview.net/articles/brent-cebul-tearing-down-black-america

Cell, J. W. (1982). *The highest stage of White supremacy.* Cambridge University Press.

Césaire, A. (1955). *Discourse on colonialism.* Présence Africaine.

Chachere, G., & Chachere, B. (1990). An illustrative estimate: The present value of the benefits from racial discrimination, 1929–1969. In R. F. America (Ed.), *The wealth of races: The present value of benefits from past injustices* (pp. 163–168). Greenwood.

Chae, D. H., Clouston, S., Hatzenbuehler, M. L., Kramer, M. R., Cooper, H. L., Wilson, S. M., Stephens-Davidowitz, S. I., Gold, R. S., & Link, B. G. (2015). Association between an internet-based measure of area racism and Black mortality. *PLOS One, 10*(4), e0122963.

Chae, D. H., Lincoln, K. D., Adler, N. E., & Syme, S. L. (2010). Do experiences of racial discrimination predict cardiovascular disease among African American men? The moderating role of internalized negative racial group attitudes. *Social Science & Medicine, 71*(6), 1182–1188.

Chae, D. H., Nuru-Jeter, A. M., Adler, N. E., Brody, G. H., Lin, J., Blackburn, E. H., & Epel, E. S. (2014). Discrimination, racial bias, and telomere length in African-American men. *American Journal of Preventive Medicine, 46*(2), 103–111.

Chae, D. H., Nuru-Jeter, A. M., Lincoln, K. D., & Francis, D. D. (2011). Conceptualizing racial disparities in health: Advancement of a socio-psychobiological approach. *Du Bois Review: Social Science Research on Race, 8*(1), 63–77.

Chae, D. H., Wang, Y., Martz, C. D., Slopen, N., Yip, T., Adler, N. E., Fuller-Rowell, T. E., Lin, J., Matthews, K. A., Brody, G. H., Spears, E. C., Puterman, E., & Epel, E. S. (2020). Racial discrimination and telomere shortening among African Americans: The coronary artery risk development in young adults (CARDIA) study. *Health Psychology, 39*(3), 209–219.

Chae, D. H., Yip, T., Martz, C. D., Chung, K., Richeson, J. A., Hajat, A., Curtis, D. S., Rogers, L. O., & LaVeist, T. A. (2021). Vicarious racism and vigilance during the COVID-19 pandemic: Mental health implications among Asian and Black Americans. *Public Health Reports, 136*(4), 508–517.

Chapleau, K. M., Oswald, D. L., & Russell, B. L. (2008). Male rape myths: The role of gender, violence, and sexism. *Journal of Interpersonal Violence, 23*(5), 600–615.

Charles, C. Z. (2003). The dynamics of racial residential segregation. *Annual Review of Sociology, 29*(1), 167–207.

Charles, K. K., & Luoh, M. C. (2010). Male incarceration, the marriage market, and female outcomes. *The Review of Economics and Statistics, 92*(3), 614–627.

Cherkas, L. F., Aviv, A., Valdes, A. M., Hunkin, J. L., Gardner, J. P., Surdulescu, G. L., Kimura, M., & Spector, T. D. (2006). The effects of social status on biological aging as measured by White-blood-cell telomere length. *Aging Cell, 5*(5), 361–365.

Chetty, R., Hendren, N., Jones, M. R., & Porter, S. R. (2018). *Race and economic opportunity in the United States* (Working Paper 24441). NBER.

Chew, P. K., & Kelley, R. E. (2006). Unwrapping racial harassment law. *Berkeley Journal of Employment and Labor Law, 27*, 49–110.

Chin, E. (2015). Commodity racism. In *The Wiley Blackwell encyclopedia of consumption and consumer studies* (pp. 1–2). Wiley.

Chiricos, T., & Eschholz, S. (2002). The racial and ethnic typification of crime and the criminal typification of race and ethnicity in local television news. *Journal of Research in Crime and Delinquency, 39*(4), 400–420.

Chiricos, T., Welch, K., & Gertz, M. (2004). Racial typification of crime and support for punitive measures. *Criminology, 42*(2), 358–390.

Chisom, R., & Washington, M. H. (1997). *Undoing racism: A philosophy of international social change*. People's Institute Press.

Cho, H., & Wilke, D. J. (2010). Gender differences in the nature of the intimate partner violence and effects of perpetrator arrest on revictimization. *Journal of Family Violence, 25*(4), 393–400.

Cho, S. K., Crenshaw, K. W., & McCall, L. (2013). Toward a field of intersectionality studies: Theory, applications, and praxis. *Signs: Journal of Women in Culture and Society, 38*(4), 785–810.

Cho, S. K., Wilson, B. D. M., & Mallory, C. (2021, January). *Black LGBT adults in the US*. Williams Institute. https://williamsinstitute.law.ucla.edu/publications/black-lgbt-adults-in-the-us

Chou, T., Asnaani, A., & Hofmann, S. G. (2012). Perception of racial discrimination and psychopathology across three U.S. ethnic minority groups. *Cultural Diversity and Ethnic Minority Psychology, 18*, 74–81.

Christ, N. M., Contractor, A. A., Wang, X., & Elhai, J. D. (2020). The mediating effect of rumination between posttraumatic stress disorder symptoms and anger reactions. *Psychological Trauma: Theory, Research, Practice, and Policy, 12*(6), 619–626.

Chung, A., Hurley, L., Januta, A., Botts, J., & Dowdell, J. (2020, August 25). Shot by cops, thwarted by judges and geography. *Reuters*. www.reuters.com/investigates/special-report/usa-police-immunity-variations

Clark, R., Anderson, N., Clark, V. R., & Williams, D. R. (1999). Racism as a stressor for African Americans: A biopsychosocial model. *American Psychologist, 54*, 805–816.

Clear, T. R. (2008). The effects of high imprisonment rates on communities. *Crime and Justice, 37*(1), 97–132.

Cleaver, E. (1968). *Soul on ice*. Dell.

Cloitre, M., Stolbach, B. C., Herman, J. L., Van der Kolk, B., Pynoos, R., Wang, J., & Petkova, E. (2009). A developmental approach to complex PTSD: Childhood and adult cumulative trauma as predictors of symptom complexity. *Journal of Traumatic Stress, 22*(5), 399–408.

Cloward, R. A., & Piven, F. F. (1971). *Regulating the poor: The functions of public welfare*. Pantheon Books.

Coates, T.-N. (2014, May 22). The case for reparations. *The Atlantic*. www.theatlantic.com/magazine/archive/2014/06/the-case-for-reparations/361631

Cobbina, J. E., Conteh, M., & Emrich, C. (2019). Race, gender, and responses to the police among Ferguson residents and protesters. *Race and Justice, 9*(3), 276–303.

Cohen, J. I. (2000). Stress and mental health: A biobehavioral perspective. *Issues in Mental Health Nursing, 21*(2), 185–202.

Coles, S. M., & Pasek, J. (2020). Intersectional invisibility revisited: How group prototypes lead to the erasure and exclusion of Black women. *Translational Issues in Psychological Science, 6*(4), 314–324.

Conley, D. (2010). *Being Black, living in the red: Race, wealth, and social policy in America*. University of California Press.

Connell, R. (1987). *Gender and power: Society, the person and sexual politics*. Stanford University Press.

Connell, R. W. (2005). *Masculinities*. Polity. (Original work published 1995)

Connor, P., Weeks, M., Glaser, J., Chen, S., & Keltner, D. (2023). Intersectional implicit bias: Evidence for asymmetrically compounding bias and the predominance of target gender. *Journal of Personality and Social Psychology, 124*(1), 22–48.

Constantine, M. G., Smith, L., Redington, R. M., & Owens, D. (2008). Racial microaggressions against Black counseling and counseling psychology faculty: A central challenge in the multicultural counseling movement. *Journal of Counseling & Development, 86*(3), 348–355.

Cook, P. W. (2009). *Abused men: The hidden side of domestic violence*. ABC-CLIO.

Cooper, B. (2021, May–July 25). Who actually gets to create Black pop culture? *Current Affairs*. www.currentaffairs.org/2021/07/who-actually-gets-to-create-black-pop-culture

Cooper, F. R. (2005). Against bipolar Black masculinity: Intersectionality, assimilation, identity performance, and hierarchy. *UC Davis Law Review, 39*, 853–906.

Cooper, H. L. (2015). War on drugs policing and police brutality. *Substance Use & Misuse, 50*(8–9), 1188–1194.

Cooper, R., & Bruenig, M. (2017). *Foreclosed: Destruction of Black wealth during the Obama presidency*. People's Policy Project. www.peoplespolicyproject.org/wp-content/uploads/2017/12/Foreclosed.pdf

Cooper, S. (2020, October 6). Is Warren Buffett funding Black lives matter? *Tablet Magazine*. www.tabletmag.com/sections/news/articles/warren-buffett-black-lives-matter

Corley, C. (2013, October 3). Wisconsin prisons incarcerate most Black men in U.S. *NPR*. www.npr.org/sections/codeswitch/2013/10/03/228733846/wisconsin-prisons-incarcerate-most-black-men-in-u-s

Cornish, A., Donevan, C., & Bior, A. (2021, October 11). Facebook is under new scrutiny for it's role in Ethiopia's conflict. *NPR*. www.npr.org/2021/10/11/1045084676/facebook-is-under-new-scrutiny-for-its-role-in-ethiopias-conflict

Correll, J., Park, B., Judd, C. M., & Wittenbrink, B. (2002). The police officer's dilemma: Using ethnicity to disambiguate potentially threatening individuals. *Journal of Personality and Social Psychology, 83*(6), 1314–1329.

Correll, J., Park, B., Judd, C. M., Wittenbrink, B., Sadler, M. S., & Keesee, T. (2007). Across the thin blue line: Police officers and racial bias in the decision to shoot. *Journal of Personality and Social Psychology*, *92*(6), 1006–1023.

Correll, J., Wittenbrink, B., Park, B., Judd, C. M., & Goyle, A. (2011). Dangerous enough: Moderating racial bias with contextual threat cues. *Journal of Experimental Social Psychology*, *47*(1), 184–189.

Corrigan, L. M. (2020). *Black feelings: Race and affect in the long sixties*. University Press of Mississippi.

Cox, O. C. (1940). Sex ratio and marital status among Negroes. *American Sociological Review*, *5*(6), 937–947.

Coxell, A. W., & King, M. B. (2010). Adult male rape and sexual assault: Prevalence, re-victimisation and the tonic immobility response. *Sexual and Relationship Therapy*, *25*(4), 372–379.

Craemer, T., Smith, T., Harrison, B., Logan, T., Bellamy, W., & Darity, W. A., Jr. (2020). Wealth implications of slavery and racial discrimination for African American descendants of the enslaved. *The Review of Black Political Economy*, *47*(3), 218–254.

Craigie, T. A., Myers, S. L., & Darity, W. A. (2018). Racial differences in the effect of marriageable males on female family headship. *Journal of Demographic Economics*, *84*(3), 231–256.

Crenshaw, K. (1989). Demarginalizing the intersection of race and sex: A Black feminist critique of antidiscrimination doctrine, feminist theory and antiracist politics. *University of Chicago Legal Forum*, 139–167.

Crenshaw, K. (1991). Mapping the margins: Identity politics, intersectionality, and violence against women. *Stanford Law Review*, *43*(6), 1241–1299.

Crenshaw, K. W. (2010). Close encounters of three kinds: On teaching dominance feminism and intersectionality. *Tulsa Law Review*, 46(1), 151–189.

Crockford, K. (2020, June 16). *How is face recognition surveillance technology racist?* ACLU of Oregon. www.aclu-or.org/en/news/how-face-recognition-surveillance-technology-racist

Crosby, A. E., & Molock, S. D. (2006). Introduction: Suicidal behaviors in the African American community. *Journal of Black Psychology*, *32*(3), 253–261.

Cross, W. E., Jr. (1971). The Negro-to-Black conversion experience. *Black World*, *20*(9), 13–27.

Cross, W. E., Jr. (1991). *Shades of Black: Diversity in African-American identity*. Temple University Press.

Cross, W. E., Jr., & Vandiver, B. J. (2001). Nigrescence theory and measurement: Introducing the cross racial identity scale (CRIS). In J. G. Ponterotto, J. M. Casas, L. A. Suzuki, & C. M. Alexander (Eds.), *Handbook of multicultural counseling* (2nd ed., pp. 371–393). Sage Publications.

Crowder, A. (2014). *Opening the door: A treatment model for therapy with male survivors of sexual abuse*. Routledge.

Cruse, H. (1967). *The crisis of the Negro intellectual: A historical analysis of the failure of Black leadership*. Quill.

Crutchfield, R. D., Skinner, M. L., Haggerty, K. P., McGlynn, A., & Catalano, R. F. (2012). Racial disparity in police contacts. *Race and Justice*, *2*(3), 179–202.

Cullen, J. (2018, July 20). *The history of mass incarceration | Brennan center for justice*. www.brennancenter.org/our-work/analysis-opinion/history-mass-incarceration

Curry, T. J. (2014). Michael Brown and the need for a genre study of Black male death and dying. *Theory & Event*, *17*(3).

Curry, T. J. (2017a). *The man-not: Race, class, genre and the dilemmas of Black manhood*. Temple University Press.

Curry, T. J. (2017b). This nigger's broken: Hyper-masculinity, the buck, and the role of physical disability in White anxiety toward the Black male body. *Journal of Social Philosophy*, *48*(3), 321–343.

Curry, T. J. (2018). Killing boogeymen: Phallicism and the misandric mischaracterizations of Black males in theory. *Res Philosophica*, *95*(2), 235–272.

Curry, T. J. (2019). Expendables for whom: Terry Crews and the erasure of Black male victims of sexual assault and rape. *Women Studies in Communication*, *42*(3), 287–307.

Curry, T. J. (2020). Conditioned for death: Analysing Black mortalities from covid-19 and police killings in the United States as a syndemic interaction. *Comparative American Studies an International Journal*, *17*(3–4), 257–270.

Curry, T. J. (2021a, April). II – must there be an empirical basis for the theorization of racialized subjects in race-gender theory? In *Proceedings of the Aristotelian society* (Vol. 121, No. 1, pp. 21–44). Oxford University Press.

Curry, T. J. (2021b). Decolonizing the intersection: Black Male studies as a critique of intersectionality's indebtedness to subculture of violence theory. In R. Beshara (Ed.), *Critical psychology praxis* (pp. 132–154). Routledge.

Curry, T. J. (2021c). George Floyd, Jr. as a philosophical problem: Why disaggregated data should guide how philosophers theorize Black male death. *The Harvard Review of Philosophy, 28*, 171–191.

Curry, T. J. (2021d). He never mattered: Poor Black males and the dark logic of intersectional invisibility. In B. Hogan, M. Cholbi, A. Madva, & B. S. Yost (Eds.), *The movement for Black lives: Philosophical perspectives* (pp. 59–89). Oxford University Press.

Curry, T. J. (2021e). He wasn't man enough: Black Male studies and the ethnological targeting of Black men in 19th century suffragist thought. In J. R. Davidson (Ed.), *African American studies* (2nd ed., pp. 209–224). Edinburgh University Press.

Curry, T. J. (2021g). Thinking through the silence: Theorizing the rape of Jewish males during the Holocaust through survivor testimonies. *Holocaust Studies, 27*(4), 447–472.

Curry, T. J. (2022a). Disaggregating death: George Floyd and the significance of Black Male Mortality in police encounters. In G. Yancy (Ed.), *Black Men from behind the Veil: An Ontological Interrogation* (pp. 65–79). Lexington Books.

Curry, T. J. (2022b). Reconstituting the object: Black Male studies and the problem of studying Black men and boys within gender theory. In S. A. Tate (Ed.), *Palgrave handbook on critical race and gender* (pp. 525–544). Palgrave Macmillan.

Curry, T. J. (2023a). Feminism as racist backlash: How racism drove the development of nineteenth- and twentieth-century feminist theory. In A. Deshpande (Ed.), *Handbook on economics of discrimination and affirmative action* (pp. 869–895). Springer.

Curry, T. J. (2023b). He didn't want any of that: Considerations in the study and theorization of Black boys' sexual victimization in the United States. In A. K. Gill & H. Begum (Eds.), *Child sexual abuse in Black and minoritised communities* (pp. 273–301). Palgrave Macmillan.

Curry, T. J., & Curry, G. (2018). Taking it to the people: Translating empirical findings about Black men and Black families through a Black public philosophy. *Dewey Studies, 2*(1), 42–71.

Curry, T. J., & Curry, G. (2020). Critical race theory and the demography of death and dying: Crit. In V. L. Farmer & E. S. W. Farmer (Eds.), *Critical race theory in the academy* (pp. 89–106). Information Age Publishing, Inc.

Curry, T. J., & Utley, E. A. (2018). She touched me: Five snapshots of adult sexual. *Kennedy Institute of Ethics Journal, 28*(2), 205–241.

Curry, T. J., & Utley, E. A. (2020). She's just a friend (with benefits). In M. C. Hopson & M. Petin (Eds.), *Reimagining Black masculinities: Race, gender, and public space* (pp. 33–52). Lexington Books.

Curtis, J. W. (2014). *The employment status of instructional staff members in higher education, Fall 2011* (pp. 54–55). American Association of University Professors.

Curtis, L. A. (1975). *Violence, race, and culture.* Lexington Books.

Cutler, D. M., & Glaeser, E. L. (1997). Are ghettos good or bad? *The Quarterly Journal of Economics, 112*(3), 827–872.

Dailey, J. E. (2000). *Before Jim Crow: The politics of race in post emancipation Virginia.* University of North Carolina Press.

Daniels, J. L. (2021, December 5). Opinion | as a Black man in America, I feel death looming every day. *The New York Times.* www.nytimes.com/2021/12/05/opinion/culture/virgil-abloh-black-mortality.html

Darity, W. A., Jr. (1980). Illusions of Black economic progress. *The Review of Black Political Economy, 10*(2), 153–168.

Darity, W. A., Jr. (1988). What's left of the economic theory of discrimination? In S. Shulman & W. Darity Jr. (Eds.), *The question of discrimination: Racial inequality in the US labor market* (pp. 335–374). University of North Carolina Press.

Darity, W. A., Jr. (1989). What's left of the economic theory of discrimination? In S. Shulman & W. Darity (Eds.), *The question of discrimination: Racial inequality in the US labor market* (pp. 335–374). Wesleyan University Press.

Darity, W. A., Jr. (1999). Who loses from unemployment. *Journal of Economic Issues, 33*(2), 491–496.

Darity, W. A., Jr. (2003). Employment discrimination, segregation, and health. *American Journal of Public Health, 93*(2), 226–231.

Darity, W. A., Jr. (2005). Stratification economics: The role of intergroup inequality. *Journal of Economics and Finance, 29*(2), 144–153.

Darity, W. A., Jr. (2008). Forty acres and a mule in the 21st century. *Social Science Quarterly, 89*(3), 656–664.

Darity, W. A., Jr. (2011). Revisiting the debate on race and culture: The new (incorrect) Harvard/Washington consensus. *Du Bois Review: Social Science Research on Race, 8*(2), 467–476.

Darity, W. A., Jr. (2021, April 30). The true cost of closing the racial wealth gap. *The New York Times*. www.nytimes.com/2021/04/30/business/racial-wealth-gap.html

Darity, W. A., Jr., Addo, F. R., & Smith, I. Z. (2021). A subaltern middle class: The case of the missing "Black bourgeoisie" in America. *Contemporary Economic Policy, 39*(3), 494–502.

Darity, W. A., Jr., Dietrich, J., & Guilkey, D. K. (1997). Racial and ethnic inequality in the United States: A secular perspective. *The American Economic Review, 87*(2), 301–305.

Darity, W. A., Jr., Dietrich, J., & Guilkey, D. K. (2001). Persistent advantage or disadvantage? Evidence in support of the intergenerational drag hypothesis. *American Journal of Economics and Sociology, 60*(2), 435–470.

Darity, W. A., Jr., & Frank, D. (2003). The economics of reparations. *American Economic Review, 93*(2), 326–329.

Darity, W. A., Jr., Guilkey, D. K., & Winfrey, W. (1996). Explaining differences in economic performance among racial and ethnic groups in the USA: The data examined. *American Journal of Economics and Sociology, 55*(4), 411–425.

Darity, W. A., Jr., & Hamilton, D. (2012). Bold policies for economic justice. *The Review of Black Political Economy, 39*(1), 79–85.

Darity, W. A., Jr., Hamilton, D., Paul, M., Aja, A., Price, A., Moore, A., & Chiopris, C. (2018). What we get wrong about closing the racial wealth gap. *Samuel DuBois Cook Center on Social Equity and Insight Center for Community Economic Development, 1*(1), 1–67.

Darity, W. A., Jr., & Mason, P. L. (1998). Evidence on discrimination in employment: Codes of color, codes of gender. *Journal of Economic Perspectives, 12*(2), 63–90.

Darity, W. A., Jr., & Mullen, A. K. (2020b). *From here to equality: Reparations for Black Americans in the twenty-first century*. UNC Press Books.

Darity, W. A., Jr., & Myers, S. L. (1983). Changes in Black family structure: Implications for welfare dependency. *The American Economic Review, 73*(2), 59–64.

Darity, W. A., Jr., & Myers, S. L., Jr. (1984a). Does welfare dependency cause female headship? The case of the Black family. *Journal of Marriage and the Family*, 765–779.

Darity, W. A., Jr., & Myers, S. L., Jr. (1984b). Public policy and the condition of Black family life. *The Review of Black Political Economy, 13*(1–2), 165–187.

Darity, W. A., Jr., & Myers, S. L., Jr. (1989). Where have all the Black men gone? *Black Excellence, 1*(2), 29–31.

Darity, W. A., Jr., & Myers, S. L., Jr. (1995). Family structure and the marginalization of Black men: Policy implications. In B. M. Tucker & C. Mitchell-Kernan (Eds.), *The decline in marriage among African Americans: Causes, consequences, and policy implications* (pp. 263–308). Russell Sage Foundation.

Darity, W. A., Jr., & Nicholson, M. J. (2005). Racial wealth inequality and the Black family. In V. C. McLoyd, N. E. Hill, & K. A. Dodge (Eds.), *African American family life: Ecological and cultural diversity* (pp. 78–85). Guilford Press.

Darity, W. "Sandy", & Mullen, K. (2020a, June 15). Black reparations and the racial wealth gap. *Brookings*. www.brookings.edu/blog/up-front/2020/06/15/black-reparations-and-the-racial-wealth-gap

Darwin, C. (1859). *On the origin of species*.

Dasgupta, N. (2013). Implicit attitudes and beliefs adapt to situations: A decade of research on the malleability of implicit prejudice, stereotypes, and the self-concept. *Advances in Experimental Social Psychology, 47*, 233–279.

Davis, A. J. (2017). Introduction. In A. J. Davis (Ed.), *Policing the Black man: Arrest, prosecution, and imprisonment* (pp. xi–xxiv). Vintage.

Davis, R., & Short, J. F., Jr. (1978). Dimensions of Black suicide: A theoretical model. *Suicide and Life-Threatening Behavior, 8*(3), 161–173.

Dawel, A., Ashhurst, C., & Monaghan, C. (2023). A three-dimensional model of emotional display rules: Model invariance, external validity, and gender differences. *Emotion*, *23*(5), 1410–1422.

DeAngelis, R. T. (2021). Systemic racism in police killings: New evidence from the mapping police violence database, 2013–2021. *Race and Justice*. https://doi.org/10.21533687211047943

Death Penalty Information Center. (n.d.). https://deathpenaltyinfo.org

De Beauvoir, S. (1949). *The second sex*. Penguin Books.

Deitch, E. A., Barsky, A., Butz, R. M., Chan, S., Brief, A. P., & Bradley, J. C. (2003). Subtle yet significant: The existence and impact of everyday racial discrimination in the workplace. *Human Relations*, *56*(11), 1299–1324.

De La Cruz-Viesca, M., Chen, Z., Ong, P. M., Hamilton, D., & Darity, W. A., Jr. (2016). *The color of wealth in Los Angeles*. Los Angeles, Duke University, The New School, and The University of California.

Delgado, R., & Stefancic, J. (1991). Images of the outsider in American law and culture: Can free expression remedy systemic social ills. *Cornell Law Review*, *77*, 1258–1297.

Deliovsky, K., & Kitossa, T. (2013). Beyond Black and White: When going beyond may take us out of bounds. *Journal of Black Studies*, *44*(2), 158–181.

Del Zotto, A. (2004). Gendercide in a historical-structural context: The case of Black male gendercide in the United States. In A. Jones (Ed.), *Gendercide and genocide* (pp. 157–171). Vanderbilt University.

DeMaris, A. (1992). Male versus female initiation of aggression: The case of courtship violence. In E. Viano (Ed.), *Intimate violence: Interdisciplinary perspectives* (pp. 111–120). Taylor & Francis.

Dennis, R. M. (1995). Social Darwinism, scientific racism, and the metaphysics of race. *Journal of Negro Education*, 243–252.

Dettling, L., Hsu, J., Jacobs, L., Moore, K. B., & Thompson, J. P. (2017). *FEDS notes*. https://www.federalreserve.gov/econres/notes/feds-notes/recent-trends-in-wealth-holding-by-race-and-ethnicity-evidence-from-the-survey-of-consumer-finances-20170927.html

DeYoung, P. A. (2015). *Understanding and treating chronic shame: A relational/neurobiological approach*. Routledge.

Dickerson, S. S., Gruenewald, T. L., & Kemeny, M. E. (2004). When the social self is threatened: Shame, physiology, and health. *Journal of Personality*, *72*(6), 1191–1216.

Din-Dzietham, R., Nembhard, W. N., Collins, R., & Davis, S. K. (2004). Perceived stress following race-based discrimination at work is associated with hypertension in African – Americans: The metro Atlanta heart disease study, 1999–2001. *Social Science & Medicine*, *58*(3), 449–461.

Dines, G. (2003). King Kong and the White woman: Hustler magazine and the demonization of Black masculinity. In G. Dines & J. M. Humez (Eds.), *Gender, race, and class in media: A text-reader* (pp. 451–461). Sage.

Dixon, T. L., Azocar, C. L., & Casas, M. (2003). The portrayal of race and crime on television network news. *Journal of Broadcasting & Electronic Media*, *47*(4), 498–523.

Dixon, T. L., & Linz, D. (2000a). Overrepresentation and underrepresentation of African Americans and Latinos as lawbreakers on television news. *Journal of Communication*, *50*(2), 131–154.

Dixon, T. L., & Linz, D. (2000b). Race and the misrepresentation of victimization on local television news. *Communication Research*, *27*(5), 547–573.

Dixon, T. L., & Linz, D. (2002). Television news, prejudicial pretrial publicity, and the depiction of race. *Journal of Broadcasting & Electronic Media*, *46*(1), 112–136.

Dohrenwend, B. P. (2000). The role of adversity and stress in psychopathology: Some evidence and its implications for theory and research. *Journal of Health and Social Behavior*, *41*, 1–19.

Dollard, J. (1937). *Caste and class in a Southern town*. Yale University Press.

Donaldson, L. (2015, August 12). When the media misrepresents Black men, the effects are felt in the real world. *The Guardian*. www.theguardian.com/commentisfree/2015/aug/12/media-misrepresents-black-men-effects-felt-real-world

Douglas, E. M., & Hines, D. A. (2011). The helpseeking experiences of men who sustain intimate partner violence: An overlooked population and implications for practice. *Journal of Family Violence*, *26*(6), 473–485.

Dovidio, J. F., & Gaertner, S. L. (1998). On the nature of contemporary prejudice: The causes, consequences and challenges of aversive racism. In S. T. Fiske & J. L. Eberhardt (Eds.), *Racism: The problem and the response* (pp. 123–134). Sage.

Dovidio, J. F., Kawakami, K., & Gaertner, S. L. (2002). Implicit and explicit prejudice and interracial interaction. *Journal of Personality and Social Psychology, 82*(1), 62–68.

Drijber, B. C., Reijnders, U. J., & Ceelen, M. (2013). Male victims of domestic violence. *Journal of Family Violence, 28*(2), 173–178.

Drummond, W. J. (1990). About face: From alliance to alienation. Blacks and the news media. *The American Enterprise, 1*(4), 22–29.

Du Bois, W. E. B. (1899a). *The Philadelphia Negro: A social study*. The University of Pennsylvania Press.

Du Bois, W. E. B. (Ed.). (1899b, May 30–31). *The Negro in business*. Report of a social study made under the direction of Atlanta University, together with the proceedings of the fourth conference for the study of the Negro problems, held at Atlanta University, Atlanta.

Du Bois, W. E. B. (1903). *The souls of Black folk*. Penguin Press.

Du Bois, W. E. B. (1935). *Black reconstruction in America 1860–1880*. Harcourt.

Du Bois, W. E. B. (1960, April 9). *Socialism and the American Negro*. http://credo.library.umass.edu/view/full/mums312-b206-i051

Dudziak, M. L. (2000). *Cold war civil rights*. Princeton University Press.

Dukes, K. N., & Gaither, S. E. (2017). Black racial stereotypes and victim blaming: Implications for media coverage and criminal proceedings in cases of police violence against racial and ethnic minorities. *Journal of Social Issues, 73*(4), 789–807.

Duncan, L. E., & Williams, L. M. (1998). Gender role socialization and male-on-male vs. female-on-male child sexual abuse. *Sex Roles, 39*(9), 765–785.

Dunham, Y., Baron, A. S., & Banaji, M. R. (2008). The development of implicit intergroup cognition. *Trends in Cognitive Sciences, 12*(7), 248–253.

Dupont, C., Armant, D. R., & Brenner, C. A. (2009, September). Epigenetics: Definition, mechanisms and clinical perspective. *Seminars in Reproductive Medicine, 27*(5), 351–357.

Durkheim, E. (1951). *Suicide: A study in sociology*. The Free Press.

Durr, M. (2015). What is the difference between slave patrols and modern day policing? Institutional violence in a community of color. *Critical Sociology, 41*(6), 873–879.

Durst, N. J. (2018). Racial gerrymandering of municipal borders: Direct democracy, participatory democracy, and voting rights in the United States. *Annals of the American Association of Geographers, 108*(4), 938–954.

Duster, T. (1997). Pattern, purpose and race in the drug war. *Crack in America: Demon Drugs and Social Justice*, 260–287.

Dworkin, A. (1974). *Woman hating*. Dutton.

Dyer, R. (1997). *White*. Routledge.

Eagly, A. H., & Kite, M. E. (1987). Are stereotypes of nationalities applied to both women and men? *Journal of Personality and Social Psychology, 53*(3), 451–462.

Eberhardt, J. L., Davies, P. G., Purdie-Vaughns, V. J., & Johnson, S. L. (2006). Looking deathworthy: Perceived stereotypicality of Black defendants predicts capital-sentencing outcomes. *Psychological Science, 17*(5), 383–386.

Ebony. (2019). www.ebony.com/news/r-kellys-brother-he-singer-molested-older-sister

Edwards, F., Esposito, M. H., & Lee, H. (2018). Risk of police-involved death by race/ethnicity and place, United States, 2012–2018. *American Journal of Public Health, 108*(9), 1241–1248.

Edwards, F., Lee, H., & Esposito, M. (2019). Risk of being killed by police use of force in the United States by age, race – ethnicity, and sex. *Proceedings of the National Academy of Sciences, 116*(34), 16793–16798.

Egede, L. E., & Walker, R. J. (2020). Structural racism, social risk factors, and Covid-19 – a dangerous convergence for Black Americans. *New England Journal of Medicine, 383*(12), e77.

Eitle, D. (2009). Dimensions of racial segregation, hypersegregation, and Black homicide rates. *Journal of Criminal Justice, 37*(1), 28–36.

Eligon, J., & Burch, A. D. (2020). Questions of bias in COVID-19 treatment add to the mourning for Black families. *The New York Times*.

Elligan, D., & Utsey, S. (1999). Utility of an African-centered support group for African American men confronting societal racism and oppression. *Cultural Diversity and Ethnic Minority Psychology, 5*(2), 156–165.

Ellis, B. H., MacDonald, H. Z., Lincoln, A. K., & Cabral, H. J. (2008). Mental health of Somali adolescent refugees: The role of trauma, stress, and perceived discrimination. *Journal of Consulting and Clinical Psychology*, *76*(2), 184–193.

Ellison, C. G. (1992). Military background, racial orientations, and political participation among Black adult males. *Social Science Quarterly*, *73*(2), 360–378.

Encyclopedia of Virginia. (n.d.). *An act concerning servants and slaves (1705)*. www.encyclopedia virginia.org/_An_act_concerning_Servants_and_Slaves_1705

English, D., Lambert, S. F., Evans, M. K., & Zonderman, A. B. (2014). Neighborhood racial composition, racial discrimination, and depressive symptoms in African Americans. *American Journal of Community Psychology*, *54*(3), 219–228.

Ensign, R. L., & Shifflett, S. (2021, August 7). College was supposed to close the wealth gap for Black Americans: The opposite happened. *Wall Street Journal*. www.wsj.com/articles/college-was-supposed-to-close-the-wealth-gap-for-black-americans-the-opposite-happened-11628328602

Entman, R. M. (1992). Blacks in the news: Television, modern racism and cultural change. *Journalism Quarterly*, *69*(2), 341–361.

Entman, R. M. (2006). *Young men of color in the media: Images and impacts*. Joint Center for Political and Economic Studies.

Entman, R. M., & Rojecki, A. (2000). *The Black image in the White mind: Media and race in America*. University of Chicago Press.

Epel, E. S., Blackburn, E. H., Lin, J., Dhabhar, F. S., Adler, N. E., Morrow, J. D., & Cawthon, R. M. (2004). Accelerated telomere shortening in response to life stress. *Proceedings of the National Academy of Sciences of the United States of America*, *101*, 17312–17315.

Epel, E. S., Lin, J., Wilhelm, F. H., Wolkowitz, O. M., Cawthon, R., Adler, N. E., Dolbier, C., Mendes, W. B., & Blackburn, E. H. (2006). Cell aging in relation to stress arousal and cardiovascular disease risk factors. *Psychoneuroendocrinology*, *31*, 277–287.

Epp, C. R., Maynard-Moody, S., & Haider-Markel, D. P. (2014). *Pulled over: How police stops define race and citizenship*. University of Chicago Press.

Essed, P. (1991). *Understanding everyday racism: An interdisciplinary theory* (Vol. 2). Sage.

Eyerman, R. (2001). *Cultural trauma: Slavery and the formation of African American identity*. Cambridge University Press.

Eyerman, R. (2004). Cultural trauma: Slavery and the formation of African American identity. In J. C. Alexander, R. Eyerman, B. Giesen, N. J. Smelser, & P. Sztompka (Eds.), *Cultural trauma and collective identity* (pp. 60–111). University of California Press.

Eyerman, R. (2012). Harvey Milk and the trauma of assassination. *Cultural Sociology*, *6*(4), 399–421.

Eyerman, R. (2015). *Is this America? Katrina as cultural trauma*. University of Texas Press.

Fairlie, R. W., & Sundstrom, W. A. (1999). The emergence, persistence, and recent widening of the racial unemployment gap. *ILR Review*, *52*(2), 252–270.

Falter, B. (2016). *Neoslavery: The perpetuation of slavery after the American civil war*. SUNY Open Access Repository.

Fanon, F. (1952). *Black skin/White masks*. Grove Press.

Fanon, F. (1963). *The wretched of the Earth*. Grove Press.

Farmer, M. M., & Ferraro, K. F. (2005). Are racial disparities in health conditional on socioeconomic status? *Social Science & Medicine*, *60*(1), 191–204.

Farmer, P. E., Nizeye, B., Stulac, S., & Keshavjee, S. (2006). Structural violence and clinical medicine. *PLOS Medicine*, *3*(10), e449.

Farrell, W. C., Jr., Dawkins, M. P., & Oliver, J. (1983). Genocide fears in a rural Black community: An empirical examination. *Journal of Black Studies*, *14*(1), 49–67.

Fatal Encounters. (n.d.). https://fatalencounters.org/tools-for-journalists

Fatal Force: Police Shootings Database. (n.d.). *Washington Post*. www.washingtonpost.com/graphics/investigations/police-shootings-database

FBI releases updated 2020 hate crime statistics. (2021, October 25). *Federal bureau of investigation* [Press Release]. www.fbi.gov/news/pressrel/press-releases/fbi-releases-updated-2020-hate-crime-statistics

FBI reports hate crimes at highest level in 12 years. (2021, September 9). *Equal justice initiative.* https://eji.org/news/fbi-reports-hate-crimes-at-highest-level-in-12-years

Feagin, J. R. (1991). The continuing significance of race: Antiblack discrimination in public places. *American Sociological Review, 56*(1), 101–116.

Feagin, J. R. (2004). Documenting the costs of slavery, segregation, and contemporary racism: Why reparations are in order for African Americans. *Harvard Black Letter Law Journal, 20*, 49.

Feagin, J. R. (2010). *Racist America* (Rev. ed.). Routledge.

Feagin, J. R. (2013). *Systemic racism: A theory of oppression.* Routledge.

Feagin, J. R. (2014, May 28). A legal and moral basis for reparations. *Time.* https://time.com/132034/a-legal-and-moral-basis-for-reparations

Feagin, J. R., & Bennefield, Z. (2014). Systemic racism and US health care. *Social Science & Medicine, 103*, 7–14.

Feagin, J. R., & McKinney, K. D. (2003). *The many costs of racism.* Rowman & Littlefield Publishers.

Feagin, J. R., Vera, H., & Batur, P. (1995). *White racism: The basics.* Routledge Press.

The fed – Distributional financial accounts overview. (n.d.). *The federal reserve.* www.federalreserve.gov/releases/z1/dataviz/dfa/index.html

Feimster, C. N. (2009). *Southern horrors: Women and the politics of rape and lynching.* Harvard University Press.

Fein, H. (1979). *Accounting for genocide: National responses and Jewish victimization during the holocaust.* Free Press.

Ferber, A. L. (2007). The construction of Black masculinity: White supremacy now and then. *Journal of Sport and Social Issues, 31*(1), 11–24.

Fiebert, M. S. (2014). References examining assaults by women on their spouses or male partners: An updated annotated bibliography. *Sexuality & Culture, 18*(2), 405–467.

Field, A. J., & Winfrey, W. R. (1997). Job displacement and reemployment in North Carolina: The relative experience of the Black worker. *The Review of Black Political Economy, 25*(3), 57–75.

Finkelhor, D., Ormrod, R., Turner, H., & Hamby, S. L. (2005). The victimization of children and youth: A comprehensive, national survey. *Child Maltreatment, 10*(1), 5–25.

Fins, D. (2016). *Death row U.S.A. criminal justice project of the NAACP legal defense and education fund.* www.naacpldf.org/our-thinking/death-row-usa

Firestone, S. (1970). *The dialectics of sex: The case for women's revolution.* William Morrow and Company.

Fiscella, K., & Williams, D. R. (2004). Health disparities based on socioeconomic inequities: Implications for urban health care. *Academic Medicine, 79*(12), 1139–1147.

Fischer, M. J., & Massey, D. S. (2004). The ecology of racial discrimination. *City & Community, 3*(3), 221–241.

Fishback, P. V., Rose, J., Snowden, K. A., & Storrs, T. (2021). *New evidence on redlining by federal housing programs in the 1930s* (No. w29244). National Bureau of Economic Research.

Fiske, S. T., & Stevens, L. E. (1993). *What's so special about sex? Gender stereotyping and discrimination.* Sage Publications, Inc.

Fitch, R. (1993). *The assassination of New York* (Vol. 8). Verso.

Fitzgerald, J. M., & Ribar, D. C. (2004). Welfare reform and female headship. *Demography, 41*(2), 189–212.

Fix, M., & Struyk, R. J. (1993). *Clear and convincing evidence: Measurement of discrimination in America* (Natural Field Experiments No. 0049). The Field Experiments Website.

Flaherty, C. (2017, September 7). The man-not. *Inside Higher Ed.* www.insidehighered.com/news/2017/09/07/tommy-curry-discusses-new-book-how-critical-theory-has-ignored-realities-black

Foa, E. B., Huppert, J. D., & Cahill, S. P. (2006). Emotional processing theory: An update. In B. O. Rothbaum (Ed.), *Pathological anxiety: Emotional processing in etiology and treatment* (pp. 3–24). The Guilford Press.

Foa, E. B., & Kozak, M. J. (1986). Emotional processing of fear: Exposure to corrective information. *Psychological Bulletin, 99*(1), 20–35.

Folmar, C. (2022, May 10). Just 2 percent of US businesses Black-owned: Report. *The Hill.* https://thehill.com/business-a-lobbying/business-lobbying/3482794-just-2-percent-of-us-businesses-black-owned-report

Foner, P. S. (1975). *History of Black Americans: From Africa to the emergence of the cotton kingdom.* Greenwood Press.

Fontes, D. (2007). Male victims of domestic violence. In J. Hamel & T. L. Nicholls (Eds.), *Family interventions in domestic violence: A handbook of gender-inclusive theory and treatment* (pp. 303–318). Springer Publishing Company.

Fontes, L. A., Cruz, M., & Tabachnick, J. (2001). Views of child sexual abuse in two cultural communities: An exploratory study among African Americans and Latinos. *Child Maltreatment, 6*(2), 103–117.

Forman, T. A., Williams, D. R., Jackson, J. S., & Gardner, C. (1997). Race, place, and discrimination. *Perspectives on Social Problems, 9*, 231–264.

Forman, T. A., Williams, D. R., Jackson, J. S., & Gardner, C. (1997). Race, place, and discrimination. In C. Gardner (Ed.), *Perspectives on social problems* (pp. 231–261). JAI Press.

Foster, T. A. (2011). The sexual abuse of Black men under American slavery. *Journal of the History of Sexuality, 20*(3), 445–464.

Foster, T. A. (2019). *Rethinking Rufus: Sexual violations of enslaved men* (Vol. 2). University of Georgia Press.

Foston, N. A. (2003). Behind the pain nobody talks about: Sexual abuse of Black boys. *Ebony, 58*(8), 126–130.

Fox, G. L., & Benson, M. L. (2006). Household and neighborhood contexts of intimate partner violence. *Public Health Reports, 121*(4), 419–427.

Fox, J. A., & Zawitz, M. W. (2006). *Homicide trends in the United States.* Government Printing Office.

Frampton, T. W. (2018). The Jim Crow Jury. *Vanderbilt Law Review, 71*, 1593–1654.

Francis, M. (2017). *Megan. Ida B. Wells and the economics of racial violence. Items: Insights from the social sciences.* SSRC.

Franklin, A. J. (2004). *From brotherhood to manhood: How Black men rescue their relationships and dreams from the invisibility syndrome.* Wiley.

Franklin, C. W. (1982). Black male-White male perceptual conflict. *The Western Journal of Black Studies, 6*(1), 2–9.

Franklin, C. W. (1984). *The changing definition of masculinity.* Plenum Press.

Franklin, C. W. (1986). Conceptual and logical issues in theory and research related to Black masculinity. *The Western Journal of Black Studies, 10*(4), 161–166.

Franklin, C. W. (1994). Ain't I a man? The efficacy of Black masculinities for men's studies in the 1990's. In R. G. Majors & J. U. Gordon (Eds.), *The American Black male: His present status and his future* (pp. 285–299). Burnham Incorporated Pub.

Franklin, F. E. (1939). *The Negro family in the United States.* University of Chicago Press.

Franklin, J. D., Smith, W. A., & Hung, M. (2014). Racial battle fatigue for Latina/o students: A quantitative perspective. *Journal of Hispanic Higher Education, 13*(4), 303–322.

Frazier, E. F. (1927, June). The pathology of race prejudice. *The Forum, 77*(60), 856–862.

Frazier, E. F. (1939). *The Negro family in the United States.* The University of Chicago Press.

Frazier, E. F. (1955). The new Negro middle class. *E. Franklin Frazier on Race Relations,* 257–266.

Frazier, E. F. (1957). *Black bourgeoisie.* The Free Press & The Falcon's Wing Press.

Frazier, E. F. (1962, February). The failure of the Negro intellectual. *Negro Digest,* 26–36.

Fredrickson, G. M. (1971). *The Black image in the White mind: The debate on Afro-American character and destiny, 1817–1914.* Harper and Row.

Freire, P. (1970). *Pedagogy of the oppressed.* Continuum.

French, B. H., Teti, M., Suh, H. N., & Serafin, M. R. (2019). A path analysis of racially diverse men's sexual victimization, risk-taking, and attitudes. *Psychology of Men & Masculinities, 20*(1), 1–11.

French, B. H., Tilghman, J. D., & Malebranche, D. A. (2015). Sexual coercion context and psychosocial correlates among diverse males. *Psychology of Men & Masculinity, 16*(1), 42–53.

Friend, D. J., Cleary Bradley, R. P., Thatcher, R., & Gottman, J. M. (2011). Typologies of intimate partner violence: Evaluation of a screening instrument for differentiation. *Journal of Family Violence, 26*(7), 551–563.

Frijda, N. H. (1986). *The emotions.* Cambridge University Press.

Frijda, N. H. (2016). The evolutionary emergence of what we call "emotions". *Cognition and Emotion, 30*(4), 609–620.

Fruen, L., & Smith, J. (2020, January 3). R. Kelly's brothers name the man they say abused the singer as a child. *Mail Online.* www.dailymail.co.uk/news/article-7847117/R-Kellys-brothers-elderly-neighbor-say-abused-singer-age-eight.html

Fuller, N. (1969). *The united independent compensatory code system/concept: A textbook/workbook for thought, speech, and/or action, for victims of racism (White supremacy).* Library of Congress.

Fullilove, M. T. (2001). Root shock: The consequences of African American dispossession. *Journal of Urban Health, 78*(1), 72–80.

Gabrielson, R., Sagara, E., & Jones, R. G. (2014). Deadly force, in Black and White. *ProPublica.* www.propublica.org/article/deadly-force-in-black-and-white.

Gaertner, S. L., & Dovidio, J. F. (1986). The aversive form of racism. In J. F. Dovidio & S. L. Gaertner (Eds.), *Prejudice, discrimination, and racism* (pp. 61–89). Academic Press.

Gaertner, S. L., & Dovidio, J. F. (2000). The aversive form of racism. In C. Stangor (Ed.), *Stereotypes and prejudice: Essential readings* (pp. 289–304). Psychology Press.

Galatzer-Levy, I. R., & Bryant, R. A. (2013). 636,120 ways to have posttraumatic stress disorder. *Perspectives on Psychological Science, 8*(6), 651–662.

Gallup Organization of Princeton. (1997). *Black/White relations in the United States; a gallup poll social audit.* Princeton University Press.

Galovski, T. E., Peterson, Z. D., Beagley, M. C., Strasshofer, D. R., Held, P., & Fletcher, T. D. (2016). Exposure to violence during Ferguson protests: Mental health effects for law enforcement and community members. *Journal of Traumatic Stress, 29*(4), 283–292.

Gans, H. J. (1999). The possibility of a new racial hierarchy in the twenty-first century United States. In M. Lamont (Ed.), *The cultural territories of race: Black and White boundaries* (pp. 371–390). University of Chicago Press.

Garcia-Rojas, C. (2016, March 3). The surveillance of blackness: From the trans-Atlantic slave trade to contemporary surveillance technologies. *Truthout.* https://truthout.org/articles/the-surveillance-of-blackness-from-the-slave-trade-to-the-police

Gary, L. E. (1995). African American men's perceptions of racial discrimination: A sociocultural analysis. *Social Work Research, 19*, 207–217.

Gary, L. E., Beatty, L., Berry, G., & Price, M. (1983). *Stable Black families: Final report.* Institute for Urban Affairs.

Gaston, S., Brunson, R. K., & Grossman, L. S. (2020). Are minorities subjected to, or insulated from, racialized policing in majority – minority community contexts? *The British Journal of Criminology, 60*(6), 1416–1437.

GBD 2019 Police Violence US Subnational Collaborators. (2021). Fatal police violence by race and state in the USA, 1980–2019: A network meta-regression. *The Lancet, 398*(10307), 1239–1255.

Gee, G. C., Walsemann, K. M., & Brondolo, E. (2012). A life course perspective on how racism may be related to health inequities. *American Journal of Public Health, 102*(5), 967–974.

Geller, A., Fagan, J., Tyler, T., & Link, B. G. (2014). Aggressive policing and the mental health of young urban men. *American Journal of Public Health, 104*(12), 2321–2327.

Gendlin, E. T. (1981). *Focusing* (Rev. ed.). Bantam.

Gendlin, E. T. (1996). *Focusing-oriented psychotherapy: A manual of the experiential method.* Guilford Press.

Geronimus, A. T., Hicken, M. T., Keene, D., & Bound, J. (2006). "Weathering" and age patterns of allostatic load scores among Blacks and Whites in the United States. *American Journal of Public Health, 96*(5), 826–833.

Geronimus, A. T., Hicken, M. T., Pearson, J. A., Seashols, S. J., Brown, K. L., & Cruz, T. D. (2010). Do U.S. Black women experience stress related accelerated biological aging? *Human Nature, 21*, 19–38.

Geronimus, A. T., & Korenman, S. (1992). The socioeconomic consequences of teen childbearing reconsidered. *The Quarterly Journal of Economics, 107*(4), 1187–1214.

Ghandnoosh, N. (2014). *Race and punishment: Racial perceptions of crime and support for punitive policies.* The Sentencing Project.

Ghavami, N., & Peplau, L. A. (2012). An intersectional analysis of gender and ethnic stereotypes: Testing three hypotheses. *Psychology of Women Quarterly*, *37*(1), 113–127.

Gibbs, J. T. (1988). The new morbidity: Homicide, suicide, accidents, and life- threatening behaviors. In J. T. Gibbs (Ed.), *Young, Black, and male in America: An endangered species* (pp. 258–293). Auburn House Publishing Company.

Gilbert, P., & Procter, S. (2006). Compassionate mind training for people with high shame and self-criticism: Overview and pilot study of a group therapy approach. *Clinical Psychology & Psychotherapy: An International Journal of Theory & Practice*, *13*(6), 353–379.

Gilens, M. (1996). "Race coding" and White opposition to welfare. *American Political Science Review*, *90*(3), 593–604.

Gilens, M., & Page, B. I. (2014). Testing theories of American politics: Elites, interest groups, and average citizens. *Perspectives on Politics*, *12*(3), 564–581.

Gilliam, W. S., Maupin, A. N., Reyes, C. R., Accavitti, M., & Shic, F. (2016). Do early educators' implicit biases regarding sex and race relate to behavior expectations and recommendations of preschool expulsions and suspensions. *Yale University Child Study Center*, *9*(28), 1–16.

Gillon, S. M. (2018, June 8). Why the 1967 Kerner report on urban riots suppressed its own expert findings. *HISTORY*. www.history.com/news/race-riots-kerner-commission-findings-suppressed-lbj

Gilmore, R. W. (1999). Globalisation and US prison growth: From military Keynesianism to post-Keynesian militarism. *Race & Class*, *40*(2–3), 171–188.

Gilmore, R. W. (2007). *Golden gulag: Prisons, surplus, crisis, and opposition in globalizing California*. University of California Press.

Giroux, H. (1997). Rewriting the discourse of racial identity: Towards a pedagogy and politics of whiteness. *Harvard Educational Review*, *67*(2), 285–321.

Glick, P., & Fiske, S. T. (1996). The ambivalent sexism inventory: Differentiating hostile and benevolent sexism. *Journal of Personality and Social Psychology*, *70*(3), 491–512.

Glick, P., & Fiske, S. T. (1997). Hostile and benevolent sexism: Measuring ambivalent sexist attitudes toward women. *Psychology of Women Quarterly*, *21*(1), 119–135.

Goff, P. A., Eberhardt, J. L., Williams, M. J., & Jackson, M. C. (2008). Not yet human: Implicit knowledge, historical dehumanization, and contemporary consequences. *Journal of Personality and Social Psychology*, *94*(2), 292–306.

Goff, P. A., Jackson, M. C., Di Leone, B. A. L., Culotta, C. M., & DiTomasso, N. A. (2014). The essence of innocence: Consequences of dehumanizing Black children. *Journal of Personality and Social Psychology*, *106*(4), 526–545.

Goffman, E. (1959). *The presentation of self in everyday life*. Doubleday.

Goldberg, D. T. (Ed.). (1990). *Anatomy of racism*. University of Minnesota Press.

Goldenberg, D. T., Stephenson, R., Freeland, R., Finneran, C., & Hadley, C. (2016). "Struggling to be the alpha": Sources of tension and intimate partner violence in same-sex relationships between men. *Culture, Health & Sexuality*, *18*(8), 875–889.

Goldsmith, A. H., Veum, J. R., & Darity, W. A., Jr. (1996). The psychological impact of unemployment and joblessness. *The Journal of Socio-Economics*, *25*(3), 333–358.

Goldsmith, A. H., Veum, J. R., & Darity, W. A., Jr. (1997). The impact of psychological and human capital on wages. *Economic Inquiry*, *35*(4), 815–829.

Goldsmith, A. H., Veum, J. R., & Darity, W. A., Jr. (2000). Working hard for the money? Efficiency wages and worker effort. *Journal of Economic Psychology*, *21*(4), 351–385.

Goldstein, R. (1997, September 2). What's sex got to do with it? The assault on Abner Louima may have been attempted murder: But it was also rape. *The Village Voice*, *42*(35), 57.

Goodwill, J. R., Taylor, R. J., & Watkins, D. C. (2021). Everyday discrimination, depressive symptoms, and suicide ideation among African American men. *Archives of Suicide Research*, *25*(1), 74–93.

Goodwin, M. (2013). The death of affirmative action? *Wisconsin Law Review*, 715–726.

Gooley, R. L. (1989). The role of Black women in social change. *The Western Journal of Black Studies*, *13*(4), 165–172.

Gordon, L. R. (1995). Sartrean bad faith and antiblack racism. In S. G. Crowell (Ed.), *The prism of the self: Philosophical essays in honor of Maurice Natanson* (Vol. 19, pp. 107–129). Springer.

Gottschalk, P. (1997). Inequality, income growth, and mobility: The basic facts. *Journal of Economic Perspectives*, *11*(2), 21–40.

Graetz, N., Boen, C. E., & Esposito, M. H. (2022). Structural racism and quantitative causal inference: A life course mediation framework for decomposing racial health disparities. *Journal of Health and Social Behavior*, *63*(2), 232–249.

Graham, M. (2021, June 18). *Benign neglect, reparations, and Juneteenth*. Actify Press. https://actifypress.com/benign-neglect-reparations-and-juneteenth

Graham, S., & Lowery, B. S. (2004). Priming unconscious racial stereotypes about adolescent offenders. *Law and Human Behavior*, *28*(5), 483–504.

Gramlich, J. (2022, January 19). *Recent surge in U.S. drug overdose deaths has hit Black men the hardest*. Pew Research Center. www.pewresearch.org/fact-tank/2022/01/19/recent-surge-in-u-s-drug-overdose-deaths-has-hit-black-men-the-hardest

Graves, K. N., Kaslow, N. J., & Frabutt, J. M. (2010). A culturally-informed approach to trauma, suicidal behavior, and overt aggression in African American adolescents. *Aggression and Violent Behavior*, *15*(1), 36–41.

Greenberg, L. S. (2015). *Emotion-focused therapy: Coaching clients to work through their feelings* (2nd ed.). American Psychological Association.

Greenberg, L. S. (2021). *Changing emotion with emotion*. American Psychological Association.

Greenberg, L. S., & Bolger, E. (2001). An emotion-focused approach to the overregulation of emotion and emotional pain. *Journal of Clinical Psychology*, *57*(2), 197–211.

Greenberg, L. S., & Iwakabe, S. (2011). Emotion-focused therapy and shame. In R. L. Dearing & J. P. Tangney (Eds.), *Shame in the therapy hour* (pp. 69–90). American Psychological Association.

Greenberg, L. S., & Paivio, S. C. (1997). *Working with emotions in psychotherapy*. Guilford Press.

Greene, G. (2020, January 13). Tyler perry on his childhood: "It was a living hell" – page 2 of 2 – blackdoctor.org – where wellness & culture connect. *BlackDoctor.Org*. https://blackdoctor.org/tyler-perry-molestation-it-was-a-living-hell

Greene, K., & Bogo, M. (2002). The different faces of intimate violence: Implications for assessment and treatment. *Journal of Marital and Family Therapy*, *28*(4), 455–466.

Greenwald, A. G., & Krieger, L. H. (2006). Implicit bias: Scientific foundations. *California Law Review*, *94*(4), 945–967.

Greenwald, A. G., McGhee, D. E., & Schwartz, J. L. K. (1998). Measuring individual differences in implicit cognition: The implicit association test. *Journal of Personality and Social Psychology*, *74*(6), 1464–1480.

Greenwald, A. G., Poehlman, T. A., Uhlmann, E. L., & Banaji, M. R. (2009). Understanding and using the implicit association test: III. meta-analysis of predictive validity. *Journal of Personality and Social Psychology*, *97*(1), 17–41.

Gregory, V. L., Jr., & Tucker Edmonds, J. L. (2023). Cultural trauma scale (CuTs): Parsimonious principal component analysis, independent Black American male sample. *Journal of Aggression, Maltreatment & Trauma*, 1–18.

Grodsky, E., & Pager, D. (2001). The structure of disadvantage: Individual and occupational determinants of the Black-White wage gap. *American Sociological Review*, 542–567.

Grosfoguel, R. (2016). What is racism? *Journal of World-Systems Research*, *22*(1), 9–15.

Gross, S. R., O'Brien, B., Hu, C., & Kennedy, E. H. (2014). Rate of false conviction of criminal defendants who are sentenced to death. *Proceedings of the National Academy of Sciences*, *111*(20), 7230–7235.

Gross, S. R., Possley, M., & Stephens, K. (2017). *Race and wrongful convictions in the United States*. National Registry of Exonerations.

Grossman, J. R. (1997). *A chance to make good: African Americans 1900–1929*. Oxford University Press.

Grother, P., Ngan, M., & Hanaoka, K. (2019). *Face recognition vendor test (FRVT) part 2: Identification*. National Institute of Standards and Technology/U.S. Department of Commerce.

Gul, P., & Kupfer, T. R. (2019). Benevolent sexism and mate preferences: Why do women prefer benevolent men despite recognizing that they can be undermining? *Personality and Social Psychology Bulletin*, *45*(1), 146–161.

Gura, D. (2021, May 27). You can still count the number of Black CEOs on one hand. *NPR*. www.npr.org/2021/05/27/1000814249/a-year-after-floyds-death-you-can-still-count-the-number-of-black-ceos-on-one-ha

Hacker, H. M. (1951). Women as a minority group. *Social Forces*, 60–69.

Hadden, S. E. (2001). *Slave patrols: Law and violence in Virginia and the Carolinas*. Harvard University Press.

Hagan, J., & Dinovitzer, R. (1999). Collateral consequences of imprisonment for children, communities, and prisoners. *Crime and Justice, 26*, 121–162.

Hahn, J. D. (2021, July 7). Jeff Bezos net worth jumps to $211 billion, making him the richest person ever. *PEOPLE.Com*. https://people.com/human-interest/jeff-bezos-net-worth-jumps-to-211-billion-making-him-the-richest-person-ever

Haiphong, D. (2022, March 30). *Madeleine Albright is dead, but intersectional imperialism is alive and well*. Black Agenda Report. www.blackagendareport.com/madeleine-albright-dead-intersectional-imperialism-alive-and-well

Hall, R. E. (2012). The feminization of social welfare: Implications of cultural tradition vis-à-vis male victims of domestic violence. *Journal of Sociology & Social Welfare, 39*, 7–27.

Hall, S. (1981). The Whites of their eyes: Racist ideologies and the media. *Silver Linings: Some Strategies for the Eighties*, 28–52.

Hamel, J. (2007). Domestic violence: A gender-inclusive conception. In J. Hamel & T. L. Nicholls (Eds.), *Family interventions in domestic violence: A handbook of gender-inclusive theory and treatment* (pp. 3–26). Springer Publishing Company.

Hamilton, D., Austin, A., & Darity, Jr., W. (2011). *Occupational segregation and the lower wages of Black men* (Briefing Paper). Economic Policy Institute.

Hamilton, D., & Chiteji, N. (2013). Wealth. In P. L. Mason (Ed.), *Encyclopedia of race and racism*. Macmillan Reference.

Hamilton, D., Darity, W. A., Jr., Price, A. E., Sridharan, V., & Tippett, R. (2015). *Umbrellas don't make it rain: Why studying and working hard isn't enough for Black Americans* (Vol. 779, pp. 780–781). The New School.

Hamilton, D., Goldsmith, A. H., & Darity, W. A., Jr. (2009). Shedding "light" on marriage: The influence of skin shade on marriage for Black females. *Journal of Economic Behavior & Organization, 72*(1), 30–50.

Hamilton, T. G. (2019). *Immigration and the remaking of Black America*. Russell Sage Foundation.

Hammond, W. P., Fleming, P. J., & Villa-Torres, L. (2016). Everyday racism as a threat to the masculine social self: Framing investigations of African American male health disparities. In Y. Wong & S. R. Wester (Eds.), *APA handbook of men and masculinities* (pp. 259–283). American Psychological Association.

Hammond, W. P., & Mattis, J. S. (2005). Being a man about it: Manhood meaning among African American men. *Psychology of Men & Masculinity, 6*(2), 114–126.

Hampton, R. L. (1980). Institutional decimation, marital exchange, and disruption in Black families. *The Western Journal of Black Studies, 4*(2), 132–139.

Hampton, R. L., Carrillo, R., & Kim, J. (2005). Domestic violence in African American communities. In N. J. Sokoloff & C. E. Pratt (Eds.), *Domestic violence at the margins: Readings on race, class, gender, and culture* (pp. 127–141). Rutgers University Press.

Hardy, K. V., & Laszloffy, T. A. (1995). Therapy with African Americans and the phenomenon of rage. *Session: Psychotherapy in Practice, 1*(4), 57–70.

Hare, N. (1971). The frustrated masculinity of the Negro male. *Negro Digest*, 5–9.

Harkinson, J. (2015, December 2). America's 100 richest families control more wealth than the entire Black population. *Mother Jones*. www.motherjones.com/politics/2015/12/report-100-people-more-wealth-african-american-population

Harnois, C. E. (2010, March). Race, gender, and the Black women's standpoint. In *Sociological forum* (Vol. 25, pp. 68–85). Blackwell Publishing Ltd.

Harnois, C. E. (2014). Complexity within and similarity across: Interpreting Black men's support of gender justice amidst cultural representations that suggest otherwise. In B. C. Slatton & K. Spates (Eds.), *Hyper sexual, hyper masculine? Gender, race and sexuality in the identities of contemporary Black men* (pp. 85–102). Routledge.

Harrell, C. J. P. (1999). *Manichean psychology: Racism and the minds of people of African descent*. Howard University Press.

Harrell, C. J. P. (2000). A multidimensional conceptualization of racism-related stress: Implications for the well-being of people of color. *American Journal of Orthopsychiatry, 70*, 42–57.

Harriot, M. (2020, August 26). *The great White heist (The other reason for reparations)*. www.colorlines.com/articles/great-white-heist-other-reason-reparations

Harris, A. P. (1990). Race and essentialism in feminist legal theory. In *Feminist legal theory*. Routledge.

Harris, A. P. (1999). Gender, violence, race, and criminal justice. *Stanford Law Review, 52*, 777.

Harris, C. I. (1993). Whiteness as property. *Harvard Law Review, 106*(8), 1707–1791.

Harris, K. M., & Schorpp, K. M. (2018). Integrating biomarkers in social stratification and health research. *Annual Review of Sociology, 44*, 361–386.

Harris, L. T. (2013). *Feel the heat: The unrelenting challenge of young, Black male unemployment*. Center for Law and Social Policy. http://www.clasp.org/resources-and-publications/files/Feel-the-Heat_Web.pdf

Harris, L. T., & Fiske, S. T. (2006). Dehumanizing the lowest of the low: Neuroimaging responses to extreme out-groups. *Psychological Science, 17*(10), 847–853.

Harris, V., & Ordona, T. (1990). Developing unity among women of color: Crossing the barriers of internalized racism and cross-racial hostility. *Making Face, Making Soul/Haciendo Caras: Creative and Critical Perspectives by Feminists of Color*, 304–316.

Harrington, C. (2021). What is "toxic masculinity" and why does it matter?. Men and masculinities, 24(2), 345–352.

Harrison, P. M., & Beck, A. J. (2006). *Prisoners in 2005*. U.S. Bureau of Justice Statistics. https://bjs.ojp.gov/library/publications/prisoners-2005

Hartfield, J. A., Griffith, D. M., & Bruce, M. A. (2018). Gendered racism is a key to explaining and addressing police-involved shootings of unarmed Black men in America. In M. A. Bruce & D. F. Hawkins (Eds.), *Inequality, crime, and health among African American males* (pp. 155–170). Emerald Publishing Limited.

Hausmann, L. R., Jeong, K., Bost, J. E., & Ibrahim, S. A. (2008). Perceived discrimination in health care and health status in a racially diverse sample. *Medical Care, 46*(9), 905–914.

Hawkins, D. F. (1987). Beyond anomalies: Rethinking the conflict perspective on race and criminal punishment. *Social Forces, 65*(3), 719–745.

Heard-Garris, N. J., Cale, M., Camaj, L., Hamati, M. C., & Dominguez, T. P. (2018). Transmitting trauma: A systematic review of vicarious racism and child health. *Social Science & Medicine, 199*, 230–240.

Heard-Garris, N. J., Ekwueme, P. O., Gilpin, S., Sacotte, K. A., Perez-Cardona, L., Wong, M., & Cohen, A. (2021). Adolescents' experiences, emotions, and coping strategies associated with exposure to media-based vicarious racism. *JAMA Network Open, 4*(6), e2113522.

Helms, J. E. (1990). *Black and White racial identity: Theory, research, and practice*. Greenwood Press.

Helms, J. E. (1992). *A race is a nice thing to have: A guide to being a White person or understanding the White persons in your life*. Content Communications.

Helms, J. E. (1995). *An update of Helm's White and people of color racial identity models*. In Versions were presented at the Psychology and Societal Transformation Conference, University Western Cape, South Africa, January 1994, and at a Workshop Entitled "Helm's Racial Identity Theory," Annual Multicultural Winter Roundtable, Teachers College – Columbia University, February 1994. Sage Publications, Inc., Thousand Oaks.

Helms, J. E. (2017). The challenge of making whiteness visible: Reactions to four whiteness articles. *The Counseling Psychologist, 45*(5), 717–726.

Helms, J. E., Nicolas, G., & Green, C. E. (2012). Racism and ethnoviolence as trauma: Enhancing professional and research training. *Traumatology, 18*(1), 65–74.

Helper, R. (1969). *Racial policies and practices of real estate brokers*. University of Minnesota Press.

Helzer, J. E., Robins, L. N., & McEvoy, L. (1987). Post-traumatic stress disorder in the general population. *New England Journal of Medicine, 317*(26), 1630–1634.

Hendin, H. (1969). *Black suicide*. Basic Books.

Henry, P. J., & Sears, D. O. (2008). Symbolic and modern racism. In J. H. Moore (Ed.), *Encyclopedia of race and racism* (pp. 111–112, Vol. 3, 1st ed.). Macmillan.

Herman, J. L. (1992). *Trauma and recovery: The aftermath of violence – from domestic abuse to political terror.* Basic Books.

Herman, J. L. (2011). Posttraumatic stress disorder as a shame disorder. In R. L. Dearing & J. P. Tangney (Eds.), *Shame in the therapy hour* (pp. 261–275). American Psychological Association.

Hernandez, J. T., Lodico, M., & DiClemente, R. J. (1993). The effects of child abuse and race on risk taking in male adolescence. *Journal of the National Medical Association, 85*(5), 593–597.

Hernton, C. C. (1965). *Sex and racism in America.* Double-day and Co.

Heron, M., Hoyert, D. L., Murphy, S. L., Xu, J., Kochanek, K. D., & Tejada-Vera, B. (2009). Deaths: Final data for 2006. *National Vital Statistics Reports, 57*, 1–135.

Herring, C., Thomas, M. E., Durr, M., & Horton, H. D. (1998). Does race matter? The determinants and consequences of self-reports of discrimination victimization. *Race and Society, 1*(2), 109–123.

Herrnstein, R. J., & Murray, C. A. (1994). *The bell curve: Intelligence and class structure in American life.* Free Press.

Hersh, S. M. (1978, March 17). C. I. A. Reportedly recruited Blacks for surveillance of panther party. *The New York Times.* www.nytimes.com/1978/03/17/archives/cia-reportedly-recruited-blacks-for-surveillance-of-panther-party.html

Hetey, R. C., & Eberhardt, J. L. (2014). Racial disparities in incarceration increase acceptance of punitive policies. *Psychological Science, 25*(10), 1949–1954.

Hickey, A. M. (2006). The sexual savage: Race science and the medicalization of Black masculinity. In C. Faircloth & D. Rosenfeld (Eds.), *Medicalized masculinities* (pp. 165–182). Temple University Press.

Hill, K. (2020, December 29). Another arrest, and jail time, due to a bad facial recognition match. *The New York Times.* www.nytimes.com/2020/12/29/technology/facial-recognition-misidentify-jail.html

Hill, K. (2023, August 6). Eight months pregnant and arrested after false facial recognition match. *The New York Times.* https://www.nytimes.com/2023/08/06/business/facial-recognition-false-arrest.html

Hilsa, D., & Vanatta, S. (2019). Du Boisian double consciousness and the appropriation of Black male bodies in Jordan Peele's get out. *Civil American, 4*(1), 1–11.

Himmelstein, K. E., Lawrence, J. A., Jahn, J. L., Ceasar, J. N., Morse, M., Bassett, M. T., Wispelwey, B. P., Darity, W. A., Jr., & Venkataramani, A. S. (2022). Association between racial wealth inequities and racial disparities in longevity among US adults and role of reparations payments, 1992 to 2018. *JAMA Network Open, 5*(11), e2240519.

Hines, D. A., & Douglas, E. M. (2010a). A closer look at men who sustain intimate terrorism by women. *Partner Abuse, 1*(3), 286–313.

Hines, D. A., & Douglas, E. M. (2010b). Intimate terrorism by women towards men: Does it exist? *Journal of Aggression, Conflict and Peace Research, 2*(3), 36–56.

Hines, D. A., & Douglas, E. M. (2018). Influence of intimate terrorism, situational couple violence, and mutual violent control on male victims. *Psychology of Men & Masculinity, 19*(4), 612–623.

Hines, D. A., & Finkelhor, D. (2007). Statutory sex crime relationships between juveniles and adults: A review of social scientific research. *Aggression and violent behavior, 12*(3), 300–314.

Hines, D. A., & Malley-Morrison, K. (2001). Psychological effects of partner abuse against men: A neglected research area. *Psychology of Men & Masculinity, 2*(2), 75–85.

Hinton, E. (2015). "A war within our own boundaries": Lyndon Johnson's great society and the rise of the carceral state. *The Journal of American History, 102*(1), 100–112.

Hinton, E., Henderson, L., & Reed, C. (2018). *An unjust burden: The disparate treatment of Black Americans in the criminal justice system* (pp. 1–20). Vera Institute of Justice.

Hipple, N. K., Huebner, B. M., Lentz, T. S., McGarrell, E. F., & O'Brien, M. (2020). The case for studying criminal nonfatal shootings: Evidence from four Midwest cities. *Justice Evaluation Journal, 3*(1), 94–113.

Hirsch, A. R. (1983). *Making the second ghetto: Race and housing in Chicago 1940–1960.* University of Chicago Press.

Hlavka, H. R. (2016). Speaking of stigma and the silence of shame: Young men and sexual victimization. *Men and Masculinities, 20*(4), 482–505.

Ho, K. (2015). Supermanagers, inequality, and finance. *HAU: Journal of Ethnographic Theory, 5*(1), 481–488.

Hochschild, J. L. (1995). *Facing up to the American dream.* Princeton University Press.

Hoffman, J. S., Shandas, V., & Pendleton, N. (2020). The effects of historical housing policies on resident exposure to intra-urban heat: A study of 108 US urban areas. *Climate*, *8*(1), 12.

Hoffman, K. M., Trawalter, S., Axt, J. R., & Oliver, M. N. (2016). Racial bias in pain assessment and treatment recommendations, and false beliefs about biological differences between Blacks and Whites. *Proceedings of the National Academy of Sciences*, *113*(16), 4296–4301.

Hoffman, S. D., Foster, E. M., & Furstenberg, F. F., Jr. (1993). Reevaluating the costs of teenage childbearing. *Demography*, 1–13.

Hoffower, H. (2019, October 18). There are 618,000 millennial millionaires in the US, and they're on track to inherit even more wealth from the richest generation ever. *Business Insider*. www.businessinsider.com/millennial-millionaires-baby-boomer-inheritance-wealth-transfer-2019-10

Hoffower, H., & Berger, C. (2023, October 28). *The 'great wealth transfer' isn't $72 trillion but $129 trillion, Bank of America says—And the government gave most of it to baby boomers*. Fortune. https://fortune.com/2023/10/28/great-wealth-transfer-baby-boomers-bank-of-america-millennials-government-policy

Hofschneider, A. (2020, February 27). Guam residents compensated for war atrocities decades later. *ABC News*. https://abcnews.go.com/Lifestyle/wireStory/islanders-suffered-1940s-war-atrocities-guam-paid-69250203

Hoggard, L. S., Powell, W., Upton, R., Seaton, E., & Neblett, Jr., E. W. (2019). Racial discrimination, personal growth initiative, and African American men's depressive symptomatology: A moderated mediation model. *Cultural Diversity and Ethnic Minority Psychology*, *25*(4), 472–482.

Holbrook, C., Fessler, D. M., & Navarrete, C. D. (2016). Looming large in others' eyes: Racial stereotypes illuminate dual adaptations for representing threat versus prestige as physical size. *Evolution and Human Behavior*, *37*(1), 67–78.

Hollingsworth, D. W., Cole, A. B., O'Keefe, V. M., Tucker, R. P., Story, C. R., & Wingate, L. R. (2017). Experiencing racial microaggressions influences suicide ideation through perceived burdensomeness in African Americans. *Journal of Counseling Psychology*, *64*(1), 104–111.

Holman, E. A., Garfin, D. R., Lubens, P., & Silver, R. C. (2020). Media exposure to collective trauma, mental health, and functioning: Does it matter what you see? *Clinical Psychological Science*, *8*(1), 111–124.

Holman, E. A., Garfin, D. R., & Silver, R. C. (2014). Media's role in broadcasting acute stress following the Boston Marathon bombings. *Proceedings of the National Academy of Sciences*, *111*(1), 93–98.

Holmes, W. C., & Slap, G. B. (1998). Sexual abuse of boys: Definition, prevalence, correlates, sequelae, and management. *JAMA*, *280*(21), 1855–1862.

Holzer, H. J. (2007). *Reconnecting young Black men: What policies would help?* National Urban League.

Holzer, H. J., & Offner, P. (2006). Trends in employment outcomes of young Black men, 1979–2000. In R. B. Mincy (Ed.), *Black males left behind* (pp. 11–37). The Urban Institute.

hooks, B. (1990). *Yearning: Race, gender, and cultural politics*.

hooks, B. (1995). *Killing rage: Ending racism*. Henry Holt and Co.

hooks, B. (2004). *We real cool: Black men and masculinity*. Psychology Press.

Horne, G. (2018). *The apocalypse of settler colonialism: The roots of slavery, White supremacy, and capitalism in 17th century North America and the Caribbean*. New York University Press.

Houle, J. N., & Light, M. T. (2014). The home foreclosure crisis and rising suicide rates, 2005 to 2010. *American Journal of Public Health*, *104*(6), 1073–1079.

Howard, G. R. (2016). *We can't teach what we don't know: White teachers, multiracial schools*. Teachers College Press.

Howard, S., & Borgella, A. M. (2020). Are Adewale and Ngochi more employable than Jamal and Lakeisha? The influence of nationality and ethnicity cues on employment-related evaluations of Blacks in the United States. *The Journal of social psychology*, *160*(4), 509–519.

Huang, B., Jiang, C., & Zhang, R. (2014). Epigenetics: The language of the cell? *Epigenomics*, *6*(1), 73–88.

Hu-DeHart, E. (1997). Affirmative action-some concluding thoughts. *University of Colorado Law Review*, *68*, 1209–1216.

Hudson, D. L., Eaton, J., Lewis, P., Grant, P., Sewell, W., & Gilbert, K. (2016a). "Racism?!? . . . Just look at our neighborhoods" views on racial discrimination and coping among African American men in Saint Louis. *The Journal of Men's Studies*, *24*(2), 130–150.

Hudson, D. L., Neighbors, H. W., Geronimus, A. T., & Jackson, J. S. (2012). The relationship between socioeconomic position and depression among a US nationally representative sample of African Americans. *Social Psychiatry and Psychiatric Epidemiology, 47*(3), 373–381.

Hudson, D. L., Neighbors, H. W., Geronimus, A. T., & Jackson, J. S. (2016b). Racial discrimination, John Henryism, and depression among African Americans. *Journal of Black Psychology, 42*(3), 221–243.

Hughes, T., McCabe, S. E., Wilsnack, S. C., West, B. T., & Boyd, C. J. (2010). Victimization and substance use disorders in a national sample of heterosexual and sexual minority women and men. *Addiction, 105*(12), 2130–2140.

Hunter, A. G., & Davis, J. E. (1992). Constructing gender: An exploration of Afro-American men's conceptualization of manhood. *Gender & Society, 6*(3), 464–479.

Hunter, A. G., & Davis, J. E. (1994). Hidden voices of Black men: The meaning, structure, and complexity of manhood. *Journal of Black Studies, 25*(1), 20–40.

Hunter, A. G., & Sellers, S. L. (1998). Feminist attitudes among African American women and men. *Gender & Society, 12*(1), 81–99.

Hurwitz, J., & Peffley, M. (1998). *Perception and prejudice: Race and politics in the United States*. Yale University Press.

Hussen, A. (2013). "Black rage" and "useless pain": Affect, ambivalence, and identity after King. *South Atlantic Quarterly, 112*(2), 303–318.

Hutchinson, E. O. (1994). *The assassination of the Black male image*. Simon and Schuster.

Hvistendahl, M. (2021, January 30). How the LAPD and Palantir use data to justify racist policing. *The Intercept*. https://theintercept.com/2021/01/30/lapd-palantir-data-driven-policing

Hyland, S., Langton, L., & Davis, E. (2015, November). *Police use of nonfatal force, 2002–11* (Special Report NCJ249216). Bureau of Justice Statistics. www.bjs.gov/content/pub/pdf/punf0211.pdf

Ialongo, N., McCreary, B. K., Pearson, J. L., Koenig, A. L., Wagner, B. M., Schmidt, N. B., Poduska, J., & Kellam, S. G. (2002). Suicidal behavior among urban, African American young adults. *Suicide and Life-Threatening Behavior, 32*(3), 256–271.

Ifatunji, M. A., & Forman, T. A. (2006). *Education and discrimination: A test of some mediating mechanisms*. Presented at the annual meeting of the Association of Black Sociologists, Montreal, Canada.

Ifatunji, M. A., & Harnois, C. E. (2016). An explanation for the gender gap in perceptions of discrimination among African Americans: Considering the role of gender bias in measurement. *Sociology of Race and Ethnicity, 2*(3), 263–288.

Jackman, M. R. (1994). *The velvet glove*. University of California Press.

Jackson, B. A. (2018). Beyond the cool pose: Black men and emotion management strategies. *Sociology Compass, 12*(4), e12569.

Jackson, F. M., James, S. A., & Owens, T. C. (2017). Anticipated negative police- youth encounters and depressive symptoms among pregnant African American women: A brief report. *Journal of Urban Health, 94*(2), 259–265.

Jackson, J., Weidman, N. M., & Rubin, G. (2005). The origins of scientific racism. *The Journal of Blacks in Higher Education, 50*(50), 66–79.

Jackson, K. T. (1985). *Crabgrass frontier: The suburbanization of the United States*. Oxford University Press.

Jacobs, D., Brewer, M., & Klein-Benheim, M. (1999). Suicide assessment: An overview and recommended protocol. In D. G. Jacobs (Ed.), *The Harvard medical school guide to suicide assessment and intervention* (pp. 3–39). San Francisco: Jossey-Bass.

Jaima, A. R. (2021). Don't talk to White people: On the epistemological and rhetorical limitations of conversations with White people for anti-racist purposes: An essay. *Journal of Black Studies, 52*(1), 77–97.

James, J. (1999). Black revolutionary icons and "neoslave" narratives. *Social Identities, 5*(2), 135–159.

James, S. A. (1994). John Henryism and the health of African-Americans. *Culture, Medicine and Psychiatry, 18*(2), 163–182.

James, S. A., Hartnett, S. A., & Kalsbeek, W. D. (1983). John Henryism and blood pressure differences among Black men. *Journal of Behavioral Medicine, 6*(3), 259–278.

James, S. A., LaCroix, A. Z., Kleinbaum, D. G., & Strogatz, D. S. (1984). John Henryism and blood pressure differences among Black men. II: The role of occupational stressors. *Journal of Behavioral Medicine, 7*(3), 259–275.

Janoff-Bulman, R. (1992). *Shattered assumptions: Towards a new psychology of trauma.* Free Press.

Jaynes, G. D. E., & Williams, Jr, R. M. (1989). *A common destiny: Blacks and American society.* National Academy Press.

Jean, Y. S., & Feagin, J. R. (1998). The family costs of White racism: The case of African American families. *Journal of Comparative Family Studies, 29*(2), 297–312.

Jiang, C., Mitran, A., Miniño, A., & Ni, H. (2015). *Racial and gender disparities in suicide among young adults aged 18–24: United States, 2009–2013* (pp. 114–127). National Center for Health Statistics.

Joe, S., & Kaplan, M. S. (2001). Suicide among African American men. *Suicide and Life-Threatening Behavior, 31*(Suppl to Issue 1), 106–121.

Joe, S., Scott, M. L., & Banks, A. (2018). What works for adolescent Black males at risk of suicide: A review. *Research on Social Work Practice, 28*(3), 340–345.

Joe, T., & Yu, P. (1984). *The "flip-side" of Black families headed by women: The economic status of Black men.* Center for the Study of Social Policy.

Johnson, A., & Martin, N. (2020, December 22). How covid-19 hollowed out a generation of young Black men. *ProPublica.* www.propublica.org/article/how-covid-19-hollowed-out-a-generation-of-young-black-men

Johnson, M. P. (2006). Conflict and control: Gender symmetry and asymmetry in domestic violence. *Violence Against Women, 12*(11), 1003–1018.

Johnson, M. P. (2008). *A typology of domestic violence: Intimate terrorism, violent resistance, and situational couple violence.* Northeastern University Press.

Johnson, M. P., & Ferraro, K. J. (2000). Research on domestic violence in the 1990s: Making distinctions. *Journal of Marriage and Family, 62*(4), 948–963.

Johnson, P. D. (2006). Counseling African American men: A contextualized humanistic perspective. *Counseling and Values, 50*(3), 187–196.

Johnson, P. D. (2016). Somebodiness and its meaning to African American men. *Journal of Counseling & Development, 94*(3), 333–343.

Johnson, R., & Leighton, P. S. (1995). Black genocide? Preliminary thoughts on the plight of America's poor Black men. *Journal of African American Men, 1*(1), 3–21.

Johnson, T. H. (2018). Challenging the myth of Black male privilege. *Spectrum: A Journal on Black Men, 6*(2), 21–42.

Johnston, R., Poulsen, M., & Forrest, J. (2007). Ethnic and racial segregation in US metropolitan areas, 1980–2000: The dimensions of segregation revisited. *Urban Affairs Review, 42*(4), 479–504.

Jones, A. (2000). Gendercide and genocide. *Journal of Genocide Research, 2*(2), 185–211.

Jones, A. (2006). Straight as a rule: Heteronormativity, gendercide, and the noncombatant male. *Men and Masculinities, 8*(4), 451–469.

Jones, D. (2021, September 4). Facebook apologizes after its AI labels Black men as "primates". *NPR.* www.npr.org/2021/09/04/1034368231/facebook-apologizes-ai-labels-black-men-primates-racial-bias

Jones, J. H. (1981). *Bad blood: The Tuskegee syphilis experiment.* The Free Press.

Jones, J. M. (1972). *Prejudice and racism.* Addison Wesley.

Jones, J. M. (1997). *Prejudice and racism* (2nd ed.). McGraw-Hill.

Jones, J. M. (2013). US death penalty support lowest in more than 40 years. *Gallup Politics, 29.*

Jones, J. M., & Carter, R. T. (1996). Racism and White racial identity: Merging realities. In B. Bowser & R. Hunt (Eds.), *Impacts of racism on White Americans* (2nd ed., pp. 1–23). Sage.

Jones, J. M., & Mosher, W. D. (2013). *Fathers' involvement with their children: United States, 2006–2010* (National Health Statistics Reports, No. 71). National Center for Health Statistics.

Jones, L. K., & Cureton, J. L. (2014). Trauma Redefined in the DSM-5: Rationale and implications for counseling practice. *Professional Counselor, 4*(3), 257–271.

Jones-Eversley, S. D., Rice, J., Adedoyin, A. C., & James-Townes, L. (2020). Premature deaths of young Black males in the United States. *Journal of Black Studies, 51*(3), 251–272.

Jones-Rogers, S. E. (2019). *They were her property.* Yale University Press.

Junn, J. (2017). The Trump majority: White womanhood and the making of female voters in the US. *Politics, Groups, and Identities, 5*(2), 343–352.

Kaba, A. J. (2005a). Progress of African Americans in higher education attainment: The widening gender gap and its current and future implications. *Education Policy Analysis Archives/Archivos Analíticos de Políticas Educativas, 13*, 1–32.

Kaba, A. J. (2005b). The gradual shift of wealth and power from African American males to African American females. *Journal of African American Studies, 9*(3), 33–44.

Kaba, A. J. (2008). Race, gender and progress: Are Black American women the new model minority? *Journal of African American Studies, 12*(4), 309–335.

Kaba, A. J. (2011). Black American females as geniuses. *Journal of African American Studies, 15*(1), 120–124.

Kang, J. (2009). *Implicit bias: A primer for the courts.* Prepared for the National Campaign to Ensure the Racial and Ethnic Fairness of America's State Courts.

Kang, J. (2012). Communications law: Bits of bias. In J. D. Levinson & R. J. Smith (Eds.), *Implicit racial bias across the law* (pp. 132–145). Cambridge University Press.

Kang, J., Bennett, M., Carbado, D., Casey, P., Dasgupta, N., Faigman, D., Godsil, R., Greenwald, A., Levinson, J., & Mnookin, J. (2012). Implicit bias in the courtroom. *UCLA Law Review, 59*(5), 1124–1186.

Kanno-Youngs, Z. (2020, June 19). U. S. Watched George Floyd protests in 15 cities using aerial surveillance. *The New York Times.* www.nytimes.com/2020/06/19/us/politics/george-floyd-protests-surveillance.html

Kaplan, G., Ranjit, N., & Burgard, S. (2008). Lifting gates – lengthening lives: Did civil rights policies improve the health of African-American women in the 1960's and 1970's? In R. F. Schoeni, J. S. House, G. A. Kaplan, & H. Pollack (Eds.), *Making Americans healthier: Social and economic policy as health policy* (pp. 145–169). Russell Sage Foundation.

Kaplan, H. (2021, August 27). Two-faced relationship between CIA and feminism | Column. *Daily Sabah.* www.dailysabah.com/opinion/columns/two-faced-relationship-between-cia-and-feminism

Karakatsanis, A. (2022, July 20). *Police departments spend vast sums of money creating "copaganda".* Economic Hardship Reporting Project. https://economichardship.org/2022/07/police-departments-spend-vast-sums-of-money-creating-copaganda

Kardiner, A. (1941). *The traumatic neuroses of war.*

Kardiner, A., & Ovesey, L. (1951). *The mark of oppression; a psychosocial study of the American Negro.* W. W. Norton & Company.

Kashdan, T. B., Barrett, L. F., & McKnight, P. E. (2015). Unpacking emotion differentiation: Transforming unpleasant experience by perceiving distinctions in negativity. *Current Directions in Psychological Science, 24*(1), 10–16.

Katz, J. (1988). *Seductions of crime: Moral and sensual attractions in doing evil.* Basic.

Katznelson, I. (2005). *When affirmative action was White: An untold history of racial inequality in twentieth-century America.* WW Norton & Company.

Kaufman, G. (1996). *The psychology of shame: Theory and treatment of shame-based syndromes* (2nd ed.). Springer Publishing Company.

Kearney, M. S., & Levine, P. (2017, March 13). *The "marriage premium for children" depends on family resources.* Brookings. www.brookings.edu/blog/social-mobility-memos/2017/03/13/the-marriage-premium-for-children-depends-on-family-resources

Keilholtz, B. M., & Spencer, C. M. (2022). Couples therapy and intimate partner violence: Considerations, assessment, and treatment modalities. *Practice Innovations, 7*(2), 124–137.

Kellerman, N. P. (2001). Psychopathology in children of Holocaust survivors: A review of the research literature. *Israel Journal of Psychiatry and Related Sciences, 38*(1), 36–46.

Kendi, I. X. (2016). *Stamped from the beginning: The definitive history of racist ideas in America.* Nation Books.

Kenney, T. (2016, August 17). Racial dot map shows over half of Wisconsin's Black neighborhoods are actually prisons. *Atlanta Black Star.* https://atlantablackstar.com/2016/08/17/racial-dot-map-shows-half-wisconsins-black-neighborhoods-actually-prisons

Kernsmith, P., & Craun, S. W. (2008). Predictors of weapon use in domestic violence incidents reported to law enforcement. *Journal of Family Violence, 23*(7), 589–596.

Kessler, R. C., Berglund, P., Demler, O., Jin, R., Koretz, D., Merikangas, K. R., Rush, A. J., Walters, E. E., & Wang, P. S. (2003). The epidemiology of major depressive disorder: Results from the national comorbidity survey replication (NCS-R). *JAMA, 289*(23), 3095–3105.

Kessler, R. C., Mickelson, K. D., & Williams, D. R. (1999). The prevalence, distribution, and mental health correlates of perceived discrimination in the United States. *Journal of Health and Social Behavior, 40*, 208–230.

Kessler, R. C., Mickelson, K. D., & Zhao, S. (1997). Patterns and correlates of self-help group membership. *American Psychologist, 44*(27), 27–46.

Kessler, R. C., & Üstün, T. B. (2004). The world mental health (WMH) survey initiative version of the world health organization (WHO) composite international diagnostic interview (CIDI). *International Journal of Methods in Psychiatric Research, 13*(2), 93–121.

Khurana, B., Hines, D. A., Johnson, B. A., Bates, E. A., Graham-Kevan, N., & Loder, R. T. (2021). Injury patterns and associated demographics of intimate partner violence in men presenting to US emergency departments. *Aggressive Behavior, 48*(3), 298–308.

Kijakazi, K., Atkins, R. M. B., Paul, M., Price, A. E., Hamilton, D., & Darity, W. A., Jr. (2016). *The color of wealth in the nation's capital.* Duke University Press.

Kimberley, M. (2021, October 6). *Thousands of police killings are unreported.* Black Agenda Report. www.blackagendareport.com/thousands-police-killings-are-unreported

Kinder, D. R., & Sears, D. O. (1981). Prejudice and politics: Symbolic racism versus racial threats to the good life. *Journal of Personality and Social Psychology, 40*(3), 414–431.

King, M. L., Jr. (1967). *Where do we go from here: Chaos or community?* Harper & Row Publishers, Inc.

Kirschenman, J., & Neckerman, K. M. (1991). We'd love to hire them, but . . .: The meaning of race for employers. In C. Jencks & P. E. Peterson (Eds.), *The urban underclass* (pp. 203–232). Brookings Institution.

Kitossa, T. (2020). *Anti-Black sexual racism: Linking White police violence, COVID-19, and popular culture* (Symposium Paper). Intervention Symposium – Black Humanity: Bearing Witness to COVID-19, Online.

Klaus, P. A., & Maston, C. T. (2008). *Criminal victimization in the united states 2006.* Statistical Tables National Crime Victimization Survey.

Klein, A. (2021, November 26). One in 10 US Black men put in solitary confinement before turning 32. *New Scientist.* www.newscientist.com/article/2299131-one-in-10-us-black-men-put-in-solitary-confinement-before-turning-32

Klein, B., Ogbunugafor, C. B., Schafer, B. J., Bhadricha, Z., Kori, P., Sheldon, J., Kaza, N., Sharma, A., Wang, E. A., Eliassi-Rad, T., & Hinton, E. (2023). COVID-19 amplified racial disparities in the US criminal legal system. *Nature*, 1–7.

Klein, C. (2016, May 24). 10 things you may not know about Nat Turner's rebellion. *History.* www.history.com/news/10-things-you-may-not-know-about-nat-turners-rebellion

Kline, P. M., Rose, E. K., & Walters, C. R. (2021). *Systemic discrimination among large US employers* (No. w29053). National Bureau of Economic Research.

Klonoff, E. A., & Landrine, H. (1999). Cross-validation of the schedule of racist events. *Journal of Black Psychology, 25*(2), 231–254.

Klonoff, E. A., & Landrine, H. (2000). Is skin color a marker for racial discrimination? Explaining the skin color – hypertension relationship. *Journal of Behavioral Medicine, 23*(4), 329–338.

Klonoff, E. A., Landrine, H., & Ullman, J. B. (1999). Racial discrimination and psychiatric symptoms among Blacks. *Cultural Diversity and Ethnic Minority Psychology, 5*(4), 329–339.

Knox, D., Lowe, W., & Mummolo, J. (2020). Administrative records mask racially biased policing. *American Political Science Review, 114*(3), 619–637.

Koball, H. (1998). Have African American men become less committed to marriage? Explaining the twentieth century racial cross-over in men's marriage timing. *Demography, 35*(2), 251–258.

Koebler, J., Cox, J., & Pearson, J. (2020, May 29). Customs and border protection is flying a predator drone over Minneapolis. *Vice.* www.vice.com/en/article/5dzbe3/customs-and-border-protection-predator-drone-minneapolis-george-floyd

Koerth, M. (2020, August 3). Many Americans are convinced crime is rising in the U.S. They're wrong. *FiveThirtyEight.* https://fivethirtyeight.com/features/many-americans-are-convinced-crime-is-rising-in-the-u-s-theyre-wrong

Kounalakis, M. (2015, October 25). The feminist was a spook. *Chicagotribune.com.* www.chicagotribune.com/opinion/commentary/ct-gloria-steinem-cia-20151025-story.html

Kraus, M. W., Rucker, J. M., & Richeson, J. A. (2017). Americans misperceive racial economic equality. *Proceedings of the National Academy of Sciences*, *114*(39), 10324–10331.

Krieger, N. (2000). Discrimination and health. *Social Epidemiology*, *1*, 36–75.

Krieger, N. (2001). Theories for social epidemiology in the 21st century: An ecosocial perspective. *International Journal of Epidemiology*, *30*(4), 668–677.

Krieger, N., Chen, J. T., Waterman, P. D., Kiang, M. V., & Feldman, J. (2015). Police killings and police deaths are public health data and can be counted. *PLOS Medicine*, *12*(12), e1001915.

Krieger, N., & Sidney, S. (1996). Racial discrimination and blood pressure: The CARDIA study of young Black and White adults. *American Journal of Public Health*, *86*, 1370–1378.

Krivo, L. J., & Peterson, R. D. (1996). Extremely disadvantaged neighborhoods and urban crime. *Social Forces*, *75*(2), 619–648.

Krivo, L. J., Peterson, R. D., & Kuhl, D. C. (2009). Segregation, racial structure, and neighborhood violent crime. *American Journal of Sociology*, *114*(6), 1765–1802.

Kukucka, J., Horodyski, A. M., & Dardis, C. M. (2022). The exoneree health and life experiences (ExHaLE) study: Trauma exposure and mental health among wrongly convicted individuals. *Psychology, Public Policy, and Law*, *28*(3), 387–399.

Kutateladze, B. L., Andiloro, N. R., Johnson, B. D., & Spohn, C. C. (2014). Cumulative disadvantage: Examining racial and ethnic disparity in prosecution and sentencing. *Criminology*, *52*(3), 514–551.

La Bash, H., & Papa, A. (2014). Shame and PTSD symptoms. *Psychological Trauma: Theory, Research, Practice, and Policy*, *6*(2), 159–166.

Landrine, H., & Klonoff, E. A. (1996). The schedule of racist events: A measure of racial discrimination and a study of its negative physical and mental health consequences. *Journal of Black Psychology*, *22*(2), 144–168.

Landry, B. (1987). *The new Black middle class*. University of California Press.

Langhinrichsen-Rohling, J., Misra, T. A., Selwyn, C., & Rohling, M. L. (2012). Rates of bidirectional versus unidirectional intimate partner violence across samples, sexual orientations, and race/ethnicities: A comprehensive review. *Partner Abuse*, *3*(2), 199–230.

Lanius, R. A., Williamson, P. C., Densmore, M., Boksman, K., Neufeld, R. W., Gati, J. S., & Menon, R. S. (2004). The nature of traumatic memories: A 4-T FMRI functional connectivity analysis. *American Journal of Psychiatry*, *161*(1), 36–44.

Lauderdale, D. S., Knutson, K. L., Yan, L. L., Rathouz, P. J., Hulley, S. B., Sidney, S., & Liu, K. (2006). Objectively measured sleep characteristics among early-middle-aged adults: The CARDIA study. *American Journal of Epidemiology*, *164*(1), 5–16.

Lawrence, C. R., III (1995). The id, the ego, and equal protection: Reckoning with unconscious racism. In K. Crenshaw, N. Gotanda, G. Peller, & K. Thomas (Eds.), *Critical race theory: The key writings that formed the movement* (pp. 235–256). New Press.

Lawrence, K., & Keleher, T. (2004, November). *Chronic disparity: Strong and pervasive evidence of racial inequalities*. Race and Public Policy Conference. www.intergroupresources.com/rc/Defini tions%20of%20Racism.pdf

Lazarus, R. S., & Folkman, S. (1984). *Stress, appraisal, and coping*. Springer Publishing Company.

Lebron, D., Morrison, L., Ferris, D., Alcantara, A., Cummings, D., Parker, G., & McKay, M. (2015). *Facts matter! Black lives matter! The trauma of racism*. McSilver Institute for Poverty Policy and Research, New York University Silver School of Social Work. https://mcsilver.nyu.edu/wp-content/uploads/2020/06/trauma_of_racism_report.pdf

Lee, B. X. (2016). Causes and cures VII: Structural violence. *Aggression and Violent Behavior*, *28*, 109–114.

Lee, C. C. (1999). Counseling African American men. In L. E. Davis (Ed.), *Working with African American males: A guide to practice* (pp. 39–53). Sage Publications, Inc.

Leland, J. (2021, August 20). Why an East Harlem street is 31 degrees hotter than central park west. *The New York Times*. www.nytimes.com/2021/08/20/nyregion/climate-inequality-nyc.html

Lemelle, A. J., Jr. (1994). Betcha cain't reason with "em": Bad Black boys in America. In B. P. Bowser (Ed.), *Black male adolescents: Parenting and education in community context* (pp. 91–128). University Press of America.

Lemelle, A. J., Jr. (1995). The political sociology of Black masculinity and tropes of domination. *Journal of African American Men, 1*(1), 87–101.

Lemelle, A. J., Jr. (2001). Patriarchal reversals of Black male prestige: Effects of the intersection of race, gender and educational class. *Journal of African American Men*, 29–46.

Lemelle, A. J., Jr. (2010). *Black masculinity and sexual politics*. Routledge.

Leonhardt, D. (2020, June 25). Opinion | the Black-White wage gap is as big as it was in 1950. *The New York Times*. www.nytimes.com/2020/06/25/opinion/sunday/race-wage-gap.html

Levin, S. (2021, September 8). Revealed: LAPD officers told to collect social media data on every civilian they stop. *The Guardian*. www.theguardian.com/us-news/2021/sep/08/revealed-los-angeles-police-officers-gathering-social-media

Levin, S. (2022, May 10). Revealed: 93% of districts in major US cities unaffordable to Black residents. *The Guardian*. www.theguardian.com/world/2022/may/10/us-major-cities-unaffordable-black-residents

Levin, S., Sinclair, S., Veniegas, R. C., & Taylor, P. L. (2002). Perceived discrimination in the context of multiple group memberships. *Psychological Science, 13*(6), 557–560.

Levine, D. S., Himle, J. A., Abelson, J. M., Matusko, N., Dhawan, N., & Taylor, R. J. (2014). Discrimination and social anxiety disorder among African-Americans, Caribbean Blacks, and non-Hispanic Whites. *The Journal of Nervous and Mental Disease, 202*(3), 224–230.

Levine, R. S., Foster, J. E., Fullilove, R. E., Fullilove, M. T., Briggs, N. C., Hull, P. C., Husaini, B. A., & Hennekens, C. H. (2001). Black-White inequalities in mortality and life expectancy, 1933–1999: Implications for healthy people 2010. *Public Health Reports, 116*(5), 474–483.

Lewan, T., & Barclay, D. (2001, December 9). Inquiry, Black landowners cheated. *Sunday Herald-Sun (Durham, NC)*, pp. Al, A3.

Lewis, T. T., Aiello, A. E., Leurgans, S., Kelly, J., & Barnes, L. L. (2010). Self-reported experiences of everyday discrimination are associated with elevated C-reactive protein levels in older African-American adults. *Brain, Behavior, and Immunity, 24*(3), 438–443.

Lewis, T. T., Barnes, L. L., Bienias, J. L., Lackland, D. T., Evans, D. A., & Mendes de Leon, C. F. (2009). Perceived discrimination and blood pressure in older African American and White adults. *Journals of Gerontology Series A: Biomedical Sciences and Medical Sciences, 64*(9), 1002–1008.

Lewis, T. T., Everson-Rose, S. A., Powell, L. H., Matthews, K. A., Brown, C., Karavolos, K., Sutton-Tyrrell, K., Jacobs, E., & Wesley, D. (2006). Chronic exposure to everyday discrimination and coronary artery calcification in African-American women: The SWAN heart study. *Psychosomatic Medicine, 68*(3), 362–368.

Lewis, T. T., Kravitz, H. M., Janssen, I., & Powell, L. H. (2011). Self-reported experiences of discrimination and visceral fat in middle-aged African-American and Caucasian women. *American Journal of Epidemiology, 173*(11), 1223–1231.

Lewis, T. T., Troxel, W. M., Kravitz, H. M., Bromberger, J. T., Matthews, K. A., & Hall, M. H. (2013). Chronic exposure to everyday discrimination and sleep in a multiethnic sample of middle-aged women. *Health Psychology, 32*(7), 810–819.

Lichter, D. T., LeClere, F. B., & McLaughlin, D. K. (1991). Local marriage markets and the marital behavior of Black and White women. *American Journal of Sociology, 96*(4), 843–867.

Lieberson, S. (1980). *A piece of the pie: Black and White immigrants since 1880*. University of California Press.

Light-Allende, K. (2004). *Relationship violence: Women perpetrators*. University of La Verne.

Lindberg, L. D., Maddow-Zimet, I., & Marcell, A. V. (2019). Prevalence of sexual initiation before age 13 years among male adolescents and young adults in the United States. *JAMA Pediatrics, 173*(6), 553–560.

Lindsey, M. A., Sheftall, A. H., Xiao, Y., & Joe, S. (2019). Trends of suicidal behaviors among high school students in the United States: 1991–2017. *Pediatrics, 144*(5).

Link, B. G., & Phelan, J. C. (2001). Conceptualizing stigma. *Annual Review of Sociology, 27*(1), 363–385.

Lipscomb, A. E., Emeka, M., Bracy, I., Stevenson, V., Lira, A., Gomez, Y. B., & Riggins, J. (2019). Black male hunting! A phenomenological study exploring the secondary impact of police induced trauma on the Black man's psyche in the United States. *Journal of Sociology and Social Work, 7*(1), 11–18.

Lipsitz, G. (1998). *The possessive investment in whiteness: How White people profit from identity politics.* Temple University Press.

Liptak, A. (2008, April 23). U.S. prison population dwarfs that of other nations. *The New York Times.* www.nytimes.com/2008/04/23/world/americas/23iht-23prison.12253738.html

Livingston, R. W., & Pearce, N. A. (2009). The teddy-bear effect: Does having a baby face benefit Black chief executive officers? *Psychological Science, 20*(10), 1229–1236.

Livingstone Smith, D., & Panaitiu, I. (2015). Aping the human essence: Simianization as dehumanization. In W. D. Hund, C. W. Mills, & S. Sebastiani (Eds.), *Simianization: Apes, gender, class, and race* (Vol. 6, pp. 77–104). LIT Verlag Münster.

Lloyd, C. (2020, July 15). Black adults disproportionately experience microaggressions. *Gallup.com.* https://news.gallup.com/poll/315695/black-adults-disproportionately-experience-microaggressions.aspx

Loo, C. M. (1994). Race-related PTSD: The Asian American Vietnam veteran. *Journal of Traumatic Stress, 7*(4), 637–656.

Loo, C. M., Fairbank, J. A., & Chemtob, C. M. (2005). Adverse race-related events as a risk factor for posttraumatic stress disorder in Asian American Vietnam veterans. *The Journal of Nervous and Mental Disease, 193*(7), 455–463.

Lundman, R. J. (2003, September). The newsworthiness and selection bias in news about murder: Comparative and relative effects of novelty and race and gender typifications on newspaper coverage of homicide. In *Sociological forum* (Vol. 18, No. 3, pp. 357–386). Kluwer Academic Publishers-Plenum Publishers.

Lynching in America report. (2017). *Equal justice initiative.* https://eji.org/reports/lynching-in-america

Mabry, J. B., & Kiecolt, K. J. (2005). Anger in Black and White: Race, alienation, and anger. *Journal of Health and Social Behavior, 46*(1), 85–101.

Mac, R., Haskins, C., Sacks, B., & McDonald, L. (2021, April 6). How a facial recognition tool found its way into hundreds of us police departments, schools, and taxpayer-funded organizations. *BuzzFeed News.* www.buzzfeednews.com/article/ryanmac/clearview-ai-local-police-facial-recognition

MacAskill, E. (2017, May 5). The CIA has a long history of helping to kill leaders around the world. *The Guardian.* www.theguardian.com/us-news/2017/may/05/cia-long-history-kill-leaders-around-the-world-north-korea

MacKinnon, C. A. (1989). *Toward a feminist theory of the state.* Harvard University Press.

Macrae, C. N., Bodenhausen, G. V., & Milne, A. B. (1995). The dissection of selection in person perception: Inhibitory processes in social stereotyping. *Journal of Personality and Social Psychology, 69*(3), 397–407.

Maercker, A., Brewin, C. R., Bryant, R. A., Cloitre, M., van Ommeren, M., Jones, L. M., Humayan, A., Kagee, A., Llosa, A. E., Rousseau, C., Somasundaram, D. J., Souza, R., Suzuki, Y., Weissbecker, I., Wessely, S. C., First, M. B., & Reed, G. M. (2013). Diagnosis and classification of disorders specifically associated with stress: Proposals for ICD-11. *World Psychiatry, 12*(3), 198–206.

Majors, R., & Billson, J. M. (1993). *Cool pose: The dilemma of Black manhood in America.* Simon and Schuster.

Malcolm describes the difference between the "house Negro" and the "field Negro". (1963, January 23). https://ccnmtl.columbia.edu/projects/mmt/mxp/speeches/mxa17.html

Malley-Morrison, K., & Hines, D. A. (2004). *Family violence in a cultural perspective: Defining, understanding, and combating abuse.* Sage.

Malley-Morrison, K., & Hines, D. A. (2007). Attending to the role of race/ethnicity in family violence research. *Journal of Interpersonal Violence, 22*(8), 943–972.

Malley-Morrison, K., Hines, D. A., West, D., Tauriac, J. J., & Arai, M. (2007). Domestic violence in ethno-cultural minority groups. In J. Hamel & T. L. Nicholls (Eds.), *Family interventions in domestic violence: A handbook of gender-inclusive theory and treatment* (pp. 319–337). Springer Publishing Company.

Maner, J. K., Kenrick, D. T., Becker, D. V., Robertson, T. E., Hofer, B., Neuberg, S. L., Delton, A. W., Butner, J., & Schaller, M. (2005). Functional projection: How fundamental social motives can bias interpersonal perception. *Journal of Personality and Social Psychology, 88*(1), 63–78.

Mann, C. R. (1988). Getting even? Women who kill in domestic encounters. *Justice Quarterly*, *5*(1), 33–51.

Marable, M. (1979). The politics of Black land tenure: 1877–1915. *Agricultural History*, *53*(1), 142–152.

Marable, M. (1983). *How capitalism underdeveloped Black America: Problems in race, political economy, and society*. South End Press.

Marable, M. (2007). Katrina's unnatural disaster: A tragedy of Black suffering and White denial. In J. James (Ed.), *Warfare in the American homeland: Policing and prison in a penal democracy* (pp. 305–314). Duke University Press.

Marcin, T. (2018, April 4). 40 percent of Whites think Black people just need to try harder, poll finds. *Newsweek*. www.newsweek.com/forty-percent-whites-think-black-people-just-need-try-harder-equality-poll-872646

March, D. S., Gaertner, L., & Olson, M. A. (2021). Danger or dislike: Distinguishing threat from negative valence as sources of automatic anti-Black bias. Journal of Personality and Social Psychology, 121(5), 984–1004.

March, D. S. (2023). Perceiving a danger within: black Americans associate black men with physical threat. Social Psychological and Personality Science, 14(8), 942–951.

Mare, R. D., & Winship, C. (1991). Socioeconomic change and the decline of marriage for Blacks and Whites. In C. Jencks & P. E. Peterson (Eds.), *The urban underclass* (pp. 175–202). Brookings Institution.

Marger, M. (2003). *Race and ethnic relations: American and global perspectives* (6th ed.). Wadsworth/Thomson Learning.

Marriott, D. (2000). *On Black men*. Columbia University Press.

Martin, E. (2017). Hidden consequences: The impact of incarceration on dependent children. *NIJ Journal*, *278*, 1–7.

Mason, M., Schuller, A., & Skordalakes, E. (2011). Telomerase structure function. *Current Opinion in Structural Biology*, *21*, 92–100.

Mason, P. (2006). *Reproducing racism: Reconstructing the political economy of race and persistent stratification economics* (Working Paper). Florida State University.

Massey, D. S. (2015, June). The legacy of the 1968 fair housing act. *Sociological Forum*, *30*, 571–588.

Massey, D. S., Albright, L., Casciano, R., Derickson, E., & Kinsey, D. N. (2013). *Climbing Mount Laurel*. Princeton University Press.

Massey, D. S., & Denton, N. A. (1989). Hypersegregation in US metropolitan areas: Black and Hispanic segregation along five dimensions. *Demography*, *26*(3), 373–391.

Massey, D. S., & Denton, N. A. (1993). *American apartheid: Segregation and the making of the underclass*. Harvard University Press.

Massey, D. S., & Kanaiaupuni, S. M. (1993). Public housing and the concentration of poverty. *Social Science Quarterly*, *74*(1), 109–122.

Massey, D. S., & Lundy, G. (2001). Use of Black English and racial discrimination in urban housing markets: New methods and findings. *Urban Affairs Review*, *36*(4), 452–469.

Massey, D. S., Rothwell, J., & Domina, T. (2009). The changing bases of segregation in the United States. *The Annals of the American Academy of Political and Social Science*, *626*(1), 74–90.

Massey, D. S., & Tannen, J. (2015). A research note on trends in Black hypersegregation. *Demography*, *52*(3), 1025–1034.

Massey, D. S., Wagner, B., Donnelly, L., McLanahan, S., Brooks-Gunn, J., Garfinkel, I., Mitchell, C., & Notterman, D. A. (2018). Neighborhood disadvantage and telomere length: Results from the Fragile families study. *The Russell Sage Foundation Journal of the Social Sciences*, *4*, 28–42.

Massie, V. M. (2016, May 25). White women benefit most from affirmative action – And are among its fiercest opponents. *Vox*. www.vox.com/2016/5/25/11682950/fisher-supreme-court-white-women-affirmative-action

Maston, C. T., Klaus, P. A., & Robinson, J. E. (2011, May). *Criminal victimization in the United States – statistical tables*. Bureau of Justice Statistics. https://bjs.ojp.gov/library/publications/criminal-victimization-united-states-statistical-tables

Matias, C. E., & Leonardo, Z. (2016). *Feeling White: Whiteness, emotionality, and education.* Sense Publishers.

Matsumoto, D. (1993). Ethnic differences in affect intensity, emotion judgments, display rule attitudes, and self-reported emotional expression in an American sample. *Motivation and Emotion, 17,* 107–123.

Mauer, M. (2017). Incarceration rates in an international perspective. In *Oxford research encyclopedia of criminology and criminal justice.* Oxford University Press.

Mauer, M., & King, R. S. (2007). *Uneven justice: State rates of incarceration by race and ethnicity.* The Sentencing Project.

Mays, V. M., Cochran, S. D., & Barnes, N. W. (2007). Race, race-based discrimination, and health outcomes among African Americans. *Annual Review of Psychology, 58,* 201–225.

Mbembé, J. A. (2003). Necropolitics. *Public Culture, 15*(1), 11–40.

Mbilishaka, A. M., Mbande, A., Gulley, C., & Mbande, T. (2021). Faded fresh tapers and line-ups: Centering barbershop hair stories in understanding gendered racial socialization for Black men. *Psychology of Men & Masculinities, 22*(1), 166–176.

McCleod, M. (1984). Women against men: An examination of domestic violence based on the analysis of official data and national victimisation data. *Justice Quarterly, 1*(2), 171–193.

McClintock, A. (1994). Soft soaping empire: Commodity racism and imperial advertising. In G. Robertson (Ed.), *Travellers' tales: Narratives of home and displacement* (pp. 131–154). Routledge.

McConahay, J. B. (1982). Self-interest versus racial attitudes as correlates of anti-busing attitudes in Louisville: Is it the buses or the Blacks? *The Journal of Politics, 44*(3), 692–720.

McConahay, J. B. (1986). Modern racism, ambivalence, and the modern racism scale. In J. F. Dovidio & S. L. Gaertner (Eds.), *Prejudice, discrimination, and racism* (pp. 91–125). Academic Press.

McConnaughy, C. M. (2017). *Black men, White women, and demands from the state: How race and gender jointly shape the public's expectations of protesters and legitimate state response.* http://www.dannyhayes.org/uploads/6/9/8/5/69858539/mcconnaughy_race_gender_protest_workshop_june 2017.pdf

McConnaughy, C. M., & White, I. K. (2011, March). *Racial politics complicated: The work of gendered race cues in American politics.* New Research on Gender in Political Psychology Conference. https://www.semanticscholar.org/paper/Racial-Politics-Complicated-%3A-The-Work-of-Gendered-McConnaughy-White/d5736007c5833f60a406d319801ae85da2a74855

McConnell, A. R., & Liebold, J. M. (2001). Relations among the implicit association test, discriminatory behavior, and explicit measures of attitudes. *Journal of Experimental Social Psychology, 37*(5), 435–442.

McCord, C., & Freeman, H. P. (1990). Excess mortality in Harlem. *The New England Journal of Medicine, 322,* 1606–1667.

McDaniel, A., DiPrete, T. A., Buchmann, C., & Shwed, U. (2011). The Black gender gap in educational attainment: Historical trends and racial comparisons. *Demography, 48*(3), 889–914.

McDonald, M. M., Navarrete, C. D., & Sidanius, J. (2011). Developing a theory of gendered prejudice. In R. M. Kramer, G. J. Leonardelli, & R. W. Livingston (Eds.), *Social cognition, social identity, and intergroup relations: A Festschrift in honor of Marilynn B. Brewer* (pp. 189–220). Psychology Press.

McDougal, S., III, & George, C., III (2016). "I wanted to return the favor": The experiences and perspectives of Black social fathers. *Journal of Black Studies, 47*(6), 524–549.

McEwen, B. S. (1998). Protective and damaging effects of stress mediators. *The New England Journal of Medicine, 338,* 171–179.

McEwen, B. S., & Stellar, E. (1993). Stress and the individual: Mechanisms leading to disease. *Archives of Internal Medicine, 153,* 2093–2101.

McFarlane, A. C. (1988). The aetiology of post-traumatic stress disorders following a natural disaster. *The British Journal of Psychiatry, 152*(1), 116–121.

McGuffey, C. S. (2008). "Saving masculinity": Gender reaffirmation, sexuality, race, and parental responses to male child sexual abuse. *Social Problems, 55*(2), 216–237.

McIntosh, P. (1988). White privilege and male privilege. In M. S. Kimmel & A. L. Ferber (Eds.), *Privilege: A reader.* Westview Press.

McIntosh, P. (1998). White privilege: Unpacking the invisible knapsack. In M. McGoldrick (Ed.), *Re-visioning family therapy: Race, culture, and gender in clinical practice* (pp. 147–152). Guilford.

McKim, K. (2021, November 10). The financial literacy gap doesn't exist. *Fortune*. https://fortune.com/2021/11/10/financial-literacy-gap-doesnt-exist-wealth-gap-inequality

McLanahan, S., & Booth, K. (1989). Mother-only families: Problems, prospects, and politics. *Journal of Marriage and the Family*, 557–580.

McLanahan, S., & Sandefur, G. D. (1994). *Growing up with a single parent: What hurts, what helps*. Harvard University Press.

McLoyd, V. C., & Lozoff, B. (2001). Racial and ethnic trends in children's and adolescents' behavior and development. *America Becoming: Racial Trends and Their Consequences*, *2*, 311–350.

McMahon, J. M., & Kahn, K. B. (2017). When sexism leads to racism: Threat, protecting women, and racial bias. *Sex Roles*, *78*(9), 591–605.

McMichael, A. J. (1999). Prisoners of the proximate: Loosening the constraints on epidemiology in an age of change. *American Journal of Epidemiology*, *149*(10), 887–897.

McNeely, R. L., Cook, P. W., & Torres, J. B. (2001). Is domestic violence a gender issue, or a human issue? *Journal of Human Behavior in the Social Environment*, *4*(4), 227–251.

McNeely, R. L., & Robinson-Simpson, G. (1987). The truth about domestic violence: A falsely framed issue. *Social Work*, *32*(6), 485–490.

McNeely, R. L., & Torres, J. B. (2009). Reflections on racial differences in perceptions of intimate partner violence: Black women have to be strong. *Social Justice in Context*, *4*(1), 129–136.

McQuail, D. (2000). *Mass communication theory*. Sage Publications.

McRae, E. G. (2018). *Mothers of massive resistance: White women and the politics of White supremacy*. Oxford University Press.

Medeiros, R. A., & Straus, M. A. (2006). Risk factors for physical violence between dating partners: Implications for gender-inclusive prevention and treatment of family violence. In J. Hamel & T. L. Nicholls (Eds.), *Family interventions in domestic violence: A handbook of gender-inclusive theory and treatment* (pp. 59–85). Springer Publishing Company.

Melton, H. C., & Belknap, J. (2003). He hits, she hits: Assessing gender differences and similarities in officially reported intimate partner violence. *Criminal Justice and Behavior*, *30*(3), 328–348.

Mendel, M. P. (1995). *The male survivor*. Sage.

Mereish, E. H., N'cho, H. S., Green, C. E., Jernigan, M. M., & Helms, J. E. (2016). Discrimination and depressive symptoms among Black American men: Moderated-mediation effects of ethnicity and self-esteem. *Behavioral Medicine*, *42*(3), 190–196.

Metzl, J. M. (2010). *The protest psychosis: How schizophrenia became a Black disease*. Beacon Press.

Metzl, J. M. (2013). Structural health and the politics of African American masculinity. *American Journal of Men's Health*, *7*(Suppl 4), 68S–72S.

Mies, M., Bennholdt-Thomsen, C., & von Werlhof, V. (1988). *Women: The last colony*. Zed.

Migliaccio, T. A. (2001). Marginalizing the battered male. *The Journal of Men's Studies*, *9*(2), 205–226.

Mihalic, S. W., & Elliott, D. (1997). If violence is domestic, does it really count? *Journal of Family Violence*, *12*(3), 293–311.

Miller, E. (1991). *Men at risk*. Jamaica Publishing House.

Miller, E. (2004). Male marginalization revisited. In B. E. Bailey & E. Leo-Rhynie (Eds.), *Gender in the 21st century: Caribbean perspectives, visions and possibilities* (pp. 99–133). Ian Randle Publishers.

Miller, J. G. (1996). *Search and destroy: African-American males in the criminal justice system*. Cambridge University Press.

Miller, S. (2020, June 11). *Black workers still earn less than their White counterparts*. SHRM. www.shrm.org/resourcesandtools/hr-topics/compensation/pages/racial-wage-gaps-persistence-poses-challenge.aspx

Miller, W. I. (1998). *The anatomy of disgust*. Harvard University Press.

Miller, W. R., & Seligman, M. E. (1973). Depression and the perception of reinforcement. *Journal of Abnormal Psychology*, *82*(1), 62–73.

Milloy, C. (2018, June 5). Perspective | to fight racism, stop trying to fix people: Fix the system that supports racism. *Washington Post*. www.washingtonpost.com/local/to-fight-racism-stop-trying-to-fix-people-fix-the-system-that-supports-racism/2018/06/05/bb9e5c1c-6835-11e8-9e38-24e693b38637_story.html

Mitchell, T. W. (2001). From Reconstruction to deconstruction: Undermining Black landownership, political independence, and community through partition sales of tenancies in common. *Northwestern University Law Review*, *95*, 505.

Mixon, G. (2005). *The Atlanta riot: Race, class, and violence in a new South city*. University of Florida Press.

Mlotek, A. E., & Paivio, S. C. (2017). Emotion-focused therapy for complex trauma. *Person-Centered & Experiential Psychotherapies*, *16*(3), 198–214.

Moffitt, T. E., Caspi, A., Rutter, M., & Silva, P. A. (2001). *Sex differences in antisocial behaviour: Conduct disorder, delinquency and violence in the Dunedin longitudinal study*. Cambridge University Press.

Monaghan, P. (2010). Telomeres and life histories: The long and the short of it. *Annals of the New York Academy of Sciences*, *1206*, 130–142.

Mong, S. N., & Roscigno, V. J. (2010). African American men and the experience of employment discrimination. *Qualitative Sociology*, *33*(1), 1–21.

Moore, A. (2014, August 5). The decadent veil: Black America's wealth illusion. *HuffPost*. www.huffpost.com/entry/the-decadent-veil-black-income-inequality_b_5646472

Moore, A. (2015a, October 26). *The five biggest U.S. Landowners own more land than all of Black America combined* [video]. Black America Web. https://blackamericaweb.com/2015/10/26/the-five-biggest-u-s-landowners-own-more-land-than-all-of-black-america-combined-video

Moore, A. (2015b, November 10). Only 5% of African American households have more than $350,000 in net worth. *EURweb*. https://eurweb.com/2015/11/10/only-5-of-african-american-households-have-more-than-350000-in-net-worth

Moore, A. (2015c, February 17). The Black male incarceration problem is real and it's catastrophic. *HuffPost*. www.huffpost.com/entry/black-mass-incarceration-statistics_b_6682564

Moore, A. (2017, December 17). Newsweek is dead wrong on Black poverty. *HuffPost*. www.huffpost.com/entry/newsweek-is-dead-wrong-on-black-poverty_b_5a36f332e4b0e1b4472ae7b0

Moore, A. (2018a, April 16). Commentary: What we get wrong about closing the racial wealth gap. *Fortune*. https://fortune.com/2018/04/16/racial-inequality-wealth-gap-black-african-americans

Moore, A. (2018b, May 21). Are more African American men incarcerated than all women are imprisoned globally? *EURweb*. https://eurweb.com/2018/05/21/are-more-african-american-men-incarcerated-than-all-women-are-imprisoned-globally-watch

Moore, A., & Bruenig, M. (2017, September 30). *Without the family car Black family wealth hardly exists*. People's Policy Project. https://www.peoplespolicyproject.org/2017/09/30/without-the-family-car-black-wealth-barely-exists/

Moore, L. D., Le, T., & Fan, G. (2013). DNA methylation and its basic function. *Neuropsychopharmacology*, *38*(1), 23–38.

Moreton-Robinson, A. (2005). Patriarchal whiteness, self determination and indigenous women: The invisibility of structural privilege and the visibility of oppression. In B. Hocking (Ed.), *Unfinished constitutional business: Re-thinking indigenous self-determination* (pp. 61–73). Aboriginal Studies Press.

Morgan, E. S. (1975). *American slavery, American freedom*. WW Norton & Company.

Morgan, R. E. (2017). *Race and Hispanic origin of victims and offenders, 2012–15*. Bureau of Justice Statistics. https://bjs.ojp.gov/content/pub/pdf/rhovo1215.pdf

Morgan-Smith, K. (2019, March 20). Las Vegas police officer video taped Black men's genitals and shared with friends. *TheGrio*. https://thegrio.com/2019/03/20/las-vegas-police-officer-video-taped-black-mens-genitals-and-shared-with-friends

Morris, W. (2016, October). Last taboo: Why pop culture just can't deal with Black male sexuality. *The New York Times Magazine*. www.nytimes.com/interactive/2016/10/30/magazine/black-male-sexuality-last-taboo.html?_r=0

Moses, A. D. (2002). Conceptual blockages and definitional dilemmas in the "racial century": Genocides of indigenous peoples and the Holocaust. *Patterns of Prejudice*, *36*(4), 7–36.

Moss, P., & Tilly, C. (2001). *Stories employers tell: Race, skill, and hiring in America*. Russell Sage Foundation.

Motley, R., & Banks, A. (2018). Black males, trauma, and mental health service use: A systematic review. *Perspectives on Social Work: The Journal of the Doctoral Students of the University of Houston Graduate School of Social Work*, *14*(1), 4–19.

Motley, R. O., Jr., Chen, Y. C., Johnson, C., & Joe, S. (2020). Exposure to community-based violence on social media among Black male emerging adults involved with the criminal justice system. *Social Work Research, 44*(2), 87–97.

Mouzon, D. M., Taylor, R. J., Nguyen, A. W., Ifatunji, M. A., & Chatters, L. M. (2020). Everyday discrimination typologies among older African Americans: Gender and socioeconomic status. *The Journals of Gerontology: Series B, 75*(9), 1951–1960.

Mozur, P. (2018, October 15). A genocide incited on Facebook, with posts from Myanmar's military. *The New York Times*. www.nytimes.com/2018/10/15/technology/myanmar-facebook-genocide.html

Müezzinler, A., Zaineddin, A. K., & Brenner, H. (2013). A systematic review of leukocyte telomere length and age in adults. *Ageing Research Reviews, 12*, 509–519.

Muhammad, K. G. (2010). *The condemnation of blackness: Race, crime, and the making of modern urban America*. Harvard University Press.

Mukherjee, S., Shukla, S., Woodle, J., Rosen, A. M., & Olarte, S. (1983). Misdiagnosis of schizophrenia in bipolar patients: A multiethnic comparison. *The American Journal of Psychiatry*, 1571–1574.

Mull, A. (2021, December 23). The great shoplifting freak-out. *The Atlantic*. www.theatlantic.com/health/archive/2021/12/shoplifting-holiday-theft-panic/621108

Mumford, G. (2017, October 11). Actor Terry Crews: I was sexually assaulted by Hollywood executive. *The Guardian*. www.theguardian.com/film/2017/oct/11/actor-terry-crews-sexually-assaulted-by-hollywood-executive

Muñoz, A. P., Kim, M., Chang, M., Jackson, R., Hamilton, D., & Darity, W. A. (2015). *The color of wealth in Boston*. SSRN.

Murphy, C. (2021, January 21). How nations heal. *Boston Review*. https://bostonreview.net/articles/colleen-murphy-transitional-justice

Murry, V. M., Brown, P. A., Brody, G. H., Cutrona, C. E., & Simons, R. L. (2001). Racial discrimination as a moderator of the links among stress, maternal psychological functioning, and family relationships. *Journal of Marriage and the Family, 63*, 915–926.

Mustillo, S., Krieger, N., Gunderson, E. P., Sidney, S., McCreath, H., & Kiefe, C. I. (2004). Self-reported experiences of racial discrimination and Black – White differences in preterm and low-birth weight deliveries: The CARDIA study. *American Journal of Public Health, 94*(12), 2125–2131.

Mutua, A. D. (2012). Multidimensionality is to masculinities what intersectionality is to feminism. *Nevada Law Journal, 13*, 341–367.

Myrdal, A. (1944). A parallel to the Negro problem. In G. Myrdal (Ed.), *An American dilemma: The Negro problem and modern democracy* (pp. 1073–1078). Harpers and Brothers Publishers.

Myrdal, G. (1944). *An American dilemma; the Negro problem and modern democracy* (2 Vols.). Harper & Brothers.

Nash, G. B. (1988). *Forging freedom: The formation of Philadelphia's Black community, 1720–1840*. Harvard University Press.

Nathanson, D. L. (1992). *Shame and pride: Affect, sex, and the birth of the self*. WW Norton & Company.

National Partnership for Women & Families. (2020, September). *Quantifying America's gender wage gap by race/ethnicity*. National Partnership for Women & Families.

The National Registry of Exonerations. (n.d.). *Exoneration registry*. www.law.umich.edu/special/exoneration/Pages/about.aspx

Navarrete, C. D., McDonald, M. M., Molina, L. E., & Sidanius, J. (2010). Prejudice at the nexus of race and gender: An outgroup male target hypothesis. *Journal of Personality and Social Psychology, 98*(6), 933–945.

Navarrete, C. D., Olsson, A., Ho, A. K., Mendes, W. B., Thomsen, L., & Sidanius, J. (2009). Fear extinction to an out-group face: The role of target gender. *Psychological Science, 20*(2), 155–158.

Neal, C. (1934). https://www.justice.gov/crt/case-document/claude-neal-notice-close-file

Neal, M. A. (2020, October 6). Pop culture helped turn police officers into rock stars – and Black folks into criminals. *LEVEL*. https://level.medium.com/pop-culture-helped-turn-police-officers-into-rock-stars-and-black-folks-into-criminals-1ac9e3faffa1

Neborsky, R. J. (2003). A clinical model for the comprehensive treatment of trauma using an affect experiencing-attachment theory approach. *Healing Trauma: Attachment, Mind, Body, and Brain*, 282–321.

Neckerman, K. M., & Kirschenman, J. (1991). Hiring strategies, racial bias, and inner-city workers. *Social Problems*, *38*(4), 433–447.

Needham, B. L., Carroll, J. E., Diez-Roux, A. V., Fitzpatrick, A. L., Moore, K., & Seeman, T. E. (2014). Neighborhood characteristics and leukocyte telomere length: The multi-ethnic study of atherosclerosis. *Health & Place*, *28*, 167–172.

Neiwert, D. (2017, October 23). *White supremacists' favorite myths about Black crime rates take another hit from BJS study*. Southern Poverty Law Center. www.splcenter.org/hatewatch/2017/10/23/white-supremacists-favorite-myths-about-black-crime-rates-take-another-hit-bjs-study

Nellis, A. (2016). *The color of justice: Racial and ethnic disparity in state prisons*. The Sentencing Project.

Neville, H. A., Awad, G. H., Brooks, J. E., Flores, M. P., & Bleumel, J. (2013). Color-blind racial ideology: Theory, training, and measurement implications in psychology. *American Psychologist*, *68*(6), 455–466.

Neville, H. A., Spanierman, L., & Doan, B. T. (2006). Exploring the association between color-blind racial ideology and multicultural counseling competencies. *Cultural Diversity and Ethnic Minority Psychology*, *12*(2), 275–290.

Neville, H. A., Worthington, R. L., & Spanierman, L. B. (2001). Race, power, and multicultural counseling psychology: Understanding White privilege and color-blind racial attitudes. In J. G. Ponterotto, J. M. Casas, L. A. Suzuki, & C. M. Alexander (Eds.), *Handbook of multicultural counseling* (pp. 257–288). Sage.

Newheiser, A.-K., & Olson, K. R. (2012). White and Black American children's implicit intergroup bias. *Journal of Experimental Social Psychology*, *48*(1), 264–270.

Newman, L. M. (1999). *White women's rights: The racial origins of feminism in the United States*. Oxford University Press on Demand.

Newman, L. M. (2007). Women's rights, race, and imperialism in US history, 1870–1920. In J. T. Campbell, M. P. Guterl, & R. G. Lee (Eds.), *Race, nation, and empire in American history* (pp. 295–343). UNC Press Books.

Newport, F. (1999, December 9). Racial profiling is seen as widespread, particularly among young Black men. *Gallup.com*. https://news.gallup.com/poll/3421/Racial-Profiling-Seen-Widespread-Particularly-Among-Young-Black-Men.aspx

Newton, H. P. (1967). Fear and doubt. *Essays from the Minister of Defense*, *15*, 15–18.

Newton, H. P. (1973). *Revolutionary suicide*. Harcourt Brace Jovanovich Inc.

Newton, H. P. (1980). *War against the Panthers: A study of repression in America* [Doctoral dissertation, University of California].

Noël, R. A. (2014, November). *Income and spending patterns among Black households: Beyond the numbers*. U.S. Bureau of Labor Statistics. www.bls.gov/opub/btn/volume-3/income-and-spending-patterns-among-black-households.htm

Nolen-Hoeksema, S., Wisco, B. E., & Lyubomirsky, S. (2008). Rethinking rumination. *Perspectives on Psychological Science*, *3*(5), 400–424.

Norgaard, R. B. (1995). *Development betrayed, the end of progress and a coevolutionary revisioning of the future*. Routledge.

Norris, F. H. (1992). Epidemiology of trauma: Frequency and impact of different potentially traumatic events on different demographic groups. *Journal of Consulting and Clinical Psychology*, *60*(3), 409–418.

Nosek, B. A., Banaji, M. R., & Greenwald, A. G. (2002). Harvesting implicit group attitudes and beliefs from a demonstration web site. *Group Dynamics: Theory, Research, and Practice*, *6*(1), 101–115.

Nosek, B. A., Greenwald, A. G., & Banaji, M. R. (2005). Understanding and using the implicit association test: II. Method variables and construct validity. *Personality and Social Psychology Bulletin*, *31*(2), 166–180.

Ocampo, N. (2020, June 12). How much NBA players actually make after taxes and agent fees. *ClutchPoints*. https://clutchpoints.com/how-much-nba-players-actually-make-after-taxes-and-agent-fees

O'Connor, J. (1973). *The fiscal crisis of the state*. Transaction Publishers.

O'Connor, R. C. (2011a). The integrated motivational- volitional model of suicidal behavior. *Crisis*, *32*(6), 295–298.

O'Connor, R. C. (2011b). Toward an integrated motivational – volitional model of suicidal behavior. In R. C. O'Connor, S. Platt, & J. Gordon (Eds.), *International handbook of suicide prevention: Research, policy and practice* (pp. 181–198). Wiley Blackwell.

Ogungbure, A. (2018). Homoeroticism, phallicism and the racialization of Black/Brown males: A historiography of sexual racism in America. *Inter-American Journal of Philosophy, 9*(2), 1–23.

Ogungbure, A. (2019a). The political economy of Niggerdom: WEB Du Bois and Martin Luther King Jr. on the racial and economic discrimination of Black males in America. *Journal of Black Studies, 50*(3), 273–297.

Ogungbure, A. (2019b, Spring). The wages of sin is death: Martin Luther King Jr.'s rhetorics of Black manhood and the contemporary discourse on Black male death. *APA Newsletter on Philosophy and the Black Experience, 18*(2), 16–23.

Oh, H., Stickley, A., Koyanagi, A., Yau, R., & DeVylder, J. E. (2019). Discrimination and suicidality among racial and ethnic minorities in the United States. *Journal of Affective Disorders, 245*, 517–523.

Øktedalen, T., Hagtvet, K. A., Hoffart, A., Langkaas, T. F., & Smucker, M. (2014). The trauma related shame inventory: Measuring trauma-related shame among patients with PTSD. *Journal of Psychopathology and Behavioral Assessment, 36*(4), 600–615.

Øktedalen, T., Hoffart, A., & Langkaas, T. F. (2015). Trauma-related shame and guilt as time-varying predictors of posttraumatic stress disorder symptoms during imagery exposure and imagery rescripting – a randomized controlled trial. *Psychotherapy Research, 25*(5), 518–532.

Oleson, J. C. (2016). The new eugenics: Black hyper-incarceration and human abatement. *Social Sciences, 5*(4), 66.

Oliver, M. B. (1994). Portrayals of crime, race, and aggression in "reality-based" police shows: A content analysis. *Journal of Broadcasting & Electronic Media, 38*(2), 179–192.

Oliver, M. L., & Shapiro, T. M. (2006). *Black wealth/White wealth: A new perspective on racial inequality*. Routledge. (Original work published 1997)

Oluwayomi, A. (2020). The man-not and the inapplicability of intersectionality to the dilemmas of Black manhood. *The Journal of Men's Studies, 28*(2), 183–205.

Operario, D., & Fiske, S. T. (2001). Ethnic identity moderates perceptions of prejudice: Judgments of personal versus group discrimination and subtle versus blatant bias. *Personality and Social Psychology Bulletin, 27*(5), 550–561.

Ore, E. J. (2019). *Lynching: Violence, rhetoric, and American identity*. University Press of Mississippi.

Orth, U., Berking, M., & Burkhardt, S. (2006). Self-conscious emotions and depression: Rumination explains why shame but not guilt is maladaptive. *Personality and Social Psychology Bulletin, 32*(12), 1608–1619.

Ortiz, P. (2005). *Emancipation betrayed: The hidden history of Black organizing and White violence in Florida from reconstruction to the bloody election of 1920*. University of California Press.

Owens, J. (2023). Seeing behavior as Black, Brown, or White: Teachers' racial/ethnic bias in perceptions of routine classroom misbehavior. *Social Psychology Quarterly, 86*(3), 298–311.

Oyewùmí, O. (1997). *The invention of women: Making an African sense of Western gender discourses*. University of Minnesota Press.

Pager, D. (2003). The mark of a criminal record. *American Journal of Sociology, 108*(5), 937–975.

Pager, D. (2007). The use of field experiments for studies of employment discrimination: Contributions, critiques, and directions for the future. *The Annals of the American Academy of Political and Social Science, 609*(1), 104–133.

Pager, D., Bonikowski, B., & Western, B. (2009). Discrimination in a low-wage labor market: A field experiment. *American Sociological Review, 74*(5), 777–799.

Paivio, S. C. (1999). Experiential conceptualization and treatment of anger. *Journal of Clinical Psychology, 55*(3), 311–324.

Paivio, S. C., & Carriere, M. (2007). Contributions of emotion-focused therapy to the understanding and treatment of anger and aggression. *Anger, Aggression and Interventions for Interpersonal Violence*, 143–164.

Paivio, S. C., & Pascual-Leone, A. (2010). *Emotion-focused therapy for complex trauma: An integrative approach*. American Psychological Association.

Palmetto, N., Davidson, L. L., & Rickert, V. I. (2013). Predictors of physical intimate partner violence in the lives of young women: Victimization, perpetration, and bidirectional violence. *Violence and Victims, 28*(1), 103–121.

Paradies, Y., Ben, J., Denson, N., Elias, A., Priest, N., Pieterse, A., Gupta, A., Kelaher, M., & Gee, G. (2015). Racism as a determinant of health: A systematic review and meta-analysis. *PLOS One, 10*(9), e0138511.

Parham, T. A. (1989). Cycles of psychological nigrescence. *The Counseling Psychologist, 17*(2), 187–226.

Park, M., Verhoeven, J. E., Cuijpers, P., Reynolds, C. F., III, & Penninx, B. W. J. H. (2015). Where you live may make you old: The association between perceived poor neighborhood quality and leukocyte telomere length. *PLOS One, 10*, e0128460.

Pascual-Leone, A., Gilles, P., Singh, T., & Andreescu, C. A. (2012). Problem anger in psychotherapy: An emotion-focused perspective on hate, rage, and rejecting anger. *Journal of Contemporary Psychotherapy, 43*(2), 83–92.

Pass, M., Benoit, E., & Dunlop, E. (2014). "I just be myself": Contradicting hyper masculine and hyper sexual stereotypes among low-income Black men in New York city. In B. C. Slatton & K. Spates (Eds.), *Hyper-sexual, hyper-masculine? Gender, race, and sexuality in the identities of contemporary Black men* (pp. 165–181). Ashgate, Routledge.

Patterson, E. J., & Wildeman, C. (2015). Mass imprisonment and the life course revisited: Cumulative years spent imprisoned and marked for working-age Black and White men. *Social Science Research, 53*, 325–337.

Patterson, O. (1982). *Slavery and social death: A comparative study*. Harvard University Press.

Patterson, W. L. (Ed.). (1952). *We charge genocide: The historic petition to the United Nations for relief from a crime of the United States government against the Negro people*. Civil Rights Congress.

Pavkov, T. W., Lewis, D. A., & Lyons, J. S. (1989). Psychiatric diagnoses and racial bias: An empirical investigation. *Professional Psychology: Research and Practice, 20*(6), 364–368.

Pawasarat, J., & Quinn, L. M. (2013). *Wisconsin's mass incarceration of African American males: Workforce challenges for 2013*. ETI Publications. https://dc.uwm.edu/eti_pubs/9

Paymar, M., & Pence, E. (1993). *Education groups for men who batter: The Duluth model*. Springer Publishing Company.

Pearlin, L. I. (1989). The sociological study of stress. *Journal of Health and Social Behavior*, 241–256.

Pedulla, D. S. (2014). The positive consequences of negative stereotypes: Race, sexual orientation, and the job application process. *Social Psychology Quarterly, 77*(1), 75–94.

Percheski, C., & Gibson-Davis, C. (2020). A penny on the dollar: Racial inequalities in wealth among households with children. *Socius, 6*. https://doi.org/10.2378023120916616

Pérez Huber, L., & Solorzano, D. G. (2015). Racial microaggressions as a tool for critical race research. *Race Ethnicity and Education, 18*(3), 297–320.

Perroud, N., Rutembesa, E., Paoloni-Giacobino, A., Mutabaruka, J., Mutesa, L., Stenz, L., Malafosse, A., & Karege, F. (2014). The Tutsi genocide and transgenerational transmission of maternal stress: Epigenetics and biology of the HPA axis. *The World Journal of Biological Psychiatry, 15*(4), 334–345.

Perry, I. (2021, May 24). Stop hustling Black death. *The Cut*. www.thecut.com/article/samaria-rice-profile.html

Pettit, B. (2012). *Invisible men: Mass incarceration and the myth of Black progress*. Russell Sage Foundation.

Pettit, B., & Western, B. (2004). Mass imprisonment and the life course: Race and class inequality in US incarceration. *American Sociological Review, 69*(2), 151–169.

Pew Research Center Parenting in America: Outlook, Worries, Aspirations are Strongly Linked to Financial Situation. (2015, December 17). https://www.pewresearch.org/social-trends/2015/12/17/parenting-in-america/

Phelan, J. C., Link, B. G., & Tehranifar, P. (2010). Social conditions as fundamental causes of health inequalities: Theory, evidence, and policy implications. *Journal of Health and Social Behavior, 51*(Suppl 1), S28–S40.

Phillips, D., & Pon, G. (2018). Anti-Black racism, bio-power, and governmentality: Deconstructing the suffering of Black families involved with child welfare. *Journal of Law and Social Policy, 28*, 81–100.

Philpott, T. L. (1978). *The slum and the ghetto: Neighborhood deterioration and middle-class reform, Chicago, 1800–1930.* Oxford University Press.

Pierce, C. M (1970). Offensive mechanisms. In F. B. Barbour (Ed.), *The Black seventies* (pp. 265–282). Porter Sargent.

Pierce, C. M (1974). Psychiatric problems of the Black minority. In G. Caplan & S. Arieti (Eds.), *American handbook of psychiatry* (pp. 512–523). Basic Books.

Pierce, C. M. (1975a). The mundane extreme environment and its effect on learning. In S. G. Brainard (Ed.), *Learning disabilities: Issues and recommendations for research* (pp. 111–119). National Institute of Education, Department of Health, Education, and Welfare.

Pierce, C. M. (1975b). Poverty and racism as they affect children. In I. Berlin (Ed.), *Advocacy for child mental health* (pp. 92–109). Brunner/Mazel.

Pierce, C. M. (1988). Stress in the workplace. In A. F. Coner-Edwards & J. Spurlock (Eds.), *Black families in crisis: The middle class* (pp. 27–35). Brunner/Mazel.

Pierce, C. M. (1992, May 4). *Public health and human rights: Racism, torture, and terrorism.* Paper presented at the annual meeting of the Presidential Seminar at the American Psychiatric Association, Washington, DC.

Pierce, C. M. (1995). Stress analogs of racism and sexism: Terrorism, torture, and disaster. In C. Willie, P. Rieker, B. Kramer, & B. Brown (Eds.), *Mental health, racism and sexism* (pp. 277–293). University of Pittsburg Press.

Pierre, M. R., & Mahalik, J. R. (2005). Examining African self-consciousness and Black racial identity as predictors of Black men's psychological well-being. *Cultural Diversity and Ethnic Minority Psychology, 11*(1), 28–40.

Pieterse, A. L., & Carter, R. T. (2007). An examination of the relationship between general life stress, racism-related stress, and psychological health among Black men. *Journal of Counseling Psychology, 54*(1), 101–109.

Piketty, T. (2014). *Capital in the 21st century.* Harvard University Press.

Pinkney, A. (1984). *The myth of Black progress.* Cambridge University Press Archive.

Pittman, C. T. (2011). Getting mad but ending up sad: The mental health consequences for African Americans using anger to cope with racism. *Journal of Black Studies, 42*(7), 1106–1124.

Plant, E. A., Goplen, J., & Kunstman, J. W. (2011). Selective responses to threat: The roles of race and gender in decisions to shoot. *Personality and Social Psychology Bulletin, 37*(9), 1274–1281.

Poe, J. (2019, July 10). Louisville housing policies cater to developers at the expense of Black residents. *Courier Journal.* www.courier-journal.com/story/opinion/contributors/2019/07/10/gentrification-just-devastating-redlining-in-louisville/1683332001

Polanco-Roman, L., & Miranda, R. (2013). Culturally related stress, hopelessness, and vulnerability to depressive symptoms and suicidal ideation in emerging adulthood. *Behavior Therapy, 44*(1), 75–87.

Porter, E. (2021, June 28). Black workers stopped making progress on pay: Is it racism? *The New York Times.* www.nytimes.com/2021/06/28/business/economy/black-workers-racial-pay-gap.html

Poteat, T., Millett, G. A., Nelson, L. E., & Beyrer, C. (2020). Understanding COVID-19 risks and vulnerabilities among Black communities in America: The lethal force of syndemics. *Annals of Epidemiology, 47,* 1–3.

Powell, L. (2023, August 29). Who are the NFL owners? *Washington Post.* https://www.washingtonpost.com/sports/interactive/2023/nfl-owners-illustrated

Powell, M. (2009, June 7). Bank accused of pushing mortgage deals on Blacks. *The New York Times.* www.nytimes.com/2009/06/07/us/07baltimore.html

Pratto, F., Sidanius, J., Stallworth, L. M., & Malle, B. F. (1994). Social dominance orientation: A personality variable predicting social and political attitudes. *Journal of Personality and Social Psychology, 67,* 741–763.

Previous editions of the code of ethics. (n.d.). *National association of realtors.* www.nar.realtor/about-nar/governing-documents/code-of-ethics/previous-editions-of-the-code-of-ethics

Puar, J. K. (2007). *Terrorist assemblages: Homonationalism in queer times.* Duke University Press.

Pudloski, K. (2020, June 12). Homeowners in formerly redlined LA neighborhoods have $524,000 less home equity. *Livabl.* www.livabl.com/2020/06/formerly-redlined-la-neighborhoods-equity.html

Purdie-Vaughns, V., & Eibach, R. P. (2008). Intersectional invisibility: The distinctive advantages and disadvantages of multiple subordinate-group identities. *Sex Roles, 59*(5), 377–391.

Purnell, T., Idsardi, W., & Baugh, J. (1999). Perceptual and phonetic experiments on American English dialect identification. *Journal of Language and Social Psychology, 18*(1), 10–30.

Quijano, A. (2000). *Qué tal Raza!* Paper prepared for the Conference of Coloniality Working Group, SUNY, Binghamton.

Quillian, L., & Pager, D. (2001). Black neighbors, higher crime? The role of racial stereotypes in evaluations of neighborhood crime. *American Journal of Sociology, 107*(3), 717–767.

Quillian, L., Pager, D., Hexel, O., & Midtbøen, A. H. (2017). Meta-analysis of field experiments shows no change in racial discrimination in hiring over time. *Proceedings of the National Academy of Sciences, 114*(41), 10870–10875.

Quinn, D. M. (2020). Experimental evidence on teachers' racial bias in student evaluation: The role of grading scales. *Educational Evaluation and Policy Analysis, 42*(3), 375–392.

Rachlinski, J. J., Johnson, S. L., Wistrich, A. J., & Guthrie, C. (2009). Does unconscious racial bias affect trial judges? *Notre Dame Law Review, 84*(3), 1195–1246.

Racial Inequalities in Homelessness, by the Numbers. (2020, June 1). *National alliance to end homelessness.* https://endhomelessness.org/resource/racial-inequalities-homelessness-numbers

Randall, A. E. (2015). Introduction: Gendering genocide studies. In A. E. Randall (Ed.), *Genocide and gender in the twentieth century: A comparative perspective* (pp. 1–34). Bloomsbury Publishers.

Ray, A. M., & Perry, R. R. (2020, April 15). Why we need reparations for Black Americans. *Brookings.* www.brookings.edu/policy2020/bigideas/why-we-need-reparations-for-black-americans

Reddy, C. (2011). *Freedom with violence.* Duke University Press.

Reed, A. (2021, July 23). Why Black lives matter can't be co-opted. *Nonsite.org.* https://nonsite.org/why-black-lives-matter-cant-be-co-opted

Reichel, P. L. (1988). Southern slave patrols as a transitional police type. *American Journal of Police, 7,* 51–77.

Reichelmann, A. V., & Hunt, M. O. (2021). White Americans' attitudes toward reparations for slavery: Definitions and determinants. *Race and Social Problems,* 1–13.

Reid, J. A., & Piquero, A. R. (2014). Age-graded risks for commercial sexual exploitation of male and female youth. *Journal of Interpersonal Violence, 29*(9), 1747–1777.

Resick, P. A., Nishith, P., & Griffin, M. G. (2003). How well does cognitive-behavioral therapy treat symptoms of complex PTSD? An examination of child sexual abuse survivors within a clinical trial. *CNS Spectrums, 8*(5), 340–355.

Reskin, B. (2005). Unconsciousness raising. *Regional Review, 14*(3), 32–37.

Rhode, D. L. (1989). *Justice and gender: Sex discrimination and the law.* Harvard University Press.

Rhodes, L. A. (2004). *Total confinement.* University of California Press.

Rice, L. N., & Greenberg, L. S. (1992). Humanistic approaches to psychotherapy. In D. K. Freedheim, H. J. Freudenberger, J. W. Kessler, S. B. Messer, D. R. Peterson, H. H. Strupp, & P. L. Wachtel (Eds.), *History of psychotherapy: A century of change* (pp. 197–224). American Psychological Association.

Rice, R. L. (1968). Residential segregation by law, 1910–1917. *The Journal of Southern History, 34*(2), 179–199.

Richardson, E. T., Malik, M. M., Darity, Jr., W. A., Mullen, A. K., Morse, M. E., Malik, M., Maybank, A., Bassett, M. T., Farmer, P. E., Worden, L., & Jones, J. H. (2021). Reparations for Black American descendants of persons enslaved in the US and their potential impact on SARS-CoV-2 transmission. *Social Science & Medicine, 276,* 113741.

Riethman, H. (2008). Human telomere structure and biology. *Annual Review of Genomics and Human Genetics, 9,* 1–19.

Roberts, A. L., Gilman, S. E., Breslau, J., Breslau, N., & Koenen, K. C. (2011). Race/ethnic differences in exposure to traumatic events, development of post-traumatic stress disorder, and treatment-seeking for post-traumatic stress disorder in the United States. *Psychological Medicine, 41,* 71–83.

Robinson, C. D., & Scaglion, R. (1987). The origin and evolution of the police function in society: Notes toward a theory. *Law and Society Review*, 109–153.

Rodgers, W. L., & Thornton, A. (1985). Changing patterns of first marriage in the United States. *Demography*, 265–279.

Rodríguez, D. (2006). *Forced passages: Imprisoned radical intellectuals and the US prison regime*. University of Minnesota Press.

Rodríguez, D. (2011). The Black presidential non-slave: Genocide and the present tense of racial slavery. In J. Go (Ed.), *Rethinking Obama* (Political power and social theory, Vol. 22, pp. 17–50). Emerald Group Publishing Limited.

Roediger, D. R. (1991). *The wages of whiteness: Race and the making of the American working class* (Rev. ed.). Verso.

Rogers, C. R. (1961). *On becoming a person: A therapist's view of psychotherapy*. Houghton Mifflin.

Rogers, C. R. (1980). *A way of being*. Houghton Mifflin.

Rogers, M. L. (2014). Introduction: Disposable lives. *Theory & Event*, *17*(3).

Romer, D., Jamieson, K. H., & De Coteau, N. J. (1998). The treatment of persons of color in local television news: Ethnic blame discourse or realistic group conflict? *Communication Research*, *25*(3), 286–305.

Rose, S. J. (2000). *Social stratification in the United States: The American profile poster*. New Press.

Rosin, H. (2014, April 29). When men are raped. *Slate*. https://slate.com/human-interest/2014/04/male-rape-in-america-a-new-study-reveals-that-men-are-sexually-assaulted-almost-as-often-as-women.html

Rosner, J. (2001). *Housing in the new millennium: A home without equity is just a rental with debt* (SSRN Scholarly Paper ID 1162456). Social Science Research Network. https://papers.ssrn.com/abstract=1162456

Rothman, L. (2013, October 9). Chris Brown was raped: Does it matter if he doesn't think so? *Time*. https://entertainment.time.com/2013/10/09/chris-brown-was-raped-does-it-matter-if-he-doesnt-think-so

Rothstein, R. (2017). *The color of law: A forgotten history of how our government segregated America*. Liveright Publishing.

Rovner, J. (2016). *Policy brief: Racial disparities in youth commitments and arrests*. The Sentencing Project. www.sentencingproject.org/publications/racial-disparities-in-youth-commitments-and-arrests

Roy, A. (2009). Why India cannot plan its cities: Informality, insurgence and the idiom of urbanization. *Planning Theory*, *8*(1), 76–87.

Rudman, L. A. (2004a). Social justice in our minds, homes, and society: The nature, causes, and consequences of implicit bias. *Social Justice Research*, *17*(2), 129–142.

Rudman, L. A. (2004b). Sources of implicit attitudes. *Current Directions in Psychological Science*, *13*(2), 79–82.

Rugaber, C. S. (2013, December 17). Income inequality is hurting the economy, 3 dozen economists say. *Huffington Post*.

Rugh, J. S., & Massey, D. S. (2014). Segregation in post-civil rights America: Stalled integration or end of the segregated century? *Du Bois Review: Social Science Research on Race*, *11*(2), 205–232.

Rusche, G., & Kirchheimer, O. (1939). *Punishment and social structure*. Columbia University Press.

Rush, F. (1980). *The best kept secret: Sexual abuse of children*. Prentice-Hall.

Russell, K. K. (2002). The racial hoax as crime: The law as affirmation. In S. L. Gabbidon, H. T. Greene, & V. D. Young (Eds.), *African American classics in criminology and criminal justice* (pp. 349–376). Sage.

Russell, P. E. (2000). *Prince henry "the navigator": A life*. Yale University Press.

Russell-Brown, K. (2017). Making implicit bias explicit. In A. J. Davis (Ed.), *Policing the Black man* (pp. 135–160). Pantheon Books.

Rutland, A., Cameron, L., Milne, A., & Mc- George, P. (2005). Social norms and self presentation: Children's implicit and explicit intergroup attitudes. *Child Development*, *76*(2), 451–466.

Sabin, J. A., & Greenwald, A. G. (2012). The influence of implicit bias on treatment recommendations for 4 common pediatric conditions: Pain, urinary tract infection, attention deficit hyperactivity disorder, and asthma. *American Journal of Public Health*, *102*(5), 988–995.

Sadler, M. S., Correll, J., Park, B., & Judd, C. M. (2012). The world is not Black and White: Racial bias in the decision to shoot in a multiethnic context. *Journal of Social Issues*, *68*(2), 286–313.

Sahm, C. (2020, February 3). Encouraging banks to serve the credit needs of everyone. *Equitable Growth*. http://www.equitablegrowth.org/encouraging-banks-to-serve-the-credit-needs-of-everyone

Saint-Aubin, A. F. (1994). Testeria: The dis-ease of Black men in White supremacist, patriarchal culture. *Callaloo*, *17*(4), 1054–1073.

Sampson, R. J. (1987). Urban Black violence: The effect of male joblessness and family disruption. *American Journal of Sociology*, *93*(2), 348–382.

Sampson, R. J. (2013). The place of context: A theory and strategy for criminology's hard problems. *Criminology*, *51*(1), 1–31.

Sampson, R. J., & Wilson, W. J. (1995). Toward a theory of race, crime, and urban inequality. In J. Hagan & R. D. Peterson (Eds.), *Crime and inequality* (pp. 37–54). Stanford University Press.

Samson, B. (2020, March 11). Police rape culture in the cannibal nation. *Medium*. https://bejtashsamson.medium.com/police-rape-culture-in-the-cannibal-nation-755b8ea53042

Santhanam, L. (2021, February 18). COVID-19 has already cut U.S. life expectancy by a year: For Black Americans, it's worse. *PBS NewsHour*. www.pbs.org/newshour/health/covid-19-has-already-cut-u-s-life-expectancy-by-a-year-for-black-americans-its-worse

Saphir, A. (2021, June 10). U.S. household wealth jumps to record $136.9 trillion, Fed says. *Reuters*. www.reuters.com/world/us/us-household-wealth-rose-record-1369-trillion-q1-fed-says-2021-06-10

Satterfield, J. (2022, September 9). Federal appeals court reinstates civil rights lawsuit over anal cavity search by Memphis PD. *Tennessee Lookout*. https://tennesseelookout.com/2022/09/09/federal-appeals-court-reinstates-civil-rights-lawsuit-over-anal-cavity-search-by-memphis-pd/

Sawyer, M. E. (2018). Post-truth, social media, and the "real" as phantasm. In M. Stenmark, S. Fuller, & U. Zackariasson (Eds.), *Relativism and post-truth in contemporary society: Possibilities and Challenges* (pp. 55–69). Palgrave Macmillan.

Scannell, R. J. (2018). *Electric light: Automating the carceral state during the quantification of everything*. City University of New York.

Scheingold, S. A. (2011). *The politics of law and order: Street crime and public policy*. Quid Pro Books.

Schlanger, M. (2013). Plata v. Brown and realignment: Jails, prisons, courts, and politics. *Harvard Civil Rights-Civil Liberties Law Review*, *48*, 165–216.

Schmader, T., Hall, W., & Croft, A. (2015). Stereotype threat in intergroup relations. In M. Mikulincer, P. R. Shaver, J. F. Dovidio, & J. A. Simpson (Eds.), *APA handbook of personality and social psychology* (Group processes, Vol. 2, pp. 447–471). American Psychological Association.

Schmitt, M. T., & Wirth, J. H. (2009). Evidence that gender differences in social dominance orientation result from gendered self-stereotyping and group-interested responses to patriarchy. *Psychology of Women Quarterly*, *33*(4), 429–436.

Schneider, D. (2011). Wealth and the marital divide. *American Journal of Sociology*, *117*(2), 627–667.

Schooley, R. C., Lee, D. L., & Spanierman, L. B. (2019). Measuring whiteness: A systematic review of instruments and call to action. *The Counseling Psychologist*, *47*(4), 530–565.

Schulman, G. I. (1974). Race, sex, and violence: A laboratory test of the sexual threat of the Black male hypothesis. *American Journal of Sociology*, *79*(5), 1260–1277.

Scott, D. (2000). The re-enchantment of humanism: An interview with Sylvia Wynter. *Small Axe*, *8*(120), 173–211.

Seamster, L. (2019). Black debt, White debt. *Contexts*, *18*(1), 30–35.

Seder, J. W., & Burrell, B. G. (1971). *Getting it together: Black businessmen in America*. Houghton Mifflin Harcourt Press.

Segal, S. P., Bola, J. R., & Watson, M. A. (1996). Race, quality of care, and antipsychotic prescribing practices in psychiatric emergency services. *Psychiatric Services (Washington, DC)*, *47*(3), 282–286.

Sellers, R. M., Copeland-Linder, N., Martin, P. P., & Lewis, R. L. H. (2006). Racial identity matters: The relationship between racial discrimination and psychological functioning in African American adolescents. *Journal of Research on Adolescence*, *16*(2), 187–216.

Sellers, R. M., & Shelton, J. N. (2003). The role of racial identity in perceived racial discrimination. *Journal of Personality and Social Psychology*, *84*, 1079–1092.

Sellers, R. M., Smith, M. A., Shelton, J. N., Rowley, S. A., & Chavous, T. M. (1998). Multidimensional model of racial identity: A reconceptualization of African American racial identity. *Personality and Social Psychology Review*, *2*(1), 18–39.

Sellin, T. (1928). The Negro criminal a statistical note. *The Annals of the American Academy of Political and Social Science*, *140*(1), 52–64.

Seltzer, J. A. (1994). Consequences of marital dissolution for children. *Annual Review of Sociology*, *20*(1), 235–266.

Sen, A. K. (1997). From income inequality to economic inequality. *Southern Economic Journal*, *64*(2), 384–401.

The Sentencing Project. (2017). *Fact sheet: Trends in U.S. corrections*. The Sentencing Project. https://perma.cc/G3Y4-JE3L

Sexton, J. (2008). *Amalgamation schemes: Antiblackness and the critique of multiracialism*. University of Minnesota Press.

Shapiro, F. (2001). *Eye movement desensitization and reprocessing: Basic principles, protocols, and procedures*. Guildford Press.

Shapiro, T. M. (2001). The importance of assets. Assets for the poor: The benefits of spreading asset ownership. In T. M. Shapiro & E. N. Wolff (Eds.), *Assets for the poor: The benefits of spreading asset ownership* (pp. 11–33). Russell Sage Foundation.

Shapiro, T. M. (2004). *The hidden cost of being African American: How wealth perpetuates inequality*. Oxford University Press.

Shapiro, T. M., & Kenty-Drane, J. L. (2005). The racial wealth gap. African Americans in the US economy. In C. Conrad, J. Stewart, J. Whitehead, & P. Mason (Eds.), *African Americans in the US economy* (pp. 175–181). Rowman & Littlefield Publishers.

Sharkey, P. (2009). *Neighborhoods and the Black-White mobility gap*. The Economic Mobility Project, an Initiative of The Pew Charitable Trusts.

Shear, M. D., & Hilzenrath, D. (2010, April 16). Obamas report $5.5 million in 2009 income. *The Ledger*. www.theledger.com/story/news/2010/04/16/obamas-report-55-million-in-2009-income/26264821007

Shellow, R. (Ed.). (2018). *The harvest of American racism: The political meaning of violence in the Summer of 1967*. University of Michigan Press.

Sherman, M. (2018, September 24). Intersectionality and the tragedy of the Black male. *Psychology Today*. www.psychologytoday.com/us/blog/real-men-dont-write-blogs/201809/intersectionality-and-the-tragedy-the-black-male

Shupe, A. D., Stacey, W. A., & Hazlewood, L. R. (1987). *Violent men, violent couples: The dynamics of domestic violence*. Lexington Books.

Sibrava, N. J., Bjornsson, A. S., Pérez Benítez, A. C. I., Moitra, E., Weisberg, R. B., & Keller, M. B. (2019). Posttraumatic stress disorder in African American and Latinx adults: Clinical course and the role of racial and ethnic discrimination. *American Psychologist*, *74*(1), 101–116.

Sidanius, J., Hudson, S. K. T., Davis, G., & Bergh, R. (2018). The theory of gendered prejudice: A social dominance and intersectionalist perspective. In A. Mintz & L. G. Terris (Eds.), *The Oxford handbook of behavioral political science* (pp. 1–35). Oxford University Press.

Sidanius, J., Levin, S., Liu, J., & Pratto, F. (2000). Social dominance orientation, anti-egalitarianism and the political psychology of gender: An extension and cross-cultural replication. *European Journal of Social Psychology*, *30*(1), 41–67.

Sidanius, J., Levin, S., & Pratto, F. (1998). Hierarchical group relations, institutional terror, and the dynamics of the criminal justice system. In J. L. Eberhardt & S. T. Fiske (Eds.), *Confronting racism: The problem and the response* (pp. 136–165). Sage Publications, Inc.

Sidanius, J., & Pratto, F. (1999). *Social dominance: An intergroup theory of social hierarchy and oppression*. Cambridge University Press.

Sidanius, J., & Pratto, F. (2012). Social dominance theory. In P. Van Lange, A. Kruglanski, & E. Higgins (Eds.), *Handbook of theories of social psychology* (pp. 418–438). Sage Publications Ltd.

Sidanius, J., Pratto, F., & Bobo, L. (1994). Social dominance orientation and the political psychology of gender: A case of invariance? *Journal of Personality and Social Psychology, 67*, 998–1011.

Sidanius, J., & Veniegas, R. C. (2000). Gender and race discrimination: The interactive nature of disadvantage. In S. Oskamp (Ed.), *Reducing prejudice and discrimination* (pp. 47–69). Lawrence Erlbaum Associates Publishers.

Siegel, J. (2023, March 28). A guide to understanding the hoax of the century: Thirteen ways of looking at disinformation. *Tablet*. www.tabletmag.com/sections/news/articles/guide-understanding-hoax-century-thirteen-ways-looking-disinformation

Siegel, R., Ma, J., Zou, Z., & Jemal, A. (2014). Cancer statistics, 2014. *CA: A Cancer Journal for Clinicians, 64*(1), 9–29.

Sigelman, L., & Tuch, S. A. (1997). Metastereotypes: Blacks' perceptions of Whites' stereotypes of Blacks. *The Public Opinion Quarterly, 61*(1), 87–101.

Sigelman, L., & Welch, S. (1991). *Black Americans' views of racial inequality: The dream deferred*. Cambridge University Press Archive.

Simien, E. (2007). A Black gender gap? Continuity and change in attitudes toward Black feminism. *African American Perspectives on Political Science*, 130–150.

Simon, N. M., Smoller, J. W., McNamara, K. L., Maser, R. S., Zalta, A. K., Pollack, M. H., Nierenberg, A. A., Fava, M., & Wong, K.-K. (2006). Telomere shortening and mood disorders: Preliminary support for a chronic stress model of accelerated aging. *Biological Psychiatry, 60*, 432–435.

Sims, M., Diez-Roux, A. V., Dudley, A., Gebreab, S., Wyatt, S. B., Bruce, M. A., James, S. A., Robinson, J. C., Williams, D. R., & Taylor, H. A. (2012). Perceived discrimination and hypertension among African Americans in the Jackson Heart Study. *American Journal of Public Health, 102*(S2), S258–S265.

Singer, J., Sussman, N., Martin, N., & Johnson, A. (2020, December 22). Black men have the shortest lifespans of any Americans: This theory helps explain why. *ProPublica*. www.propublica.org/article/black-men-have-the-shortest-lifespans-of-any-americans-this-theory-helps-explain-why?token=NME_NcoroUdzje1h9I_NahlDXcB6TjfG

Singer, M., Bulled, N., Ostrach, B., & Mendenhall, E. (2017). Syndemics and the biosocial conception of health. *The Lancet, 389*(10072), 941–950.

Singletary, G. (2020). Beyond PTSD: Black male fragility in the context of trauma. *Journal of Aggression, Maltreatment & Trauma, 29*(5), 517–536.

Skinner-Dorkenoo, A. L., Sarmal, A., Rogbeer, K., André, C., Patel, B., & Cha, L. (2022). Highlighting COVID-19 racial disparities can reduce support for safety precautions among White US residents. *Social Science & Medicine*, 114951.

Slavin, L. A., Rainer, K. L., McCreary, M. L., & Gowda, K. K. (1991). Toward a multicultural model of the stress process. *Journal of Counseling & Development, 70*(1), 156–163.

Slootmaeckers, J., & Migerode, L. (2018). Fighting for connection: Patterns of intimate partner violence. *Journal of Couple & Relationship Therapy, 17*(4), 294–312.

Slootmaeckers, J., & Migerode, L. (2020). EFT and intimate partner violence: A roadmap to de-escalating violent patterns. *Family Process, 59*(2), 328–345.

Smedley, A., & Smedley, B. D. (2005). Race as biology is fiction, racism as a social problem is real: Anthropological and historical perspectives on the social construction of race. *American Psychologist, 60*(1), 16–26.

Smedley, B. D., Stith, A. Y., & Nelson, A. R. (2003). Racial and ethnic disparities in diagnosis and treatment: A review of the evidence and a consideration of causes. In B. D. Smedley, A. Y. Stith, & A. R. Nelson (Eds.), *Unequal treatment: Confronting racial and ethnic disparities in health care* (pp. 417–454). National Academies Press.

Smelser, N. J. (2004). Psychological trauma and cultural trauma. *Cultural Trauma and Collective Identity, 4*, 31–59.

Smiley, C., & Fakunle, D. (2016). From "brute" to "thug:" The demonization and criminalization of unarmed Black male victims in America. *Journal of Human Behavior in the Social Environment*, *26*(3–4), 350–366.

Smith, S. G., Chen, J., Basile, K. C., Gilbert, L. K., Merrick, M. T., Patel, N., & Jang, A. (2017). *The national intimate partner and sexual violence survey (NISVS): 2010–2012 state report*. National Center for Injury Prevention and Control, Centers for Disease Control and Prevention. www.cdc.gov/violenceprevention/pdf/NISVS-StateReportBook.pdf

Smith, W. A. (2010). Toward an understanding of Black misandric microaggressions and racial battle fatigue in historically White institutions. In V. C. Polite (Ed.), *The state of the African American male in Michigan: A courageous conversation* (pp. 265–277). Michigan State University Press.

Smith, W. A., Hung, M., & Franklin, J. D. (2011). Racial battle fatigue and the miseducation of Black men: Racial microaggressions, societal problems, and environmental stress. *The Journal of Negro Education*, 63–82.

Smith, W. A., Hung, M., & Franklin, J. D. (2012). Between hope and racial battle fatigue: African American men and race-related stress. *Journal of Black Masculinity*, *2*(1), 35–58.

Smith, W. A., Mustaffa, J. B., Jones, C. M., Curry, T. J., & Allen, W. R. (2016). You make me want to holla and throw up both my hands: Campus culture, Black misandric microaggressions, and racial battle fatigue. *International Journal of Qualitative Studies in Education*, *29*(9), 1189–1209.

Smith, W. A., Yosso, T. J., & Solórzano, D. G. (2007). Racial primes and Black misandry on historically White campuses: Toward critical race accountability in educational administration. *Educational Administration Quarterly*, *43*(5), 559–585.

Smith Lee, J. R., & Robinson, M. A. (2019). "That's my number one fear in life. It's the police": Examining young Black men's exposures to trauma and loss resulting from police violence and police killings. *Journal of Black Psychology*, *45*(3), 143–184.

Sniderman, P., & Piazza, T. (1993). *The scar of race*. Harvard University Press.

Sobel, N. (2020, June 6). What is qualified immunity, and what does it have to do with police reform? *Lawfare*. www.lawfareblog.com/what-qualified-immunity-and-what-does-it-have-do-police-reform

Son Hing, L. S., Chung-Yan, G. A., Hamilton, L. K., & Zanna, M. P. (2008). A two-dimensional model that employs explicit and implicit attitudes to characterize prejudice. *Journal of Personality and Social Psychology*, *94*(6), 971–987.

Soss, J., & Weaver, V. (2017). Police are our government: Politics, political science, and the policing of race – class subjugated communities. *Annual Review of Political Science*, *20*, 565–591.

Sotero, M. (2006). A conceptual model of historical trauma: Implications for public health practice and research. *Journal of Health Disparities Research and Practice*, *1*(1), 93–108.

Soto, J. A., Dawson-Andoh, N. A., & BeLue, R. (2011). The relationship between perceived discrimination and generalized anxiety disorder among African Americans, Afro Caribbeans, and non-Hispanic Whites. *Journal of Anxiety Disorders*, *25*(2), 258–265.

South, S. J. (1996). Mate availability and the transition to unwed motherhood: A paradox of population structure. *Journal of Marriage and the Family*, 265–279.

Squires, G. D., & Chadwick, J. (2006). Linguistic profiling: A continuing tradition of discrimination in the home insurance industry? *Urban Affairs Review*, *41*(3), 400–415.

Staggers-Hakim, R. (2016). The nation's unprotected children and the ghost of Mike Brown, or the impact of national police killings on the health and social development of African American boys. *Journal of Human Behavior in the Social Environment*, *26*(3–4), 390–399.

Staples, R. (1978). Masculinity and race: The dual dilemma of Black men. *Journal of Social Issues*, 169–183.

Staples, R. (1982). *Black masculinity: The Black male's role in American society*. Black Scholar Press.

Staples, R. (1985). Changes in Black family structure: The conflict between family ideology and structural conditions. *Journal of Marriage and the Family*, 1005–1013.

Staples, R. (1987a). Black male genocide: A final solution to the race problem in America. *The Black Scholar*, *18*(3), 2–11.

Staples, R. (1987b). Social structure and Black family life: An analysis of current trends. *Journal of Black Studies*, *17*(3), 267–286.

Staub, E. (1989). *The roots of evil: The origins of genocide and other group violence.* Cambridge University Press.

Stein, M. N. (2015). *Measuring manhood: Race and the science of masculinity, 1830–1934.* University of Minnesota Press.

Stein, S. (2019). *Capital city: Gentrification and the real estate state.* Verso Books.

Steinmetz, S., & Lucca, J. (1988). Husband battering. In V. Van Hasselt (Ed.), *Handbook of family violence* (pp. 233–246). Plenum Press.

Stemple, L., Flores, A., & Meyer, I. H. (2017). Sexual victimization perpetrated by women: Federal data reveal surprising prevalence. *Aggression and Violent Behavior, 34,* 302–311.

Stemple, L., & Meyer, I. H. (2014). The sexual victimization of men in America: New data challenge old assumptions. *American Journal of Public Health, 104*(6), e19–e26.

Stern, M. J. (2019, June 5). The ruling against a cop accused of a horrific body cavity search is a rare victory for police accountability. *Slate.* https://slate.com/news-and-politics/2019/06/michigan-lawsuit-officer-daniel-mack-illegal-body-cavity-search.html

Stevenson, B. (2017). A presumption of guilt: The legacy of America's history of racial injustice. In A. J. Davis (Ed.), *Policing the Black man* (pp. 3–30). Pantheon Books.

Stewart, J. B. (1980). The political economy of Black male suicides. *Journal of Black Studies, 11*(2), 249–261.

Stewart, J. B. (1994). Neoconservative attacks on Black families and the Black male: An analysis and critique. In R. G. Majors & J. U. Gordon (Eds.), *The American Black male: His present status and his future* (pp. 39–58). Nelson-Hall Publishers.

Stewart, J. B., & Scott, J. W. (1978). The institutional decimation of Black American males. *Western Journal of Black Studies, 2*(2), 82–92.

Stewart, M. (2018, May 16). The 9.9 percent is the new American aristocracy. *The Atlantic.* www.theatlantic.com/magazine/archive/2018/06/the-birth-of-a-new-american-aristocracy/559130

Stockstill, C., & Carson, G. (2021). Are lighter-skinned Tanisha and Jamal worth more pay? White people's gendered colorism toward Black job applicants with racialized names. *Ethnic and Racial Studies, 45*(5), 896–917.

Stop-and-frisk 2011: NYCLU briefing (2012, May 9). *NYCLU.* www.nyclu.org/sites/default/files/publications/2012_Report_NYCLU_0.pdf

Storr, W. (2011, July 16). The rape of men: The darkest secret of war. *The Observer.* www.theguardian.com/society/2011/jul/17/the-rape-of-men

Straus, M. A., Hamby, S. L., Boney-McCoy, S. U. E., & Sugarman, D. B. (1996). The revised conflict tactics scales (CTS2) development and preliminary psychometric data. *Journal of Family Issues, 17*(3), 283–316.

Strobino, D. M., & Sirageldin, I. (1981). Racial differences in early marriages in the United States. *Social Science Quarterly, 62*(4), 758–766.

Strolovitch, D. Z., Wong, J. S., & Proctor, A. (2017). A possessive investment in White heteropatriarchy? The 2016 election and the politics of race, gender, and sexuality. *Politics, Groups, and Identities, 5*(2), 353–363.

Struckman-Johnson, C. (1988). Forced sex on dates: It happens to men, too. *Journal of Sex Research, 24*(1), 234–241.

Substance Abuse and Mental Health Services Administration. (2014). *SAMHSA's concept of trauma and guidance for a trauma-informed approach* (HHS Publication No. (SMA) 14–4884). Substance Abuse and Mental Health Services Administration. https://ncsacw.acf.hhs.gov/userfiles/files/SAMHSA_Trauma.pdf

Sue, D. W. (2003). *Overcoming our racism: The journey to liberation.* Jossey-Bass.

Sue, D. W. (2004). Whiteness and ethnocentric monoculturalism: Making the "invisible" visible. *American Psychologist, 59*(8), 761–769.

Sue, D. W., Capodilupo, C. M., Torino, G. C., Bucceri, J. M., Holder, A. M. B., Nadal, K. L., & Esquilin, M. (2007). Racial microaggressions in everyday life: Implications for clinical practice. *American Psychologist, 62,* 271–286.

Sullivan, B. (2021, October 18). The U.S. supreme court rules in favor of officers accused of excessive force. *NPR*. www.npr.org/2021/10/18/1047085626/supreme-court-police-quali fied-immunity-cases

Sullivan, J. F. (1990, February 19). New jersey police are accused of minority arrest campaigns. *The New York Times*. www.nytimes.com/1990/02/19/nyregion/new-jersey-police-are-accused-of-minority-arrest-campaigns.html

Sullivan, M. (1989). *Getting paid: Youth crime and work in the inner city*. Cornell University Press.

Survey of Consumer Finances. (2019). https://www.federalreserve.gov/econres/scf_2019.htm

Suzuki, M. (2002). Selective immigration and ethnic economic achievement: Japanese Americans before world war II. *Explorations in Economic History, 39*(3), 254–281.

Swaine, J., Laughland, O., & Lartey, J. (2015, June 1). Black Americans killed by police twice as likely to be unarmed as White people. *The Guardian*. www.theguardian.com/us-news/2015/jun/01/black-americans-killed-by-police-analysis

Swaine, J., & McCarthy, C. (2017, January 8). Young Black men again faced highest rate of US police killings in 2016. *The Guardian*. www.theguardian.com/us-news/2017/jan/08/the-counted-police-killings-2016-young-black-men

Sykes, B. L., Chavez, E., & Strong, J. (2021). Mass incarceration and inmate mortality in the United States – death by design? *JAMA Network Open, 4*(12), e2140349.

Sznycer, D., Xygalatas, D., Agey, E., Alami, S., An, X. F., Ananyeva, K. I., Atkinson, Q., Broitman, B. R., Conte, T. J., Flores, C., Fukushima, S., Hitokoto, H., Kharitonov, A. N., Onyishi, C. N., Onyishi, I. E., Romero, P. P., Schrock, J. M., Snodgrass, J. J., Sugiyama, L. S. . . . Tooby, J. (2018). Cross-cultural invariances in the architecture of shame. *Proceedings of the National Academy of Sciences, 115*(39), 9702–9707.

Takaki, R. (1989). *Strangers from a different shore: A history of Asian Americans*. Little, Brown and Company.

Takaki, R. (1993). *A different mirror: A history of multicultural America*. Little, Brown and Company.

Tangney, J. P., & Dearing, R. L. (2002). *Shame and guilt*. Guilford Press.

Tarba, L. R. (2015). *Relating a model of resolution of arrested anger to outcome in emotion-focused therapy of depression* [Doctoral dissertation, York University].

Tate, G. (1973). Humanistic psychology and Black psychology: A study of parallels. Humanistic psychology. In F. Richards & I. D. Welch (Eds.), *Sightings: Essays in humanistic psychology* (pp. 156–166). Shields Publishing.

Tatum, D. C. (2017). Donald Trump and the legacy of Bacon's rebellion. *Journal of Black Studies, 48*(7), 651–674.

Taylor, J., & Turner, R. J. (2002). Perceived discrimination, social stress, and depression in the transition to adulthood: Racial contrasts. *Social Psychology Quarterly*, 213–225.

Taylor, S. E. (1999). *Health psychology* (4th ed.). McGraw-Hill.

Taylor, T. R., Williams, C. D., Makambi, K. H., Mouton, C., Harrell, J. P., Cozier, Y., Palmer, J. R., Rosenberg, L., & Adams-Campbell, L. L. (2007). Racial discrimination and breast cancer incidence in US Black women: The Black women's health study. *American Journal of Epidemiology, 166*(1), 46–54.

Terborg-Penn, R. (1998). *African American women in the struggle for the vote, 1850–1920*. Indiana University Press.

Testa, M., Astone, N. M., Krogh, M., & Neckerman, K. M. (1993). Employment and marriage among inner-city fathers. In W. J. Wilson (Ed.), *The ghetto underclass: Social science perspectives* (pp. 96–108). Sage Publications, Inc.

Testa, M., & Krogh, M. (1995). The effect of employment on marriage among Black males in inner-city Chicago. In M. B. Tucker & C. Mitchell-Kernan (Eds.), *The decline in marriage among African Americans* (pp. 59–95). Russell Sage Foundation.

Thiem, K. C., Neel, R., Simpson, A. J., & Todd, A. R. (2019). Are Black women and girls associated with danger? Implicit racial bias at the intersection of target age and gender. *Personality and Social Psychology Bulletin, 45*(10), 1427–1439.

Thomas, G. (2006). Proud Flesh inter/views: Sylvia Wynter. *ProudFlesh: New Afrikan Journal of Culture, Politics and Consciousness, 4*, 1–36.

Thomas, G. (2007). *The sexual demon of colonial power: Pan-African embodiment and erotic schemes of empire*. Indiana University Press.

Thomas, H. (1997). *The slave trade: The story of the Atlantic slave trade: 1440–1870*. Simon and Schuster.

Thompson, C. E., & Carter, R. T. (1997). An overview and elaboration of Helms' racial identity development theory. In C. E. Thompson & R. T. Carter (Eds.), *Racial identity theory: Applications to individual, group, and organizational interventions* (pp. 15–32). Routledge.

Thompson, M. E. (2023). Examining the Black gender gap in educational attainment: The role of exclusionary school discipline & criminal justice contact. *Social Forces*, soad110.

Thompson, V. L. S. (1996). Perceived experiences of racism as stressful life events. *Community Mental Health Journal*, *32*(3), 223–233.

Thompson, V. L. S. (2002). Racism: Perceptions or distress among African Americans. *Community Mental Health Journal*, *38*, 111–118.

Timulak, L. (2015). *Transforming emotional pain in psychotherapy: An emotion-focused approach*. Routledge.

Todd, A. R., Simpson, A. J., Thiem, K. C., & Neel, R. (2016). The generalization of implicit racial bias to young Black boys: Automatic stereotyping or automatic prejudice? *Social Cognition*, *34*(4), 306–323.

Tolnay, S. E., & Beck, E. M. (1995). *A festival of violence: An analysis of southern lynchings, 1882–1930*. University of Illinois Press.

Toossi, M., & Joyner, L. (2018). Blacks in the labor force: United States bureau of labor statistics. *Spotlight on Statistics*, 1–21.

Tormala, T. T., & Mc Kenzie, R. (2021). Social representations of blackness in America: Stereotypes about Black immigrants and Black Americans. In H. Chu & B. Thelamour (Eds.), *Conceptual and methodological approaches to navigating immigrant ecologies* (pp. 89–106). Springer.

Travis, J., & Western, B. (2017). Poverty, violence, and Black incarceration. In A. J. Davis (Ed.), *Policing the Black man* (pp. 294–321). Pantheon Books.

Trawalter, S., Todd, A. R., Baird, A. A., & Richeson, J. A. (2008). Attending to threat: Race-based patterns of selective attention. *Journal of Experimental Social Psychology*, *44*(5), 1322–1327.

Tsai, T., & Scommegna, P. (2012). *U.S. has world's highest incarceration rate*. Population Reference Bureau. www.prb.org/us-incarceration

Turnbull, G. J. (1998). A review of post-traumatic stress disorder. Part I: Historical development and classification. *Injury*, *29*(2), 87–91.

Turner, M. A., Freiberg, F., Godfrey, E., Herbig, C., Levy, D. K., & Smith, R. R. (2002). *All other things being equal: A paired testing study of mortgage lending institutions*. The Urban Institute.

Turner, M. A., Godfrey, E., Ross, S. L., & Smith, R. R. (2003). *Other things being equal: A paired testing study of discrimination in mortgage lending* (Economics Working Papers 200309). https://digitalcommons.lib.uconn.edu/econ_wpapers/200309

Turner, S., Taillieu, T., Cheung, K., & Afifi, T. O. (2017). The relationship between childhood sexual abuse and mental health outcomes among males: Results from a nationally representative United States sample. *Child Abuse & Neglect*, *66*, 64–72.

Turney, I. C., Lao, P. J., Rentería, M. A., Igwe, K. C., Berroa, J., Rivera, A., Benavides, A., Morales, C. D., Rizvi, B., Schupf, N., Mayeux, R., Manly, J. J., & Brickman, A. M. (2022). Brain aging among racially and ethnically diverse middle-aged and older adults. *JAMA Neurology*, *80*.

Twine, F. W., & Gallagher, C. (2008). The future of whiteness: A map of the "third wave". *Ethnic and Racial Studies*, *31*(1), 4–24.

Tynes, B. M., Willis, H. A., Stewart, A. M., & Hamilton, M. W. (2019). Race-related traumatic events online and mental health among adolescents of color. *Journal of Adolescent Health*, *65*(3), 371–377.

Uhuru, A. (2021, Fall). The polemical as non-violent protest: James Baldwin and the "gendered" Black body. *APA Newsletter on Philosophy and the Black Experience*, *21*(1), 4–12.

Umberson, D. (2017). Black deaths matter: Race, relationship loss, and effects on survivors. *Journal of Health and Social Behavior*, *58*(4), 405–420.

Umfleet, L. (2005). *1898 Wilmington race riot report*. Office of Archives and History, North Carolina Department of Cultural Resources.

United States. National Advisory Commission on Civil Disorders, & United States. Kerner Commission. (1968). *Report of the national advisory commission on civil disorders.* US Government Printing Office.

Unnever, J. D., & Chouhy, C. (2021). Race, racism, and the cool pose: Exploring Black and White male masculinity. *Social Problems, 68*(2), 490–512.

Unnever, J. D., & Cullen, F. T. (2009). Empathetic identification and punitiveness: A middle-range theory of individual differences. *Theoretical Criminology, 13*(3), 283–312.

Unnever, J. D., & Cullen, F. T. (2012). White perceptions of whether African Americans and Hispanics are prone to violence and support for the death penalty. *Journal of Research in Crime and Delinquency, 49*(4), 519–544.

Üstün, T. B., Ayuso-Mateos, J. L., Chatterji, S., Mathers, C., & Murray, C. J. (2004). Global burden of depressive disorders in the year 2000. *The British Journal of Psychiatry, 184*(5), 386–392.

Utley, E. A. (2016). Humanizing Blackness: An interview with Tommy J. Curry. *Southern Communication Journal, 81*(4), 263–266.

Utsey, S. O. (1997). Racism and the psychological well-being of African American men. *Journal of African American Men*, 69–87.

Utsey, S. O. (1999). Development and validation of a short form of the index of race-related stress (IRRS) – brief version. *Measurement and Evaluation in Counseling and Development, 32*(3), 149–167.

Utsey, S. O., Bolden, M. A., & Brown, A. L. (2001). Visions of revolution from the spirit of Frantz Fanon: A psychology of liberation for counseling African Americans confronting societal racism and oppression. In J. G. Ponterotto, J. M. Casas, L. A. Suzuki, & C. M. Alexander (Eds.), *Handbook of multicultural counseling* (pp. 311–336). Sage Publications, Inc.

Utsey, S. O., Ponterotto, J. G., & Porter, J. S. (2008). Prejudice and racism, year 2008 – still going strong: Research on reducing prejudice with recommended methodological advances. *Journal of Counseling & Development, 86*(3), 339–347.

U.S. Bureau of Labor Statistics. (2019). *Characteristics of minimum wage workers, 2018.* BLS Reports. www.bls.gov/opub/reports/minimumwage/2018/pdf/home.pdf

Vaes, J., Paladino, M. P., Castelli, L., Leyens, J. P., & Giovanazzi, A. (2003). On the behavioral consequences of infrahumanization: The implicit role of uniquely human emotions in intergroup relations. *Journal of Personality and Social Psychology, 85*(6), 1016–1034.

Van der Kolk, B. A. (2003). The neurobiology of childhood trauma and abuse. *Child and Adolescent Psychiatric Clinics, 12*(2), 293–317.

Van der Kolk, B. A. (2005). Developmental trauma disorder. *Psychiatric Annals, 35*(5), 401–408.

Van der Kolk, B. A., McFarlane, A. C., & Van der Hart, O. (1996). A general approach to treatment of posttraumatic stress disorder. In B. A. Van der Kolk, A. C. McFarlane, & L. Weisaeth (Eds.), *Traumatic stress: The effects of overwhelming experience on mind, body, and society* (pp. 417–440). The Guilford Press.

Van Dijk, T. A. (1987). *Communicating racism: Ethnic prejudice in thought and talk.* Sage Publications, Inc.

Vargas, J. H. C. (2018). *The denial of antiblackness: Multiracial redemption and Black suffering.* University of Minnesota Press.

Vedder, R., Gallaway, L., & Klingaman, D. C. (1990). Black exploitation and White benefits: The civil war income revolution. In R. F. America (Ed.), *The wealth of races: The present value of benefits from past injustices* (pp. 125–138). Greenwood.

Veenstra, G. (2012). The gendered nature of discriminatory experiences by race, class, and sexuality: A comparison of intersectionality theory and the subordinate male target hypothesis. *Sex Roles, 68*(11), 646–659.

Velopulos, C. G., Carmichael, H., Zakrison, T. L., & Crandall, M. (2019). Comparison of male and female victims of intimate partner homicide and bidirectionality – an analysis of the national violent death reporting system. *Journal of Trauma and Acute Care Surgery, 87*(2), 331–336.

Voigt, L., Thornton, W. E., & Barrile, L. (1994). *Criminology and justice.* McGraw-Hill Humanities, Social Sciences & World Languages.

Voigt, R., Camp, N. P., Prabhakaran, V., Hamilton, W. L., Hetey, R. C., Griffiths, C. M., Jurgens, D., Jurafsky, D., & Eberhardt, J. L. (2017). Language from police body camera footage shows racial disparities in officer respect. *Proceedings of the National Academy of Sciences, 114*(25), 6521–6526.

Wacquant, L. (2000). The new peculiar institution': On the prison as surrogate ghetto. *Theoretical Criminology, 4*(3), 377–389.

Wacquant, L. (2005). Race as civic felony. *International Social Science Journal, 57*(183), 127–142.

Wacquant, L. (2009). The body, the ghetto and the penal state. *Qualitative Sociology, 32*(1), 101–129.

Wahba, P. (2021, February 1). Only 19: The lack of Black CEOs in the history of the Fortune 500. *Fortune.* https://fortune.com/longform/fortune-500-black-ceos-business-history

Waldinger, R. (1997). Black/immigrant competition re-assessed: New evidence from Los Angeles. *Sociological Perspectives, 40*(3), 365–386.

Waldinger, R., & Lichter, M. I. (2003). *How the other half works.* University of California Press.

Walker, R., Francis, D., Brody, G., Simons, R., Cutrona, C., & Gibbons, F. (2017). A longitudinal study of racial discrimination and risk for death ideation in African American youth. *Suicide and Life-Threatening Behavior, 47*(1), 86–102.

Walmsley, R. (2003). *World prison population list.* Home Office.

Walmsley, R. (2009). *World prison population list* (8th ed.). International Centre for Prison Studies.

Walton, Q. L., & Shepard Payne, J. (2016). Missing the mark: Cultural expressions of depressive symptoms among African-American women and men. *Social Work in Mental Health, 14*(6), 637–657.

Ward, E., & Mengesha, M. (2013). Depression in African American men: A review of what we know and where we need to go from here. *American Journal of Orthopsychiatry, 83*(2pt3), 386–397.

Ward, G. (2018). Living histories of White supremacist policing: Towards transformative justice. *Du Bois Review: Social Science Research on Race, 15*(1), 167–184.

Warner, J. (2021). Psychiatry confronts its racist past, and tries to make amends. *The New York Times,* p. 30.

Warren, C. L. (2015). Black nihilism and the politics of hope. *CR: The New Centennial Review, 15*(1), 215–248.

Warren, C. L. (2018). *Ontological terror: Blackness, nihilism, and emancipation.* Duke University Press.

Washington, H. A. (2006). *Medical apartheid: The dark history of medical experimentation on Black Americans from colonial times to the present.* Doubleday Books.

Watkins, D. C., Green, B. L., Rivers, B. M., & Rowell, K. L. (2006). Depression and Black men: Implications for future research. *Journal of Men's Health and Gender, 3*(3), 227–235.

Watson, T., & McLanahan, S. (2011). Marriage meets the joneses relative income, identity, and marital status. *Journal of Human Resources, 46*(3), 482–517.

Waytz, A., Hoffman, K. M., & Trawalter, S. (2014). A superhumanization bias in Whites' perceptions of Blacks. *Social Psychological and Personality Science, 6*(3), 352–359.

Weaver, V. M. (2007). Frontlash: Race and the development of punitive crime policy. *Studies in American Political Development, 21*(2), 230–265.

Weber, M. (1947). *The theory of social and economic organization.* Free Press.

Weber, M. (1978). *Economy and society: An outline of interpretive sociology* (Vol. 2, G. Roth & C. Wittich, Eds.). University of California Press.

Weil, J. Z., Blanco, A., & Dominguez, L. (2022, January 10). More than 1,800 congressmen once enslaved Black people: This is who they were, and how they shaped the nation. *Washington Post.* www.washingtonpost.com/history/interactive/2022/congress-slaveowners-names-list/

Weitzer, R., & Tuch, S. A. (1999). Race, class, and perceptions of discrimination by the police. *Crime & Delinquency, 45*(4), 494–507.

Welch, K. (2007). Black criminal stereotypes and racial profiling. *Journal of Contemporary Criminal Justice, 23*(3), 276–288.

Welch, K., Chiricos, T., & Gertz, M. (2002). *Racial typification of crime and punitive attitudes.* Paper presented at annual meeting of the American Society of Criminology, Chicago, IL.

Welch, S., Sigelman, L., Bledsoe, T., & Combs, M. (2001). *Race and place: Race relations in an American city.* Cambridge University Press.

Welsing, F. C. (1991). *The Isis papers: The keys to the colors.* CW Pub.

West, C. M. (2012). Partner abuse in ethnic minority and gay, lesbian, bisexual, and transgender populations. *Partner Abuse, 3*(3), 336–357.

West, C. M. (2016). Living in a web of trauma. In C. A. Cuevas & C. M. Rennison (Eds.), *The Wiley handbook on the psychology of violence* (pp. 649–665). John Wiley & Sons.

West, H. C. (2010). *Prison inmates at midyear 2009-statistical tables NCJ 230113*. Bureau of Justice Statistics, Office of Justice Programs, US Department of Justice.

West, H. C., Sabol, W. J., & Greenman, S. J. (2010). *Prisoners in 2009*. Washington, DC: US Department of Justice, Bureau of Justice Statistics.

Western, B. (2006). *Punishment and inequality in America*. Russell Sage Foundation.

Western, B., & Beckett, K. (1999). How unregulated is the US labor market? The penal system as a labor market institution. *American Journal of Sociology, 104*(4), 1030–1060.

Western, B., & Pettit, B. (2005). Black-White wage inequality, employment rates, and incarceration. *American Journal of Sociology, 111*(2), 553–578.

Western States Center. (2003). *Dismantling racism: A resource book*. http://intergroupresources.com/rc/RESOURCE%20CENTER/OWEN%27S%20CATEGORIZATION%20OF%20RC/2%20-%20Curricular%20Materials/2a%20-%20Publicly%20available/Dismantling%20Racism-%20A%20Resource%20Book%20for%20Social%20Change%20Groups%20-%20Western%20States%20Center.pdf

Whitaker, D. J., Haileyesus, T., Swahn, M., & Saltzman, L. S. (2007). Differences in frequency of violence and reported injury between relationships with reciprocal and nonreciprocal intimate partner violence. *American Journal of Public Health, 97*(5), 941–947.

White, A. M. (2008). *Ain't I a feminist? African American men speak out on fatherhood, friendship, forgiveness, and freedom*. SUNY Press.

White, J. L. (1970, September). Toward a Black psychology. *Ebony*, 43–50.

White, M. (2011). *From Jim Crow to Jay-Z: Race, rap, and the performance of masculinity*. University of Illinois Press.

White, M. J. (1980). *Urban renewal and the changing residential structure of the city*. Community and Family Study Center, University of Chicago.

Whitehouse, M. (2019, June 18). Black poverty is rooted in real estate exploitation. *Crain's Chicago Business*. www.chicagobusiness.com/opinion/black-poverty-rooted-real-estate-exploitation

Wilderson, F. B., III. (2017). Blacks and the master/slave relation. In F. B. Wilderson III, S. Hartman, S. Martinot, J. Sexton, & H. J. Spillers (Eds.), *Afro-pessimism: An introduction* (pp. 15–30). Racked & Dispatched.

Wilderson, F. B., III. (2018). "We're trying to destroy the world": Anti-blackness and police violence after Ferguson. In M. Gržinić & A. Stojnić (Eds.), *Shifting corporealities in contemporary performance: Danger, im/mobility and politics* (pp. 45–59). Palgrave Macmillan.

Wilkinson, D. (1977). The stigmatization process. In D. Y. Wilkinson & R. L. Taylor (Eds.), *The Black male in America: Perspectives on his status in contemporary society* (pp. 145–158). Nelson-Hall.

Willhelm, S. M. (1986). The economic demise of Blacks in America: A prelude to genocide? *Journal of Black Studies, 17*(2), 201–254.

Williams, D. R. (2021, May 26). Why discrimination is a health issue. *RWJF*. www.rwjf.org/en/culture-of-health/2017/10/discrimination-is-a-health-issue.html

Williams, D. R., & Collins, C. (1995). US socioeconomic and racial differences in health: Patterns and explanations. *Annual Review of Sociology, 21*(1), 349–386.

Williams, D. R., & Collins, C. (2004). Reparations: A viable strategy to address the enigma of African American health. *American Behavioral Scientist, 47*(7), 977–1000.

Williams, D. R., Gonzalez, H. M., Neighbors, H., Nesse, R., Abelson, J. M., Sweetman, J., & Jackson, J. S. (2007). Prevalence and distribution of major depressive disorder in African Americans, Caribbean Blacks, and non-Hispanic Whites: Results from the National Survey of American Life. *Archives of General Psychiatry, 64*(3), 305–315.

Williams, D. R., & Mohammed, S. A. (2013). Racism and health I: Pathways and scientific evidence. *American Behavioral Scientist, 57*, 1152–1173.

Williams, D. R., & Neighbors, H. (2001). Racism, discrimination and hypertension: Evidence and needed research. *Ethnicity & Disease, 11*(4), 800–816.

Williams, D. R., Neighbors, H. W., & Jackson, J. S. (2003). Racial/ethnic discrimination and health: Findings from community studies. *American Journal of Public Health, 93*(2), 200–208.

Williams, D. R., & Williams-Morris, R. (2000). Racism and mental health: The African American experience. *Ethnicity and Health, 5*, 243–268.

Williams, E. (1994). *Capitalism and slavery*. The University of North Carolina Press.

Williams, H. S. (2016). Uses of the interstitial as power: Black, bisexual men building maroon health. In L. D. Follins & J. M. Lassiter (Eds.), *Black LGBT health in the United States: The intersection of race, gender, and sexual orientation* (pp. 39–54). Lexington Books.

Williams, J. E., & Holmes, K. A. (1981). *The second assault: Rape and public attitudes*. Greenwood Press.

Williams, M. T., Gooden, A. M., & Davis, D. (2012). African Americans, European Americans, and pathological stereotypes: An African-centered perspective. In G. R. Hayes & M. H. Bryant (Eds.), *Psychology of culture* (pp. 25–46). Nova Science Publishers.

Williams, O., III, Pieterse, A. L., DeLoach, C., Bolden, M. A., Ball, J., & Awadalla, S. (2010). Beyond health disparities: Examining power disparities and industrial complexes from the views of Frantz Fanon (part 1). *Journal of Pan African Studies, 3*(8), 151–179.

Williams, R. B. (2017). Wealth privilege and the racial wealth gap: A case study in economic stratification. *The Review of Black Political Economy, 44*(3–4), 303–325.

Williams-Myers, A. J. (1995). *Destructive impulses: An examination of an American secret in race relations: White violence*. University Press of America.

Williams-Washington, K. N. (2010). Historical trauma. In R. L. Hampton, T. P. Gullotta, & R. L. Crowel (Eds.), *Handbook of African American health* (pp. 31–50). The Guilford Press.

Willoughby, C. D. (2018). Running away from Drapetomania: Samuel A. Cartwright, medicine, and race in the Antebellum South. *Journal of Southern History, 84*(3), 579–614.

Wilson, J. P., Hugenberg, K., & Rule, N. O. (2017a). Racial bias in judgments of physical size and formidability: From size to threat. *Journal of Personality and Social Psychology, 113*(1), 59–80.

Wilson, J. P., Remedios, J. D., & Rule, N. O. (2017b). Interactive effects of obvious and ambiguous social categories on perceptions of leadership: When double-minority status may be beneficial. *Personality and Social Psychology Bulletin, 43*(6), 888–900.

Wilson, K. B., Thorpe, R. J., Jr., & LaVeist, T. A. (2017). Dollar for dollar: Racial and ethnic inequalities in health and health-related outcomes among persons with very high income. *Preventive Medicine, 96*, 149–153.

Wilson, T. D., Lindsey, S., & Schooler, T. Y. (2000). A model of dual attitudes. *Psychological Review, 107*(1), 101–126.

Wilson, W. J. (1987). *The truly disadvantaged: The inner city, the underclass, and public policy*. University of Chicago Press.

Wilson, W. J. (1996). *When work disappears: The world of the new urban poor*. Vintage.

Wilson, W. J., Aponte, R., Kirschenman, J., & Wacquant, L. (1988). The ghetto underclass and the changing structure of American poverty. In F. R. Harris & R. W. Wilkins (Eds.), *Quiet riots: Race and poverty in the United States* (pp. 123–154). Pantheon.

Wilson, W. J., & Neckerman, K. (1986). Poverty and family structure: The widening gap between evidence and public policy issues. In S. Danziger & D. Weinberg (Eds.), *Fighting poverty: What works and what doesn't* (pp. 232–259). Harvard University Press.

Wingfield, A. H. (2007). The modern mammy and the angry Black man: African American professionals' experiences with gendered racism in the workplace. *Race, Gender & Class*, 196–212.

Winkelmann, L., & Winkelmann, R. (1998). Why are the unemployed so unhappy? Evidence from panel data. *Economica, 65*(257), 1–15.

Winship, S., Pulliam, C., Shiro, A. G., Reeves, R. V., & Deambrosi, S. (2021, June 10). *Long shadows: The Black-White gap in multigenerational poverty*. Brookings. www.brookings.edu/research/long-shadows-the-black-white-gap-in-multigenerational-poverty

Wise, L. A., Palmer, J. R., Cozier, Y. C., Hunt, M. O., Stewart, E. A., & Rosenberg, L. (2007). Perceived racial discrimination and risk of uterine leiomyomata. *Epidemiology (Cambridge, MA), 18*(6), 747–757.

Witzig, R. (1996). The medicalization of race: Scientific legitimization of a flawed social construct. *Annals of Internal Medicine, 125*, 675–679.

Wolfers, J., Leonhardt, D., & Quealy, K. (2015, April 20). 1.5 million missing Black men. *The New York Times*. www.nytimes.com/interactive/2015/04/20/upshot/missing-black-men.html

Wolff, E. N. (2001). *Racial wealth disparities: Is the gap closing?* (No. 66). Public Policy Brief.

Wolfgang, M. E., & Ferracuti, F. (1967). *The subculture of violence: Towards an integrated theory in criminology.* Tavistock Publications.

Wong, E. (2019). *Digital blackface: How 21st century Internet language reinforces racism.* UC Berkeley Library. https://escholarship.org/uc/item/91d9k96z

Woodard, V. (2014). *The delectable Negro.* New York University Press.

Woods, E. T. (2019). Cultural trauma: Ron Eyerman and the founding of a new research paradigm. *American Journal of Cultural Sociology, 7*(2), 260–274.

Woodson, C. G. (1933). *The mis-education of the Negro.* The Associated Publishers.

Woodyatt, A. (2022, February 2). More than 1,000 students were sexually abused at this university: An ex-NFL player wants their stories to be heard. *CNN.* www.cnn.com/2022/01/29/sport/university-of-michigan-robert-anderson-victims-intl-spt/index.html

World Health Organization. (2019). *ICD-11: International classification of diseases* (11th revision). WHO.

Wortman, C. B., & Brehm, J. W. (1975). Responses to uncontrollable outcomes: An integration of reactance theory and the learned helplessness model. In L. Berkowitz (Ed.), *Advances in experimental social psychology* (Vol. 8, pp. 277–336). Academic Press.

Wynter, S. (1992). No humans involved: An open letter to my colleagues. *Voices of the African Diaspora, 8*(2), 13–18.

Wynter, S. (2001). Towards the sociogenic principle: Fanon, identity, the puzzle of conscious experience, and what it is like to be "Black". In A. Gomez-Moriana & M. Duran-Cogan (Eds.), *National identities and sociopolitical changes in Latin America* (pp. 30–66). Routledge.

Wynter, S. (2003). Unsettling the coloniality of being/power/truth/freedom: Towards the human, after man, its overrepresentation – an argument. *CR: The New Centennial Review, 3*(3), 257–337.

Wynter, S. (2006). On how we mistook the map for the territory, and imprisoned ourselves in our unbearable wrongness of being, of Desetre: Black studies toward the human project. In L. R. Gordon & J. A. Gordon (Eds.), *Not only the masters tools: African-American studies in theory and practice* (A Companion to African-American Studies, pp. 107–172). Paradigm Publishers.

Xiao, Y., Cerel, J., & Mann, J. J. (2021). Temporal trends in suicidal ideation and attempts among US adolescents by sex and race/ethnicity, 1991–2019. *JAMA Network Open, 4*(6), e2113513.

Yehuda, R., Daskalakis, N. P., Bierer, L. M., Bader, H. N., Klengel, T., Holsboer, F., & Binder, E. B. (2016). Holocaust exposure induced intergenerational effects on FKBP5 methylation. *Biological Psychiatry, 80*(5), 372–380.

Yetman, N. (1985). Introduction: Definitions and perspectives. In N. Yetman (Ed.), *Majority and minority: The dynamics of race and ethnicity in American life* (4th ed., pp. 1–20). Allyn & Bacon.

Yimgang, D. P., Wang, Y., Paik, G., Hager, E. R., & Black, M. M. (2017). Civil unrest in the context of chronic community violence: Impact on maternal depressive symptoms. *American Journal of Public Health, 107*(9), 1455–1462.

Yinger, J. (1995). *Closed doors, opportunities lost: The continuing costs of housing discrimination.* Russell Sage Foundation.

Ziegert, J. C., & Hanges, P. J. (2005). Employment discrimination: The role of implicit attitudes, motivation, and a climate for racial bias. *Journal of Applied Psychology, 90*(3), 553–562.

Zoellner, L. A., Rothbaum, B. O., & Feeny, N. C. (2011). PTSD not an anxiety disorder? DSM committee proposal turns back the hands of time. *Depression and Anxiety, 28*(10), 853–856.

Zurara, G. E. D., Beazley, C. A. R., & Prestage, E. (1896). *The chronicle of the discovery and conquest of Guinea.*

2013 Update: The Spillover Effects of Foreclosures. (2013, August). *Center for responsible lending.* www.responsiblelending.org/mortgage-lending/research-analysis/2013-crl-research-update-foreclosure-spillover-effects-final-aug-19-docx.pdf

2020 FBI hate crimes statistics. (2021, November 17). www.justice.gov/crs/highlights/2020-hate-crimes-statistics

INDEX

Note: Page numbers in *italics* indicate figures on the corresponding pages.

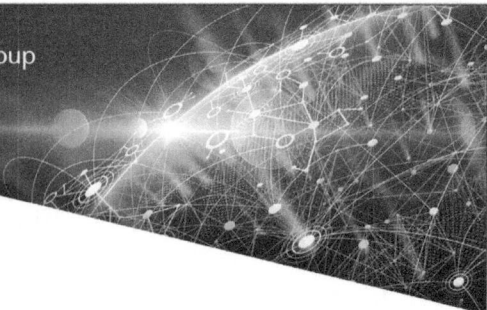